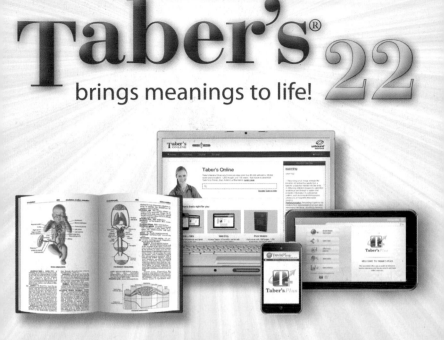
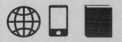

Maternal-Newborn Nursing Care

BEST EVIDENCE-BASED PRACTICES

Jamille Nagtalon-Ramos, MSN, CRNP, WHNP-BC
Associate Director
University of Pennsylvania School of Nursing
Women's Health Nurse Practitioner Program
Philadelphia, PA

Women's Health Nurse Practitioner
Hospital of the University of Pennsylvania
Department of Obstetrics and Gynecology
Philadelphia, PA

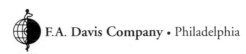
F.A. Davis Company • Philadelphia

F. A. Davis Company
1915 Arch Street
Philadelphia, PA 19103
www.fadavis.com

Copyright © 2014 by F. A. Davis Company

Printed in the United States of America

Last digit indicates print number: 10 9 8 7 6 5 4 3 2 1

Publisher, Nursing: Lisa B. Houck
Developmental Editor: Jamie Elfrank
Director of Content Development: Darlene D. Pedersen
Project Editor: Jamie Elfrank/Christina Snyder
Design and Illustration Manager: Carolyn O'Brien

As new scientific information becomes available through basic and clinical research, recommended treatments and drug therapies undergo changes. The author(s) and publisher have done everything possible to make this book accurate, up to date, and in accord with accepted standards at the time of publication. The author(s), editors, and publisher are not responsible for errors or omissions or for consequences from application of the book, and make no warranty, expressed or implied, in regard to the contents of the book. Any practice described in this book should be applied by the reader in accordance with professional standards of care used in regard to the unique circumstances that may apply in each situation. The reader is advised always to check product information (package inserts) for changes and new information regarding dose and contraindications before administering any drug. Caution is especially urged when using new or infrequently ordered drugs.

Library of Congress Cataloging-in-Publication Data

Nagtalon-Ramos, Jamille.
 Maternal-newborn nursing care / Jamille Nagtalon-Ramos. -- 1st ed.
   p. ; cm. -- (Best evidence-based practices)
 Includes bibliographical references and index.
 ISBN 978-0-8036-2246-3
 I. Title.
 [DNLM: 1. Maternal-Child Nursing--methods--Handbooks. 2. Evidence-Based Nursing--methods--Handbooks. 3. Infant, Newborn. 4. Perinatal Care--methods--Handbooks. 5. Pregnancy--Handbooks. WY 49]
 RG951
 618.2'0231--dc23
                            2013011141

This book is dedicated to one of the most compassionate nurses I know, Alissa Ferri, who served as my main inspiration for this book. While leading Alissa's orientation at her first nursing job years ago, I gave her a little notebook to serve as her "Pocket Brain" and in which to write important information she learned. I encouraged her to keep this notebook in her pocket and have it accessible at all times. While writing this book, I thought of Alissa and all my wonderful nursing students, past, present, and future, and asked myself what they would need to know in order to give the best care to their patients. I wrote this reference manual with the hope that it would serve as a reliable and handy resource, a "Pocket Brain," for nursing students as well as new-to-practice and expert nurses who share my passion in caring for women.

And, of course, this book is dedicated to Reg, my husband, who has taught me that the key to communication is listening; to my son Leo, whom I truly admire for the way he stays calm and intensely focused under pressure (especially at baseball!); to my fearless Leilani, who is always curious and who proudly refers to anatomical parts correctly and is not afraid to say "vagina!"; and to our Baby Leah, a warm snuggler who commands a room with her laughter. I dedicate this book and my heart to you.

To all the beautiful, strong, and brave women for whom I have had the privilege of caring and who allowed me to be part of their lives, this book is for you.

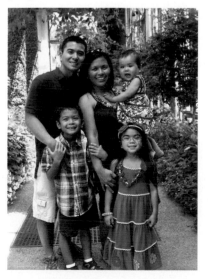

Preface

Maternal-Newborn Nursing Care: Best Evidence-Based Practices is intended to serve as a reliable reference book for nurses working in the area of women's health. This book was written with the nursing student as well as new-to-practice and experienced nurses in mind and is meant to be used as a dynamic "Pocket Brain" to help guide nurses in diverse hospital and community settings in providing safe, proficient, quality care to mothers, newborns, and their families.

Chapter content includes an examination of normal and abnormal pathophysiology of the childbearing woman and newborn and an overview of the components of care for normal and high-risk pregnant and postpartum women and neonates. Other chapters are dedicated to teaching nurses to provide culturally competent care in the women's health setting and to training nurses to recognize signs of abuse and assess, counsel, and follow up with compromised mothers. This book contains unique features, such as sample scripts for nurses who are discussing with their patients potentially sensitive situations surrounding contraception, sexually transmitted infections, and abuse as well as a chart of common medical terms translated from English to Spanish.

Nurses who share a passion for and commitment to the care of mothers and their newborns will appreciate the inclusion of concise, comprehensive assessments; discussion of disease processes; easy-to-understand tables of laboratory work-ups and values; common treatment guidelines and modalities; and the steps to implement and evaluate nursing care specific to women's health.

Reviewers

Rebecca L. Allen, RN, MNA
Assistant Professor
Clarkson College
Omaha, NE

Amy Cosimano, EdD (c), RNC
Assistant Professor
Creighton University School of Nursing
Omaha, NE

JoAnn G. Crownover, RN, MSN, CNE
Assistant Professor, Nursing
Colorado State University-Pueblo
Pueblo, CO

Laurie A. Downes, PhD, RN
Associate Professor
Elms College
Chicopee, MA

Cynthia A. Dyson, MSN, RN, BC, CNE
Assistant Professor of Nursing
Charleston Southern University
Hanahan, SC

Karen Ferguson, PhD, RNC-OB, SANE-A
Assistant Professor, Division of Nursing
Martin Methodist College
Pulaski, TN

Alissa Ferri, RN, BA, BSN
Clinical Nurse III
Hospital of the University of Pennsylvania
Philadelphia, PA

Sarah Fuchs, MS, RNC
Assistant Professor of Nursing
Jamestown College
Jamestown, ND

L. Sue Gabriel, EdD, MSN, MFS, RN, SANE-A, CFN
Associate Professor
BryanLGH College of Health Sciences, School of Nursing
Lincoln, NE

Allyssa L. Harris, RN, PhD, WHNP-BC
Clinical Instructor
Boston College
Chestnut Hill, MA

Jill Holmstrom, RN, MS
Associate Professor
Concordia College
Moorhead, MN

Judith Ingrasin, MS, RN
Assistant Professor of Nursing
Kansas City Community College
Kansas City, KS

Terri Kahle, MSN, RNC, CNE
Instructor
Southeast Missouri Hospital College of Nursing and Health Sciences
Cape Girardeau, MO

Beverly Kawa, RN, MS
Instructor
Morton College
Cicero, IL

Mona P. Klose, RN, MS, CPHQ
Assistant Professor
Jamestown College
Jamestown, ND

Michele Lamar-Suggs, BS, BSN, MSN
Clinical Nurse II
Hospital of the University of Pennsylvania
Philadelphia, PA

Deborah MacMillan, RN, CNM
Assistant Professor
Georgia College & State University
Milledgeville, GA

Dolores A. Minchhoff, RN, MSN, FNP-BC
Assistant Professor
Lancaster General College
Lancaster, PA

Pertice Moffitt, RN, BSN, MN, PhD
Senior Instructor, Nursing
Aurora College
Yellowknife, NT, Canada

Susan Olsen, RN, MSN, CNM
Clinical Assistant Professor
Georgia State University
Atlanta, GA

Anne E. Ormsby, RNC, MSN, CNE
Certified Childbirth Educator
Faculty
Trinitas School of Nursing
Elizabeth, NJ

Cynthia R. Payne, MS, RNC, NP-C, CNM
Assistant Professor
Georgia Perimeter College
Clarkston, GA

Marilyn K. Rhodes, EdD, MSN, RN, CNM
Assistant Professor
Auburn Montgomery School of Nursing
Montgomery, AL

Cynthia D. Rothenberger, MSN, RN, ACNS, BC
Assistant Professor, Nursing
Alvernia University
Reading, PA

Maria E. Satre, MSN, RN
Nursing Instructor
Capital University
Bexley, OH

Leslie Schaaf Treas, PhD, RN, NNP-BC, CPNP-PC

Paula Scherer, RNC, MSN
OB Faculty
Apollo College
Phoenix, AZ

Michelle A. Schutt, EdD, MSN, RN, CNE
Assistant Professor
Auburn Montgomery School of Nursing
Montgomery, AL

Karen Noell Shepherd, RN, MSN
Assistant Professor of Nursing
College of the Ozarks
Point Lookout, MO

Claudia Stoffel, MSN, RN, CNE
Professor
West Kentucky Community and Technical College
Paducah, KY

Lynn M. Stover, RN, BC, DSN, SANE
Associate Professor of Nursing
Armstrong Atlantic State University
Savannah, GA

Mary Tanner, PhD, RN
Associate Professor, School of Nursing
The College of St. Scholastica
Duluth, MN

Debbie Tavernier, MSN, RN
Associate Professor and Assistant Director
California State University, Stanislaus
Turlock, CA

Elizabeth J. Tipping, BSN, RNC-OB, MN
Professor
Greenville Technical College
Greenville, SC

Charlotte Ward, PhD, RN
Professor
College of the Ozarks-Armstrong
McDonald School of Nursing
Point Lookout, MO

Marilyn L. Weitzel, PhD, RN, CNL, CNE
Assistant Professor
Cleveland State University
Cleveland, OH

Jennifer Whitaker, MSN, RN
Assistant Professor of Nursing
El Paso Community College
El Paso, TX

Ruth A. Wittmann-Price, PhD, RN, CNE, Perinatal CNS
Assistant Professor
Drexel University College of Nursing and Health Professions
Philadelphia, PA
Nursing Research Coordinator
Hahnemann University Hospital
Philadelphia, PA

Marianne M. Wollyung, MSN, RN
Maternal/Child Nursing Instructor
Schuylkill Health School of Nursing
Pottsville, PA

Acknowledgments

I would like to extend my utmost gratitude to the many individuals who contributed to the development of this book, without whom this book would never have been completed.

To the very patient staff at F.A. Davis who worked tirelessly with me on this book from start to finish.

To Lisa B. Houck, Publisher, who showed faith in me and supported me throughout the process.

To Jamie Elfrank, Project Editor and Developmental Editor, whose patience, guidance, and editorial expertise helped me complete this book.

To the Potter family, Rhea, Sylvester, and Baby Micah, for taking and sharing their beautiful breastfeeding pictures with us.

To Alissa Ferri and Michele Lamar-Suggs, who joyfully read the first draft of the book and gave feedback from a staff-nurse perspective.

To my faculty colleagues at the University of Pennsylvania, School of Nursing, for instilling in me the vitality of evidence-based practice as a graduate student many years ago. Special thanks to Dr. Lynn Stringer for her guidance and mentorship, and to the Women's Health Care Studies faculty for their commitment to educating future women's health nurse practitioners and midwives.

To my colleagues at the Hospital of the University of Pennsylvania, all the nurses, nurse practitioners, doctors, midwives, CNAs, social workers, secretaries, and staff, your tireless efforts to provide world-class patient care inspire me every day. I am so proud to have been a part of this amazing team for the past 12 years.

To my grandmother, Lydia Venzon, who is a nursing pioneer in the Philippines. I continue to be in awe of her commitment to education for more than 50 years and her dedication to writing numerous nursing textbooks.

To my grandmother, Ester Nagtalon, for serving as a role model and for keeping me focused on the most important thing in life—my family.

To my mom and dad, thank you for believing in me.

To my husband, Reg, for his continued faith, love, support, and patience...and for not minding that I made a lot of Crock-Pot dinners (some delicious and some disastrous) and had our favorite Japanese and Filipino restaurants on speed dial while writing this book.

To my children, Leo, Leilani, and Leah, for their unconditional love. I can only hope that someday I will serve as an inspiration to you.

List of Tables

List of Figures

Contents in Brief

Contents

CHAPTER 2

CHAPTER 3

CHAPTER 7

CHAPTER 8

CHAPTER 9

CHAPTER 11

1 Normal Pregnancy

CHAPTER 1

Normal Pregnancy

The principal focus of nursing care during pregnancy is educating the mother and the family, assessing risks, and facilitating medical and psychosocial interventions, follow-up, and referrals. Obtaining early, adequate prenatal care is associated with good pregnancy outcomes and should be encouraged and provided for all pregnant women.

Terminology

- **Last menstrual period (LMP):** first day of the woman's last menses
- **Estimated date of delivery (EDD)/estimated date of birth (EDB)/estimated date of confinement (EDC):** expected date of the baby's birth
- **Gravidity:** total number of a woman's pregnancies including current one
- **Multigravida:** a woman who has had more than one pregnancy
- **Primigravida:** a woman who is pregnant for the first time
- **Parity:** number of pregnancies carried to the 20th week of gestation or that delivered an infant weighing more than 500 g, regardless of the outcome
- **Nullipara:** a woman who has never carried a pregnancy beyond the 20th week of gestation or carried a fetus weighing more than 500 g
- **Primipara:** a woman who has been or is currently pregnant for the first time past the 20th week of gestation
- **Multipara:** a woman who has carried a pregnancy past the 20th week of gestation or delivered an infant weighing more than 500 g more than once
- **Trimester:** length of pregnancy divided into three 3-month segments. The first trimester is from weeks 1 to 14; the second lasts from week 14 until week 28; and the last trimester refers to week 28 through delivery.

Diagnosis of Pregnancy

Presumptive Signs of Pregnancy

Presumptive signs of pregnancy are subjective signs self-reported by the patient. These may be caused by other medical conditions and are the least reliable signs of pregnancy. They include the following:

- Amenorrhea
- Breast tenderness
- Fatigue
- Nausea and vomiting
- Quickening
- Skin changes
- Urinary frequency

Probable Signs of Pregnancy

Probable signs of pregnancy are objective observations noted by the examiner. However, a pregnancy diagnosis cannot be made using these findings alone.

Probable signs of pregnancy include the following:

- **Abdominal enlargement:** increased abdominal circumference
- **Braxton Hicks contractions:** intermittent and irregular contractions that do not cause cervical dilation and effacement
- **Chadwick's sign:** discoloration of the cervix and the vagina into a deep blue-violet color caused by increased vascularity of the area
- **Goodell's sign:** softening of the cervix
- **Hegar's sign:** softening of the lower uterine segment
- **Positive pregnancy test:** human chorionic gonadotropin (hCG) in urine or serum

Positive Signs of Pregnancy

The following indicators are diagnostic of a pregnancy:

- Auscultation of fetal heartbeat
- Fetal visualization by ultrasound
- Fetal movements felt by the examiner

Duration of Pregnancy

The length of a human pregnancy is measured from the first day of the LMP to delivery, typically spanning 280 days, or 40 weeks. Calculated using the monthly calendar, a pregnancy lasts for 9 months. However, health-care providers refer to gestational age using the concept of lunar months (28 days/4 weeks), which equates to 10 months.

Gestational Age Assessment

- **Naegele's rule:** The date of delivery can be estimated using Naegele's rule, as in the following example:

First day of LMP	October	24
Subtract 3 months	– 3 months	
	July	24
Add 7 days	+	7 days
Estimated date of delivery	July	31

- **Pregnancy wheel/calculator:** This tool may be used to determine the EDD based on the first day of the LMP.

- **Ultrasound:** An ultrasound may be used to obtain an estimated gestational age. In the first trimester, an ultrasound is used to measure the fetal crown rump length (CRL). A CRL measurement is the most accurate way to date a pregnancy. In the second and third trimesters, the biparietal diameter, head circumference, abdominal circumference, and femur length are measured to obtain an estimated fetal weight and gestational age.

- **Fetal heartbeat:** Fetal heartbeats may be detected as early as 5.5 to 6 weeks via transvaginal ultrasound, 11 to 12 weeks using an electronic Doppler device, and 19 to 20 weeks using a DeLee-Hillis fetoscope.

- **Uterine sizing:** Useful especially in the first trimester. By performing a bimanual examination, experienced examiners are able to estimate the gestational age of the fetus. A nonpregnant or 5-week pregnant uterus is about the size of a small pear; the size of a 6-week pregnant uterus is comparable to a small orange; an 8-week pregnant uterus is similar in size to a large navel orange; and a 12-week pregnant uterus measures about the size of a grapefruit.

- **Fundal height measurement:** The examiner measures the size of the uterus from the pubic symphysis to the fundus (the top of the uterus). Between 16 and 38 weeks, the gestational age correlates with the measurement in centimeters, ± 3 cm.

- **Quickening:** This initial awareness of the fetus by the mother usually occurs between 16 and 22 weeks of gestation.

⭐ **BEST PRACTICES**

ROUTINE PRENATAL VISIT FREQUENCY

Following is the recommended frequency of routine prenatal visits:
- First prenatal visit, usually in the first trimester
- Monthly until 28th week of gestation
- Biweekly from 28 to 36 weeks
- Weekly from 36 weeks to delivery

More frequent visits may be required if patient is diagnosed as having a high-risk pregnancy.

GTPAL

Some facilities use the GTPAL acronym to briefly refer to a woman's obstetric history.

- **G**ravida: number of pregnancies (regardless of outcome or number of fetuses carried)
- **Term**: number of pregnancies carried to term (37 weeks)
- **Preterm**: number of pregnancies carried preterm (<37 weeks)
- **Abortions**: number of elective or spontaneous abortions before 20 weeks
- **Living**: number of living children

Initial Prenatal Visit: History and Physical Examination

Obtain a comprehensive *health history* of the mother and pertaining history of the father, the baby, and their families.

- Current pregnancy
  - LMP for clinical dating
  - Discomforts such as nausea, constipation, or urinary frequency
  - Problems such as bleeding or cramping
  - Questions or concerns
- Obstetric history
  - Number of total pregnancies
  - Number of term and preterm deliveries
  - Methods of delivery with each pregnancy (it is important to know whether the individual has had a cesarean section or forceps/vacuum-assisted delivery in the past and why) and anesthesia used, if any

---

⭐ **BEST PRACTICES**

EXAMPLES OF GRAVIDA AND PARA NOTATION

- Example 1: A woman who is currently pregnant with her second child can be referred to as gravida 2. Remember that gravidity refers to the number of pregnancies, including the present one, regardless of the outcome.
- Example 2: A woman has been pregnant three times. Her first pregnancy resulted in twins; the second and third pregnancies resulted in singletons. She can be referred to as a gravida 3. Remember that gravidity refers to the number of pregnancies, not the number of resulting fetuses.
- Example 3: A woman who had a stillborn delivery at 35 weeks and an abortion at 16 weeks can be referred to as gravida 2, para 1. Remember, parity refers to the number of pregnancies that went beyond 20 weeks, regardless of outcome.
- Example 4: A woman who is currently pregnant for the third time had a baby born at 28 weeks (currently alive and well) and an abortion at 12 weeks. Her current GTPAL is G3, T0, P1, A1, L1. Once she gives birth to her baby at term, her GTPAL will change to G3, T1, P1, A1, L2.

⭐ **BEST PRACTICES**

Most facilities have a standard form or computerized system for obtaining a patient's history. Following is a sample of a patient's concise obstetric history:

Gravida 2, Para T1P0A0L1

2005: Live male infant, 8 lb. 15 oz. @ 39 weeks via C-section for breech presentation. Spinal anesthesia. No complications.

- Complications with any of the pregnancies and deliveries, such as postpartum hemorrhage, pre-eclampsia
- Number of abortions, either spontaneous or elective
- Number of living children and their weights at delivery
- Gynecological history
  - Papanicolaou (Pap) smear history including any abnormalities and follow-up
  - Sexually transmitted disease (STD) history, treatment, and follow-up
  - Contraceptive history
- Medical history
  - Medical conditions and chronic diseases, especially ones that may affect pregnancy such as asthma, diabetes, anemia, and hypertension
  - Hospitalizations and emergency department visits
- Surgical history
  - List surgeries, indications, anesthesia used, and any complications
- Occupational history
  - Exposure to hazardous or teratogenic substances
  - Shift work
  - Heavy lifting
  - Extended periods of standing
- Religious and/or cultural beliefs, practices, and preferences
  - Primary language spoken
- Medications, including dosages, indications, and last dose taken
  - Over the counter
  - Prescription
  - Herbs, vitamins, and other supplements
- Allergies, making sure to ascertain reactions and complications
  - Medications
  - Food
  - Environmental
- Substance use and exposure history, making sure to ascertain time and day of last use, extent of use, desire, and attempts to quit
  - Tobacco
  - Alcohol
  - Illegal drugs
  - Diethylstilbestrol (DES) exposure of patient or her mother or grandmother
- Nutrition history
  - 24-hour diet recall
  - History of eating disorder, pica, or hyperemesis gravidarum

ALERT!

Diethylstilbestrol (DES) was prescribed to women in the past to prevent miscarriages and premature deliveries. Between 5 and 10 million people were exposed to DES in the United States between 1938 and 1971. All women older than 35 years of age, as well as foreign-born women, should be screened for exposure to DES in utero. Daughters of women who were prescribed DES while pregnant are at increased risk for clear cell adenocarcinoma of the vagina and the cervix, structural variations of the reproductive tract, higher incidence of ectopic pregnancies, and preterm labor (PTL) and birth.

- Abuse
  - History of sexual, mental, or physical abuse
- History of the baby's father
  - Age
  - General health
  - Medical history
  - Blood type and Rh factor (if known)
  - Occupation
  - Substance use
  - Involvement with the pregnancy

Initial Physical Examination

Prepare the patient by discussing the components of the examination. Encourage the patient to void before the examination to feel more comfortable. Ensure the patient's privacy by drawing the curtains and closing the door.

- **Vital signs:** Record respiration, pulse, temperature, and blood pressure.
- **Weight and height**
- **Skin:** Note color, presence of edema, and changes associated with pregnancy.
- **Neck:** Assess for thyroid enlargement, which may be associated with thyroid disease.
- **Breasts:** Inspect and palpate. Further evaluate nodularities.
- **Heart:** Note regularity, rate, and rhythm. Systolic murmur may be heard because of the increase in blood volume in pregnancy.
- **Abdomen:** Inspect and palpate. Measure the fundus. See Figure 1–1 for uterine growth pattern in pregnancy and Figure 1–2 for measurement of the fundal height. Obtain fetal heartbeat. Remember, fetal heartbeats can be detected by the 12th week, and sometimes the 11th week, using an electronic Doppler device, and by 20 weeks using a DeLee-Hillis fetoscope. Normal fetal heart rate is between 110 and 160 bpm.
- **Extremities:** Assess upper and lower extremities for edema. Ascertain for any tenderness in the calf.
- **Reflexes:** Assess the brachial and patellar reflexes. Hyperreflexia may be a sign of developing pre-eclampsia.
- **Pelvic examination:** Examine external and internal genitalia; obtain Pap smear and gonorrhea and chlamydia cultures, as indicated; size uterus and palpate ovaries, as indicated and as per institution policy.
- **Rectal examination:** Visually note any hemorrhoids.

Nursing Care During Subsequent Prenatal Visits

1. **Weight:** Weight should be obtained at each visit.
   - **First trimester:** *Total* of 1.1 to 4.4 lb of weight gain is normal.
   - **Second and third trimesters:** 3 to 4 lb *per month* of weight gain is normal (refer to Table 1–1).

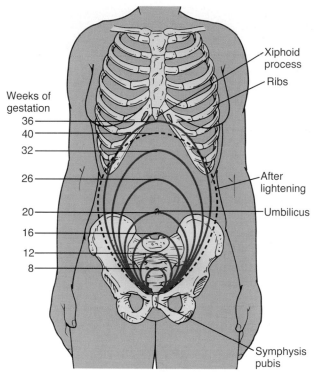

FIGURE 1-1: Uterine growth pattern. At 10–12 weeks, the fundus of the uterus may be palpated right above the pubic symphysis. At 20 weeks, the fundus may be palpated at the umbilicus. At 36 weeks, the fundus may reach the level of the xiphoid process, and at 40 weeks, decrease in height after lightening occurs.

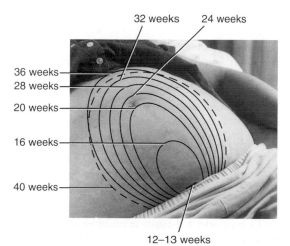

FIGURE 1-2: The height of the fundus in centimeters is a rough estimate of the gestation in weeks.

Table 1-1 Institute of Medicine's Recommendations for Weight Gain in Pregnancy According to Prepregnancy Body Mass Index

PREPREGNANCY BMI	BMI	TOTAL WEIGHT GAIN RANGE	SECOND AND THIRD TRIMESTER WEIGHT GAIN (LB/WEEK)*
Underweight	<18.5	28–40	1 (1–1.3)
Normal weight	18.5–24.9	25–35	1 (0.8–1)
Overweight	25–29.9	15–25	0.6 (0.5–0.7)
Obese	≥30	11–20	0.5 (0.4–0.6)

*Calculation based on assumption of a 1.1- to 4.4-lb total weight gain in the first trimester.
BMI, body mass index.
From Institute of Medicine. Resource Sheet, May 2009. Weight Gain During Pregnancy: Reexamining the Guidelines. Retrieved September 6, 2012, from www.iom.edu.

2. **Vital signs:** Routinely, blood pressure and pulse are taken at each visit. Temperature and respirations are deferred unless the patient does not appear well or reports symptoms such as fever, chills, palpitations, and shortness of breath.
3. **Urinalysis:** Dip urine at each visit to determine presence of the following:
   - **Protein:** Presence in urine may be sign of a urinary tract infection (UTI), kidney damage, or pre-eclampsia.
   - **Ketones:** Produced when the body starts breaking down fat for energy. May be seen in patients who have nausea and vomiting or uncontrolled diabetes.
   - **Glucose:** Presence of glucose in the urine may be normal in pregnancy, but may be indicative of gestational diabetes.
   - **Nitrites:** Presence is a strong indication of a UTI. A urine culture may be sent to confirm diagnosis.
4. **Blood tests:** Depending on the institution, nurses may be responsible for obtaining blood samples for testing. See Tables 1–2 through 1–4 for routine blood tests in pregnancy.
5. **Glucose challenge test (GCT) or glucose tolerance test (GTT)**
   - **How to perform 1-hour screening test:** Test is to be done between 24 and 28 weeks. No fasting is necessary. Administer a 50-g load of oral glucose. Patient is not allowed to eat, drink, smoke cigarettes, or chew gum while awaiting blood draw. After an hour, obtain a serum glucose sample.
     - **Normal:** <130 to 140 mg/dL
     - If >140 mg/dL, proceed to 3-hour test
   - **How to perform a 3-hour screening test:** Patient needs to fast for 12 hours before test. Obtain a fasting serum blood glucose. Administer a 100-g load of oral glucose. Patient is not allowed to eat, drink, smoke cigarettes, or chew gum while

waiting for succeeding blood draws. Serum blood glucose is obtained at 1, 2, and 3 hours after ingestion of glucose solution.

- **Results:** Positive diagnosis if two or more abnormal values (see Table 2–3 for blood glucose goals in diabetes during pregnancy.)

Table 1–2 Laboratory Testing and Procedures in Pregnancy

LABORATORY TESTING AND PROCEDURES	PURPOSE AND RESULTS
INITIAL LABORATORY TESTS	
Antibody screen	Serum test to screen for antibodies due to exposure to fetal blood
Blood type	Serum test to identify which blood group the patient belongs to: A, B, AB, or O
Complete blood count	Serum test to detect anemia, infection, or clotting disorders; if anemic, may need iron supplementation
Hepatitis B virus	Serum test to identify presence of antigen; if positive, may indicate acute or chronic infection
HIV	Serum test to screen for HIV; if positive, will need further testing for confirmation of infection
Papanicolaou smear	Cervical sampling to screen for cervical cancer; if abnormal results, further testing/biopsy may be indicated
Rh factor	Serum test to determine patient's Rh status; if patient is Rh negative and fetus is Rh positive, there may be a risk for isoimmunization
Rubella	Serum test to determine whether patient has immunity; if not immune, postpartum vaccination recommended
Syphilis	Serum test to screen for syphilis; if positive, further testing indicated for confirming diagnosis and level of treatment
Urinalysis/Urine culture	To test for the presence of bacteria, glucose, ketones, and protein in the urine; if urinary tract infection is suspected, culture may be indicated for more comprehensive diagnosis
Varicella	Serum test to determine immunity to varicella; if not immune, postpartum varicella vaccination recommended
Gonorrhea and chlamydia	Culture to detect a gonorrhea or chlamydial infection
Hemoglobin electrophoresis	Serum test to identify abnormal hemoglobinopathies such as sickle cell anemia and thalassemias
Tuberculin skin test (purified protein derivative [PPD])	Skin test to screen for tuberculosis

Table 1–3 Laboratory Tests and Procedures in Pregnancy According to Gestational Age

LABORATORY TESTING AND PROCEDURES	PURPOSE AND RESULTS
8 TO 20 WEEKS	
Genetic testing	See Table 1-4
Ultrasound	Used for dating the pregnancy and general anatomic survey of the fetus
24 TO 28 WEEKS	
Anti-D immune globulin (RhIg or RhoGAM)	Administer at ≥28 weeks if patient is Rh negative
Complete blood count	Repeat testing, if indicated, for anemia
Diabetes screen (1-hour glucose tolerance test)	Serum test to screen for gestational diabetes risk
3-Hour glucose tolerance test	If 1-hour glucose tolerance test is abnormal, 3-hour test needed for diagnosis of gestational diabetes
32 TO 36 WEEKS	
Complete blood count	Repeat testing, if indicated, for anemia
Gonorrhea and chlamydia	Repeat testing, if indicated
Group B Streptococcus (GBS)	Vaginal/rectal culture done at 35 weeks to determine colonization of GBS; if positive, antibiotic needed in labor
HIV	Centers for Disease Control and Prevention (CDC) now recommends repeat testing in third trimester
Syphilis	CDC recommends repeat testing in third trimester

6. **Screen for domestic violence (see Best Practices Box, page 232)**
7. **Danger signs in pregnancy:** Assess for danger signs in pregnancy that may indicate a problem and the need for further evaluation by a nurse practitioner, midwife, or obstetrician (see Table 1–5).

Table 1–4 Genetic Screening and Tests

LABORATORY TESTING AND PROCEDURES	PURPOSE AND RESULTS
GENETIC SCREENING	
First trimester screening	Performed between 11 and 14 weeks to detect Down syndrome and trisomy 18; screening test is a blood test in conjunction with ultrasound; blood test measures pregnancy-associated plasma protein (PAPP-A) and human chorionic gonadotropin (hCG); ultrasound examination measures the thickness of the skin at the back of the fetus's neck (nuchal translucency); Down syndrome is detected about 85% of the time
Second trimester screening (also called "multiple marker screening," "triple screen," or "quad screen")	Performed between 15 and 20 weeks to detect Down syndrome, trisomy 18, and neural tube defects; when blood test measures three substances—α-fetoprotein (AFP), estriol, and hCG—this test is referred to as a "triple screen"; with the addition of a fourth substance, Inhibin-A, the test is called a "quad screen"; Down syndrome is detected about 70% and 80% of the time when using the triple and quadruple screen tests, respectively; AFP detects neural tube defects 80% of the time
Combined first and second trimester screening	First and second trimester screening results are combined to increase accuracy of detecting Down syndrome to 85% to 96%
Cell Free Fetal DNA	A noninvasive prenatal testing for trisomy 13, 18, and 21 using cell free fetal DNA from the pregnant woman's plasma. Test can be performed as early as the 10th week of pregnancy.
GENETIC DIAGNOSTIC TESTS	
Chorionic villi sampling (CVS)	Done in the first trimester between 11 and 13 weeks; a thin collecting tube is inserted through transcervically or transabdominally, and with ultrasound guidance, cell samples from the placenta are collected for karyotyping
Amniocentesis	Done in the second trimester; a thin, long needle is inserted intra-abdominally, and with ultrasound guidance, amniotic fluid and cell samples are obtained for fetal karyotyping; amniocentesis can also be used to test for infection and ascertain fetal lung maturity
Ultrasound	A detailed ultrasound may be done to examine the fetus for features associated with chromosomal abnormalities such as Down syndrome or trisomy 18. An ultrasound may also be used to guide in procedures such as CVS and amniocentesis.

8. **Pregnancy education:** Address appropriate topics pertinent to patient's questions, complaints, and needs. Provide anticipatory guidance pertinent to patient's gestational age. See section titled "Health Promotion in Pregnancy."

GENETIC SCREENING AND COUNSELING

The American College of Obstetrics and Gynecology (ACOG) recommends that genetic screening and counseling be offered to all pregnant women regardless of age. Particular attention should be given to an expectant mother with the following history:

- Mother's age ≥35 years as of EDD
- Mother with phenylketonuria, type 1 diabetes, or other metabolic disorders
- Patient or the baby's father had a previous child with birth defects
- Canavan disease (common for Ashkenazi Jews)
- Congenital heart defect
- Cystic fibrosis
- Down syndrome
- Familial dysautonomia (common for Ashkenazi Jews)
- Hemophilia or other blood disorders
- Huntington's chorea
- Mental retardation or autism
- Muscular dystrophy
- Neural tube defect (meningomyelocele, spina bifida, or anencephaly)
- Sickle cell disease or trait (common for African descent)
- Tay-Sachs disease (common for Ashkenazi Jews, Cajun, and French Canadian descent)
- Thalassemia (common for Italian, Greek, Mediterranean, or Asian descent) or mother with a mean corpuscular volume (MCV) less than 80

Table 1–5 Danger Signs in Pregnancy

DANGER SIGN	POSSIBLE CAUSE
Vaginal bleeding	First trimester: miscarriage, implantation bleeding Second and third trimesters: placenta previa, abruption placentae, "bloody show" Anytime: sexually transmitted disease, after intercourse
Dysuria, urgency, and/or frequency	Urinary tract infection, sexually transmitted infection
Fever and chills	Infection
Intractable vomiting	Hyperemesis gravidarum
Severe headache	Pre-eclampsia, hypertension
Visual disturbances (spots before eyes, blurry vision)	Pre-eclampsia
Epigastric pain	Pre-eclampsia

Table 1–5 **Danger Signs in Pregnancy—cont'd**

DANGER SIGN	POSSIBLE CAUSE
Loss of fluid	Premature rupture of membranes
Uterine contractions, abdominal pain, pelvic pressure, backache before 37 weeks	Preterm labor, abruption placentae

Physiological Changes in Pregnancy

Various physiological changes occur during pregnancy. Many of these changes are due to the shifts in hormonal levels. It is important for the nurse to know the normal parameters of these changes to provide proper care and education to the pregnant patient.

Integumentary System

- **Increased pigmentation:** Hormonal changes cause melasma gravidarum, also called *chloasma* or the "mask of pregnancy," and the appearance of linea nigra.
- **Linea nigra:** A hyperpigmented line is found on a mother's abdomen that extends from the symphysis pubis to the top of the fundus. The line extends upward as the uterus grows during the pregnancy.
- **Hyperpigmentation:** Often is more noticeable in women with darker complexions. Encourage decreased sun exposure and the regular use of sun block.
- **Striae gravidarum:** Also known as stretch marks, striae gravidarum are commonly found on the abdomen, breasts, and buttocks. They will eventually fade to silvery lines during the postpartum period.
- **Thicker hair:** Thicker hair is most likely not a result of abundant hair growth but instead results from a portion of hair follicles being suspended from entering the telogen phase during pregnancy, meaning that hair that would naturally fall out does not. During the postpartum period, hair proceeds to the telogen phase and telogen effluvium, or hair shedding, occurs. Acknowledge to the patient that it is concerning to see hair falling out. It may take 1 to 5 months after childbirth for the full thickness of the hair to return to normal.

Musculoskeletal System

- Increased production of relaxin and progesterone hormones causes ligament laxity.
- Pubic symphysis widens, causing the mother to "waddle" when walking.
- Lumbar lordosis may occur as uterus enlarges and moves upward and outward.

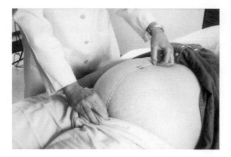

FIGURE 1-3: Fundal height measured by the healthcare provider.

Reproductive System

- **Uterus:** Pattern of growth is predictable (see Fig. 1–3). Blood flow to the uterus increases because of progesterone. Softening of the lower uterine segment occurs (Hegar's sign).
- **Cervix:** Softens (Goodell's sign) and may become deep blue-violet color because of increased vascularity of the area (Chadwick's sign). Operculum (mucous plug) forms.
- **Vagina:** Also may develop a deep-blue hue (Chadwick's sign).
- **Ovaries:** Ovulation ceases in pregnancy. The corpus luteum produces progesterone for 6 to 8 weeks. When the placenta becomes more functional, it then takes over the production of progesterone.
- **Breasts:** Because of the rise of estrogen and progesterone, enlargement and sensitivity may occur. Montgomery tubercles, which are the sebaceous glands of the areola, may also enlarge.

Cardiovascular System

- **Heart:** displaced upward to the left
- **Cardiac output:** increases as early as 5 weeks' gestation by 10% and up to 50% by 34 weeks' gestation
- **Heart rate:** increases by 10 to 15 bpm
- **Clotting factors:** levels increase for prevention of postpartum hemorrhage
- **White blood cells:** physiological leukocytosis occurs

Gastrointestinal System

- Nausea and vomiting are common, especially in first trimester because of hCG hormone. (See Common Discomforts in Pregnancy at the end of this chapter.)
- Hyperemia in the gums increases the potential for bleeding from routine oral hygienic practices such as brushing the teeth.
- Progesterone causes decreased gallbladder and stomach emptying, resulting in an increased risk for gallstones and occurrence of constipation, respectively.

Urinary System

- Increased urinary frequency and nocturia occur because of pressure of the gravid uterus on the bladder and the smooth muscle relaxation effects of progesterone.

- Dilation of ureters and renal pelves allows for bacterial ascension, which puts gravid women at an increased risk for pyelonephritis.

Endocrine System
- **Thyroid gland:** Pregnant women generally remain euthyroid. Thyroid gland may increase in size slightly. Total thyroxine (TT_4) level increases.
- **Adrenal gland:** Cortisol and aldosterone levels increase.
- **Pituitary gland:** Pituitary gland enlarges. Prolactin hormone levels increase. Follicle-stimulating hormone and luteinizing hormone decrease to undetectable levels.
- **Pancreas:** Hypoglycemia and hypoinsulinemia occur faster in response to starvation. Hyperglycemia and hyperinsulinemia occur as a response after eating.

Primary Hormones of Pregnancy

Estrogen
- Produced by placenta
- Increased levels in pregnancy cause hyperpigmentation and spider angiomas
- Stimulates enlargement of breasts and uterus
- Contributes to insulin resistance

Progesterone
- Produced by corpus luteum until 6 to 8 weeks' gestation, at which time placenta takes over production
- Vital to the maintenance of pregnancy
- Smooth muscle relaxant; helps uterus remain quiescent
- Essential in the growth of alveoli and ducts in the mammary glands in preparation for lactation

Human Placental Lactogen
- Hormone produced by the placenta
- Insulin antagonist, thus increasing blood glucose in pregnancy
- Almost at an undetectable level shortly after delivery of the placenta

Human Chorionic Gonadotropin
- Secreted by the trophoblast to maintain corpus luteum until placenta becomes functional in producing progesterone
- Detectable in urine and serum 8 to 10 days after conception
- Hormone detected by urine pregnancy tests

Relaxin
- Produced by corpus luteum and then by placenta after 6 to 8 weeks' gestation
- Relaxes pelvic muscles and joints in preparation for childbirth

Oxytocin
- Produced in hypothalamus and secreted by the posterior pituitary gland
- Induces uterine contractions in labor
- Responsible for milk ejection or "letdown" reflex during lactation

Prolactin
- Produced by the anterior pituitary gland
- Prolactin levels increase up to 10 times greater than prepregnancy levels by term
- Essential to milk production

Psychosocial Adaptations in Pregnancy

According to Reva Rubin, a nursing theorist who introduced the concept of maternal role attainment, a woman must carry out specific "developmental tasks in pregnancy" to make the transition to the role of mother.

Seeking Safe Passage
- **First trimester:** During the first trimester, the mother is focused on her own safety.
- **Second trimester:** The mother is now more aware of the infant growing inside of her and becomes very protective of the fetus. The woman will seek to gain more knowledge about the pregnancy to ensure her infant's safe passage by reading books and magazines, using television and the Internet, and obtaining medical advice from people who she believes are experts in childbearing, such as midwives, nurses, and doctors.
- **Third trimester:** Both self and baby are of utmost concern to the woman. Her attitude toward her fast-changing body image conjures doubt and a sense of vulnerability. She begins to perceive everyday events as potential threats to her and her fetus.

Acceptance of the Child by Significant Others
- **First trimester:** Focus is on reworking and reorganizing relationships in order for the important people in the woman's life to accept the idea of her pregnancy.
- **Second trimester:** Focus is redirected to the acceptance of her child into her family. The woman summons ideas of her child's relationship with her family and loved ones.
- **Third trimester:** This is a critical time wherein the woman not only wants familial acceptance for her and her baby but also tries to ascertain the level of acceptance. Is having a child of a certain sex preferred in her family? What if the infant is diagnosed with a

medical condition? Will the infant be highly welcomed by the family?

Binding-in
- **First trimester:** The woman accepts the idea of being pregnant.
- **Second trimester:** This is a vital period wherein fetal movement conjures in the woman a higher sense of determination to undertake the tasks of pregnancy in a serious manner. She feels a growing love for her infant while in utero.
- **Third trimester:** The woman starts getting tired of the pregnancy. She wants to be able to hold the infant and be done with the pregnancy.

Giving of Oneself
- **First trimester:** The mother evaluates what may be given by a child and what may be taken away.
- **Second trimester:** The woman explores the act of giving as well as finding enjoyment and pleasure from receiving. She increasingly values the gift of friendship, companionship, and acceptance.
- **Third trimester:** Patient realizes the demands of labor and delivery and starts doubting her capacity to give and whether she will be able to give enough.

Fetal Assessment

Assessment of the fetus may be prompted by certain maternal and/or pregnancy-related conditions that may affect the well-being and growth of the fetus.

Maternal Indications
- Antiphospholipid syndrome
- Hemoglobinopathies
- Hypertensive disorders
- Hyperthyroidism
- Systemic lupus erythematosus
- Type 1 diabetes mellitus

Pregnancy-Related Indications
- Decreased fetal movement
- Intrauterine growth restriction
- Isoimmunization
- Multiple gestation
- Oligohydramnios
- Polyhydramnios
- Postterm pregnancy
- Pregnancy-induced hypertension
- Previous fetal demise

Types of Fetal Assessment

Fetal Kick Counts

Two of the most widely used approaches to assess fetal movement as per ACOG are as follows.

1. Ask the woman to lie on her side and count 10 fetal movements in 2 hours. Once she has reached 10, she may discontinue the count. Obtaining 10 movements in 2 hours is considered reassuring.
2. Instruct the woman to count fetal movements for 1 hour three times a week. If the number of movements is equal to or greater than the baseline count, this would be considered reassuring.

Ultrasound

- First trimester uses
  - Assess cause of vaginal bleeding
  - Evaluate suspected ectopic pregnancy
  - Confirm intrauterine pregnancy
  - Assess gestational age
  - Confirm cardiac activity
  - Determine fetal number
  - Guide with procedures such as chorionic villus sampling or removal of an intrauterine device
- Second and third trimester uses
  - Confirm gestational age
  - Evaluate fetal anatomy
  - Assess level of amniotic fluid
  - Assess location of placenta
  - Identify fetal presentation
  - Guide with procedures such as amniocentesis
  - Evaluate suspected fetal death
  - Assess cause of vaginal bleeding
  - Evaluate cervical insufficiency

- Limited obstetric ultrasounds may be performed by registered nurses who are certified.

Nonstress Test

A nonstress test (NST) is performed to assess fetal heart rate reactivity, which indicates fetal autonomic function.

Procedure

1. Seat the patient in a reclining position or semi-Fowler's position with a lateral tilt.
2. Place two belts around her abdomen. One is to hold an external transducer in place to monitor fetal heart rate, and the other is to hold a tocodynamometer (or "toco") in place to monitor uterine activity (see Figs. 1–4 and 1–5).
3. Establish the fetal heart rate baseline (normally within 110 to 160 bpm).
4. Monitor the patient for at least 20 minutes or longer, if necessary.
5. Vibroacoustic stimulation (VAS) may be used to elicit fetal heart rate accelerations. The VAS device is placed on the patient's abdomen to provide 1 to 2 seconds of stimulation and may be repeated up to three times during the course of the NST.

Results

- Reactive
  - Two or more accelerations that peak 15 bpm above the baseline and last for 15 seconds within 20 minutes of tracing (see Fig. 1–6)
  - This is a reassuring result.
- Nonreactive
  - Tracing with *one* acceleration that peaks 15 bpm above the baseline and lasts for 15 seconds

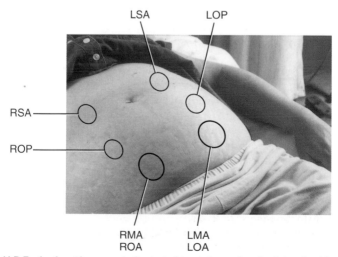

FIGURE 1-4: Placement of external transducer for obtaining fetal heart rate depends on the position of the fetus.

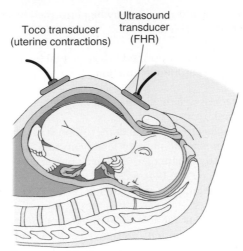

FIGURE 1-5: External fetal monitor.

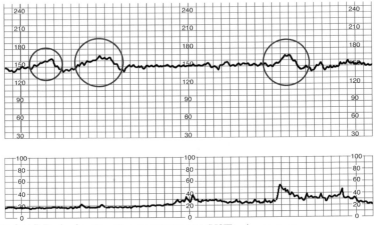

FIGURE 1-6: Reactive nonstress test (NST).

- Tracing without any accelerations
- Tracing with accelerations *less than or equal to* 15 bpm above the baseline or acceleration not lasting at least 15 seconds during period of testing
- This is a nonreassuring result and prompts further testing and evaluation (see Fig. 1–7)
- Unsatisfactory
  - Tracing unable to be interpreted
  - Repeat testing and further evaluation necessary

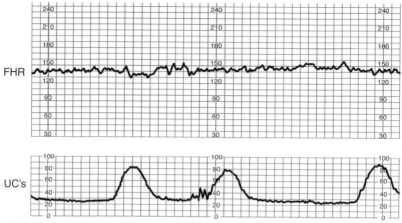

FIGURE 1-7: Top line is the fetal heart rate. Bottom line indicates the uterine contractions. This is a nonreactive nonstress test.

Contraction Stress Test

A contraction stress test checks fetal heart rate response to uterine contractions.

Procedure

1. Follow steps 1 to 3 for NST.
2. If three spontaneous contractions lasting at least 40 seconds each are present during a 10-minute period, uterine stimulation is unnecessary.
3. If during a 10-minute period fewer than three contractions lasting at least 40 seconds each are present, uterine stimulation will be induced by using intravenous oxytocin (Pitocin) or nipple stimulation. Follow hospital protocol and prescriber's orders for Pitocin infusion or procedure for nipple stimulation.

Results

- Negative
  - No late or significant variable deceleration (see Fig. 1–8)
  - Reassuring result, which indicates that the fetus will be able to tolerate labor
- Positive
  - Late decelerations following half of contractions or more
  - Fetus is suboptimally oxygenated in the presence of stress (uterine contraction).
  - Physician or midwife may offer to expedite a vaginal delivery or proceed to a cesarean section.

ALERT!

Contraindications to a contraction stress test include the following:

- PTL
- Patients at high risk for PTL
- Preterm rupture of membrane
- Classical cesarean section
- Placenta previa

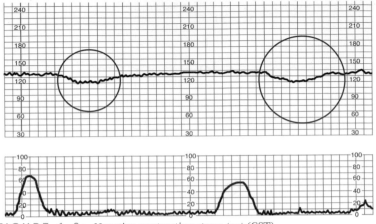

FIGURE 1-8: Negative contraction stress test (CST).

- Equivocal—suspicious
  - Intermittent late decelerations or variable decelerations that are significant
  - Further evaluation needed
- Equivocal—hyperstimulatory
  - If late decelerations are present with contractions lasting longer than 90 seconds or contractions occurring every 2 minutes, further evaluation is needed.
- Unsatisfactory
  - Fewer than three contractions lasting at least 40 seconds in 10 minutes of tracing, or tracing unable to be interpreted
  - Further evaluation needed

Biophysical Profile

The biophysical profile is composed of five parameters including an NST and four ultrasound findings. Each component is assigned a score of either 2 for normal findings or 0 if absent or abnormal findings (see Table 1–6).

Results

- **Score of 8 to 10:** normal and reassuring
- **Score of 6:** equivocal. Depending on clinical picture, repeat testing in 24 hours and perform further evaluation if necessary. Physician or midwife may suggest delivery for a term fetus.
- **Score of 0 to 4:** abnormal. Depending on clinical picture, expeditious delivery may be warranted.
- **Oligohydramnios:** If an amniotic fluid volume ≤5 cm is found, regardless of the presence of the other components, further evaluation is necessary.

AMNIOTIC FLUID INDEX

An AFI is obtained by the use of ultrasound to measure the deepest vertical pocket of amniotic fluid in each of the four abdominal quadrants. Amniotic fluid volume can be used to evaluate long-term uteroplacental function.

Table 1–6 **Components of a Biophysical Profile**

COMPONENT	NORMAL	ABNORMAL
Nonstress Test	Reactive (2 points)	Nonreactive (0 points)
Ultrasound findings below need to be obtained within 30 minutes of scanning.		
Fetal breathing	At least one episode of fetal breathing lasting 30 seconds (2 points)	No breathing, or intermittent episodes of breathing not lasting 30 seconds each (0 points)
Fetal tone	At least one episode of exten sion of a fetal extremity with return to flexion, or opening or closing of hand (2 points)	No extension with return to flexion of an extremity or opening or closing of hand (0 points)
Fetal gross body movement	At least three body or limb movements (2 points)	None or fever than three body or limb movements (0 points)
Amniotic fluid volume	A single vertical pocket of fluid ≥2 cm (2 points)	Pocket of fluid <2 cm (0 points)

Modified Biophysical Profile

A modified biophysical profile is a combination of NST interpretation and the assessment of the amniotic fluid volume

Results

- **Normal:** reactive NST and amniotic fluid index (AFI) >5 cm
- **Abnormal:** nonreactive NST and/or AFI ≤5 cm

Health Promotion in Pregnancy

- **Alcohol, tobacco, and illegal substances:** See Chapter 11 "Substance Abuse" on maternal and fetal effects of alcohol, tobacco, and illegal substances.
- **Exercise:** Patient should discuss this with the health-care provider before starting an exercise program. Generally, most women may engage in 30 minutes or more of exercise daily.
- **Medications:** Patient should consult a physician, nurse practitioner, or midwife regarding medications prescribed to you during or prior to pregnancy. Instruct the patient to make the health-care provider aware of over-the-counter, herbal, and prescription medications. Some medications are teratogenic and may cause birth defects, but others are safe.

OFFERING SUPPORT

As the nurse educating your client about exercise, you may want to offer the following advice: "You may notice that your center of gravity is off due to the growing fetus and that you tire more easily. This may place you at an increased risk for falling and causing trauma to your abdominal area. Make sure you limit exercising in hot weather or a hot room to prevent overheating. Drink plenty of fluids. Also, wear a well-supporting bra and well-fitted shoes."

RESOURCES FOR WORKPLACE SAFETY

• Occupational Safety and Health Administration: www.osha.gov
• National Institute for Occupational Safety and Health: www.cdc.gov/niosh

- **Sexual activity:** Most healthy women are able to engage in sexual intercourse throughout the pregnancy without causing the fetus any harm. Different sexual positions may have to be used to accommodate a growing abdomen and the woman's comfort and to avoid supine hypotension.
- **Travel:** It is safe for most pregnant women to travel until 36 weeks. ACOG recommends air travel within the United States up to 36 weeks' gestation (35 weeks' gestation for international air travel). Refer to individual airline restrictions for more details.
- **Work:** Patient should avoid heavy lifting and exposure to chemicals, fumes, radiation, and diseases that may be transferred through close contact. Recommend periods of rest. Encourage brief walks to promote circulation.

Nutrition

A proper diet is essential to meet the needs of the mother and her growing fetus. An increase of 100 to 300 calories per day is recommended in pregnancy.

The U.S. Department of Agriculture (USDA) has a user-friendly Web site (www.mypyramid.org/mypyramidmoms) wherein a person may search for recommended meal plans. The site calculates the number of servings from each of the six basic food groups depending on a person's age, sex, physical activity, and pregnancy or lactating status, as follows:

- **Grains:** 1 serving = 1 slice of bread, 1 cup (8 oz) cereal, $\frac{1}{2}$ cup cooked rice or pasta
- **Vegetables:** 1 serving = $\frac{1}{2}$ cup
- **Fruits:** 1 serving = 1 medium-sized piece of fruit, $\frac{1}{2}$ cup (4 oz) fruit juice
- **Milk:** 1 serving = 1 cup yogurt or cow's milk or soy milk, 1 oz cheese
- **Meat:** 1 serving = 3 oz chicken, fish, or meat
- **Oils:** 1 serving = 1 teaspoon butter, 1 tbsp. salad dressing

Primary Sources of Essential Nutrients, Vitamins, and Minerals in Pregnancy
Nutrients
- **Protein (4 calories/g):** meat, fish, eggs, beans
- **Carbohydrates (4 calories/g):** bread, cereal, rice, pasta, potatoes
- **Fat (9 calories/g):** oils, margarine, nuts, eggs, meat

Vitamins
- **Vitamin A (retinol/carotenoids):** yellow or orange vegetables, such as carrots, pumpkin, and sweet potatoes; green leafy vegetables; milk; animal sources such as liver and fish

- **Vitamin B$_1$ (thiamin):** lean meat; pork; poultry; fish; whole grains, especially wheat germ; enriched breads; cereals and pasta; dried beans
- **Vitamin B$_2$ (riboflavin):** liver, eggs, green leafy vegetables, whole-grain or enriched breads and cereals, legumes
- **Vitamin B$_6$ (pyridoxine):** bananas, beans, nuts, beef, liver, pork, whole-grain–enriched cereals
- **Vitamin B$_{12}$:** animal products only, such as fish, meat, dairy
- **Vitamin C:** green peppers, citrus fruits, strawberries, tomatoes, leafy greens
- **Vitamin D:** fortified milk and cereals, fish, cheese, butter
- **Vitamin E:** wheat germ, nuts, seeds, green leafy vegetables
- **Folic acid (vitamin B$_9$):** beans, legumes, citrus fruits, dark leafy vegetables, poultry, pork, fortified bread, cereal and pasta, liver
- **Niacin (vitamin B$_3$):** lean meat, fish, poultry, nuts, eggs

Minerals
- **Calcium:** sardines, salmon, dairy, green leafy vegetables
- **Iodine:** iodized salt, seafood
- **Iron:** spinach, liver, dried beans and fruits, eggs, dark red meat, iron-fortified cereals
- **Magnesium:** bananas, avocados, soy products, legumes, whole grains
- **Phosphorus:** milk and dairy products, meat
- **Zinc:** beef, pork, lamb, nuts, legumes, pumpkin seeds

Recommended Weight Gain in Pregnancy

The recommended total weight gain during pregnancy depends on a patient's prepregnancy body mass index (BMI). A person's BMI is a measurement of body fat based on her height and weight. BMI can be calculated as follows:

$$BMI = \frac{\text{Weight in pounds}}{(\text{Height in inches}) \times (\text{Height in inches})} \times 703$$

General Nutrition Counseling

- Encourage the patient to achieve the following nutrition goals during pregnancy:
  - Maintain a healthy weight in pregnancy.
  - Use the food pyramid guide regarding recommended amounts.
  - Eat a variety of grains (especially whole grains), fruits, and vegetables.
  - Avoid or limit caffeine intake in pregnancy.
  - Take 400 µg of folic acid supplementation for at least 1 month before pregnancy and for another 3 months into the pregnancy. This prevents neural tube defects such as spina bifida and cleft palate.

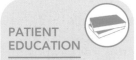
- Often, a practitioner will prescribe a prenatal vitamin, which is a supplement for vitamins and minerals, in addition to a well-balanced diet. If there is a need to increase certain vitamins and minerals, instruct the patient not to double the dose of vitamins because of the risk for toxicity.
- Fish and shellfish are wonderful sources of omega-3 fatty acids. However, caution should be taken in ingesting certain types of fish that contain high levels of mercury, which can be teratogenic to the developing fetus.
- Listeriosis is a serious infection caused by ingesting food contaminated with the *Listeria monocytogenes* bacterium. Such foods include luncheon meats and hotdogs.

Special Populations and Considerations

Certain populations of people have special needs that should be addressed by the nurse and the health-care practitioner when providing nutritional counseling.

Adolescents

- Adolescents will need extra nutrition to support their own growth needs plus those of the fetus.
- Common among adolescents are body image issues, fad diets, eating disorders, peer pressure, and others, and these may affect nutritional status.
- Patient education should be at the level of the adolescent patient.

Iron-Deficiency Anemia

The fetus uses the mother's red blood cells for growth and development. If the mother has inadequate iron stores and does not consume an iron-rich diet, this may lead to iron-deficiency anemia. Hemoglobin and hematocrit blood counts (as a component of the complete blood cell count) are obtained periodically in pregnancy to assess for anemia. If anemia is detected, nutrition counseling and supplementation is warranted. Educate on combining iron-rich foods with vitamin C to enhance absorption of iron.

Cultural/Ethnic/Religious Backgrounds

Consider the patient's background and food preferences when giving nutrition counseling and advice on meal planning. For example, a Muslim woman may be fasting for Ramadan. If Roman Catholic, she may be observing dietary restrictions for Lent.

Lactose Intolerance

Lactose intolerance is the inability to digest lactose, a sugar found in milk and milk products, because of a deficiency of the enzyme lactase. It is more common in African Americans, Hispanic Americans, American Indians, and Asian Americans than in Americans of European descent.

Pica

Some pregnant women have the urge to eat non-substantive food items such as clay, cornstarch, ice, and soil. This may affect intake of other substantial nutrients. Thorough assessment for pica when obtaining patient's nutritional history is essential. Doctor/nurse practitioner/midwife may consult a nutritionist.

Vegetarians

A major concern for vegetarians is obtaining adequate amounts of protein, calcium, iron, zinc, and vitamin B_{12}, which are all primarily found in animal products. Assess which type of vegetarian diet the patient is following.

Proteins

Animal products are primary sources for complete proteins (containing essential amino acids). Incomplete proteins are found in plant sources: grains, legumes, and nuts. However, by combining incomplete proteins (consumed together or throughout the day), complete protein can be achieved.

FISH CONSUMPTION IN PREGNANCY

Currently, according to the U.S. Environmental Protection Agency (EPA), it is safe to eat up to 12 oz per week or two average meals of the following types of fish: catfish, Pollock, shrimp, salmon, and tuna (canned light). Ingestion of albacore tuna and tuna steak should be limited to up to 6 oz per week. King mackerel, shark, swordfish, and tile fish should be avoided in pregnancy.

For more updated information regarding fish consumption, refer to the section on safe fish consumption in pregnancy on the EPA Web site (www.epa.gov).

CALCIUM CONTENT IN NONDAIRY SOURCES

- Rhubarb: 1 cup = 348 mg
- Sardines with bone: 3 oz = 325 mg
- Spinach: 1 cup = 291 mg
- Salmon: 1 cup = 181 mg
- Soy milk: 1 cup = 61 mg
- Orange: 1 medium sized = 52 mg
- Broccoli: 1 cup = 41 mg

★ BEST PRACTICES

LACTOSE INTOLERANCE

Because dairy products are the primary source of calcium, it is essential to review nondairy sources of calcium with patients who are lactose intolerant. In addition, discuss with these patients certain products that contain lactose that may not be considered dairy but may contain milk and milk products.

Following are examples of incomplete protein (plant sources) combinations that make a complete protein:
- Peanut butter on whole-grain toast
- Rice and beans
- Whole-wheat bun with sesame seeds
- Hummus made with chick peas and sesame paste
- Tortilla with refried beans
- Veggie burgers on whole-grain bun

FOOD PRODUCTS THAT MAY CONTAIN MILK AND MILK PRODUCTS

- Baked goods such as cookies
- Breakfast items such as pancakes, waffles, biscuits, doughnuts, and cereals
- Margarine
- Potato chips and other processed snacks
- Processed meats such as bacon, hot dogs, lunch meats, and sausage
- Salad dressings

AVAILABILITY AND ACCESS TO SUPPLEMENTAL NUTRITION

Low socioeconomic status may pose a barrier for pregnant women who want to obtain adequate nutrition. Referral to federal programs such as WIC (The Special Supplemental Nutrition Program for Women, Infants, and Children) and local community resources may be warranted. Under the WIC

Continued

Calcium

Some types of vegetarians do not consume milk or milk products. These patients need to be counseled on sources of nondairy calcium such as soy milk, tofu, sesame butter, almonds, and nori (dried seaweed).

Iron

Heme (well-absorbed type of iron) sources are meat, poultry, and fish. Nonheme (type of iron not as well absorbed) sources are plant products such as fruit, vegetables, grains, and nuts. Vegetarian patients need to be counseled to eat nonheme iron foods high in vitamin C, which facilitates iron absorption; for example, eating beans with tomato sauce.

Zinc

Absorption of zinc is hindered when taken with fiber-rich foods and calcium. Supplementation may be needed.

Vitamin B_{12}

Supplementation of vitamin B_{12} is necessary.

Common Discomforts in Pregnancy

First Trimester

- **Breast tenderness:** Wear a supportive bra, even at night if necessary.
- **Fatigue:** Rest as needed and consider taking naps and going to bed earlier.
- **Gingivitis**
  - Practice good oral hygiene.
  - Brush teeth and gums gently.
  - See a dentist as needed.
- **Leukorrhea**
  - May persist throughout pregnancy.

- Avoid douching.
- Wear cotton underwear.
- Wipe from front to back.
- **Nasal stuffiness and epistaxis (nosebleeds):** Use a humidifier.
- **Nausea and vomiting**
  - Avoid odors and foods that trigger nausea.
  - Before getting out of bed, eat dry toast or crackers.
  - Eat five to six small meals throughout the day.
  - Avoid fatty, greasy, spicy, gas-forming foods.
  - If intractable vomiting and weight loss occurs, a health-care provider should be notified.
- **Ptyalism (excessive secretion of saliva)**
  - Chew gum or suck on hard candy.
  - Use astringent mouthwash.
- **Urinary frequency**
  - Perform Kegel exercises.
  - Hydrate well in the daytime and limit fluid intake at night.
  - If accompanied by pain or burning, alert health-care provider.

Second Trimester
- **Heartburn**
  - Avoid fatty, greasy, spicy, gas-forming foods and large meals.
  - Remain upright after meals.
  - Avoid caffeine and tobacco.
  - Health-care provider may order antacids.
- **Varicosities**
  - Avoid standing for long periods of time, constricting clothing, or crossing legs at the knee.
  - Wear supportive hose to prevent blood pooling in the legs.
  - Elevate legs.
- **Supine hypotension:** To prevent the uterus from applying pressure on ascending vena cava, change sleeping/reclined positioned to side lying.
- **Constipation**
  - Increase fluid intake to eight 8-oz glasses daily.
  - Consume high-fiber foods such as whole-grain bread, fresh fruit, and vegetables.
  - Exercise.
- **Round ligament pain**
  - Squatting and bending knees may help alleviate cramping.
  - Apply a warm compress.

AVAILABILITY AND ACCESS TO SUPPLEMENTAL NUTRITION—cont'd

program, low-income pregnant women are eligible up to 6 weeks postpartum for supplemental, nutritious food; nutrition education; and counseling at any of the WIC agencies across the United States. For more information about WIC, visit the WIC Web site: www.fns.usda.gov/wic.

Third Trimester

- **Shortness of breath**
  - Sleep with pillows.
  - Stop smoking.
  - If symptoms worsen, contact a health-care provider.
- **Urinary frequency and urgency**
  - May return in the third trimester because of the pressure of the gravid uterus on the bladder
  - Same relief strategies as first trimester
- **Braxton Hicks contractions**
  - Breathing techniques
  - Position changes
  - Effleurage
  - Rest
- **Leg cramps**
  - Dorsiflex foot and stretch the leg for relief of cramp.
  - Apply heat to the muscle.
  - Elevate legs to improve circulation.
- **Hemorrhoids**
  - See strategies to avoid constipation.
  - Avoid straining when defecating.
  - For relief, apply topical anesthetic ointments and witch hazel pads. May also feel relief with warm soaks and use of sitz bath.

2 High-Risk Pregnancy

1cm

CHAPTER 2

High-Risk Pregnancy

Certain high-risk conditions, such as placenta previa, develop during pregnancy; other conditions that may cause problems are pre-existing conditions such as sickle cell disease. The following high-risk conditions are the most common ones seen in pregnancy.

Anemias and Hemoglobinopathies

Reference laboratory value for hemoglobin is < 11 mg/dL or hematocrit < 32%.

Iron Deficiency Anemia
- **Etiology:** diet poor in iron, short interconceptual period, and postpartum hemorrhage
- **Incidence:** Most common type of anemia worldwide. According to the World Health Organization, incidence of iron deficiency anemia is 17% in industrialized countries and 56% in developing countries.
- **Effects on pregnancy:** preterm delivery and low birth weight
- **Management:** may need iron supplements in addition to prenatal vitamins. For dietary iron counseling, see the section on nutrition in Chapter One "Normal Pregnancy." If there are enough maternal iron stores, laboratory values will return to normal around 6 weeks postpartum.

Megaloblastic Anemia
- **Etiology:** folate or vitamin B_{12} deficiency
- **Incidence:** uncommon, usually does not occur until the third trimester
- **Effects on pregnancy:** low folate level is associated with an increased risk for neural tube defect, greater risk for pre-eclampsia, prematurity, and very low birth weight.
- **Management:** Women of childbearing age should take 400 mcg folic acid supplementation for at least 1 month before pregnancy and for another 3 months into the pregnancy. A prescription for 1 g of folic acid may be given to women who are carrying multiple

fetuses, are taking anticonvulsant medications (such as phenytoin and carbamazepine), or have hemoglobinopathies. See the section on nutrition in Chapter One "Normal Pregnancy" for vitamin B_{12} dietary sources.

- Causes of vitamin B_{12} deficiency
  - **Diet:** vegetarian
  - **Coexisting medical condition:** Crohn's disease
  - **Surgery:** gastric bypass, gastrectomy, ileal bypass
  - **Medications:** metformin and proton pump inhibitors (such as lansoprazole)

Sickle Cell Anemia

Sickle cell anemia is characterized by the presence of sickle-shaped red blood cells that contain hemoglobin S. Patients with sickle cell disease are homozygous for hemoglobin S (hemoglobin SS), and those with sickle cell trait are heterozygous for hemoglobin S (hemoglobin AS).

- **Incidence:** Sickle cell anemia is common in people of African American heritage. One in 12 black adults in the United States is a carrier for the sickle cell trait.
- **Effects on pregnancy:** Women with sickle cell disease have a greater morbidity and mortality in pregnancy compared with those who are without disease. There is an increased risk for antepartum hospitalization because of preterm labor and premature rupture of membranes (PROM).
- **Laboratory tests/diagnosis:** Hemoglobin electrophoresis tests for the different types of hemoglobin that may be present in the blood. Testing should be encouraged for spouses/partners of women who are carriers of the sickle cell trait. If both prospective parents are determined to be carriers, the physician may offer prenatal diagnosis.
- **Implications in pregnancy:** During a sickle cell crisis, vaso-occlusion may occur (usually in the extremities, joints, and abdomen) and cause extreme pain.
- **Treatment and management of a sickle crisis:** Treatment and management include analgesics, oxygen, and intravenous (IV) hydration. Prevention of the crisis is key.

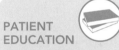

PATIENT EDUCATION

To help prevent a crisis, the patient should hydrate herself with six to eight glasses of water a day, avoid exertion in warm weather, eat a healthy diet, take a folic acid supplement to help the body make new red blood cells, and make sure to attend all scheduled prenatal visits. Symptoms, blood work, and health of mother and baby should be closely monitored.

Asthma

Asthma is a chronic lung disease characterized by inflammation and narrowing of the airway causing wheezing, chest tightness, shortness of breath, and coughing possibly triggered by allergens (such as pollen and animal dander), medical conditions (such as upper respiratory infection), and irritants (such as cigarette smoke and chemicals).

- **Incidence:** 4% to 8% in pregnancy, making this the most common medical condition that may lead to complications during pregnancy
- **Effects on pregnancy:** in about 30% of patients with asthma, the condition becomes worse during pregnancy.
- **Management:** Strict assessment and monitoring of asthma using a peak flow meter at each prenatal visit is recommended. Instruct patient to monitor fetal activity and, if there is a decrease, to alert her health-care practitioner (HCP) immediately. Ultrasound surveillance for fetal growth may be advised by the physician for patients with poorly controlled asthma. Avoid allergens and irritants. Educate patient on smoking cessation and proper use of medications prescribed by HCP.

> **WHY IS ASTHMA IMPORTANT?**
>
> Poor control of asthma in pregnancy leads to maternal hypoxia, which may cause poor maternal and fetal outcomes. Moderate-to-severe asthma requiring medication is associated with an infant who is small for gestational age, reduction of gestational age at delivery, and pre-eclampsia.

- Treatment goal for asthma control is defined by the National Asthma Education and Prevention Program Expert Panel as follows:
  - Minimal or no chronic symptoms day or night
  - Minimal or no exacerbations
  - No limitations on activities
  - Maintenance of (near) normal pulmonary functions
  - Minimal use of short-acting inhaled $beta_2$-agonist
  - Minimal or no adverse effects from medications

Bleeding Disorders

The following conditions may cause abnormal bleeding in pregnancy.

Spontaneous Abortion (Miscarriage)

Abortion is the delivery of a fetus before the 20th week of gestation.

- **Signs and symptoms:** Typically, bleeding occurs followed by abdominal cramping pain.
- **Etiology:** About half of early spontaneous abortions are due to chromosomal abnormalities such as trisomies. Other factors include infection (e.g., *Chlamydia trachomatis* and *Listeria monocytogenes*), endocrine (e.g., thyroid autoantibodies), environmental factors (e.g., tobacco use), and uterine factors (fibroids).
- **Incidence:** 15% to 25% of pregnancies. An estimated 80% of these miscarriages happen within the first 12 weeks of gestation.

- Types of spontaneous abortion
  - **Threatened:** first-trimester bleeding in the absence of fluid or tissue loss
  - **Inevitable:** cervical dilation in the setting of rupture of membranes most often followed by contractions and the expulsion of placental or fetal tissue or both
  - **Incomplete:** characterized by bleeding through a dilated internal cervical os; placental or fetal tissue or both, either completely or partially remain in utero and may need to be extracted by ring forceps or evacuated by suction and curettage
  - **Complete:** placental or fetal tissue or both is completely and spontaneously delivered
  - **Missed:** retained placental or fetal tissue, or both, from a failed intrauterine pregnancy
  - **Induced abortion:** an elective medical or surgical termination of a pregnancy before viability

Ectopic Pregnancy

An ectopic pregnancy refers to the implantation of the blastocyst outside the uterine cavity.
- **Locations of implantation:** fallopian tube (98% of the time), ovary, cervix, and abdomen
- Risk factors
  - Infection such as chlamydia and gonorrhea
  - History of infertility
  - Smoking
  - Prior ectopic pregnancy
  - Diethylstilbestrol exposure
  - Advanced maternal age
- Symptoms
  - Pregnancy-associated symptoms such as nausea and vomiting and breast tenderness
  - Shoulder pain
  - Vaginal bleeding may or may not be present
  - Pain in the lower abdomen and/or pelvis
- Physical examination findings
  - Abdominal tenderness
  - Cervical motion tenderness
  - Uterine enlargement
  - Softening of the uterus
  - Fever
- Diagnosis
  - Transvaginal ultrasound
  - Serum beta-human chorionic gonadotropin (hCG)
- Management
  - Medical management with the use of methotrexate
  - Surgical management

Abruptio Placentae or Placental Abruption

Abruptio placentae or placental abruption refers to placental detachment from the uterus (see Fig. 2–1).

- **Incidence:** 1 in 75 to 226 deliveries
- **Signs and symptoms:** vaginal bleeding (although in 10%–20% of cases, no vaginal bleeding occurs; instead, occult uterine bleeding is present), abdominal pain, uterine contractions, uterine tenderness, nonreassuring fetal heart rate patterns, fetal death
- **Risk factors:** cocaine abuse, history of abruption in a previous pregnancy, maternal hypertension (chronic, gestational, or pre-eclampsia), increased parity and/or age of mother, PROM, tobacco use, placental abnormalities, inherited thrombophilia, quick decompression of uterine cavity secondary to spontaneous rupture of membranes of a woman with polyhydramnios or after the delivery of the first child in a multifetal pregnancy
- **Management:** Depending on the gestational age and severity of the abruption at the time of the diagnosis, timing and mode of delivery will be determined by the managing HCP. Close laboratory monitoring of hemoglobin, hematocrit, coagulation studies, and fibrinogen level is warranted. Ensure that the patient has a large-bore IV catheter. In case of severe bleeding, immediate IV access for fluids, blood products, or both for transfusion may be necessary. Alert the charge nurse and the operating room team regarding the patient's plan of care.

Placenta Previa

Placenta previa occurs when the placenta is located over the cervical os, covering the os either partially or fully (see Fig. 2–2).

- **Incidence:** 4 in 1000 deliveries
- **Signs and symptoms:** painless vaginal bleeding
- **Classifications:** complete placenta previa refers to a placenta covering the cervical os, and a marginal placenta previa is defined as a placenta covering only about 2 to 3 cm of the cervical os

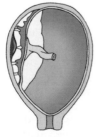 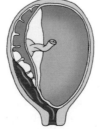 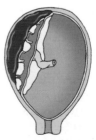

| Partial separation (concealed hemorrhage) | Partial separation (apparent hemorrhage) | Complete separation (concealed hemorrhage) |

FIGURE 2-1: Placental abruption.

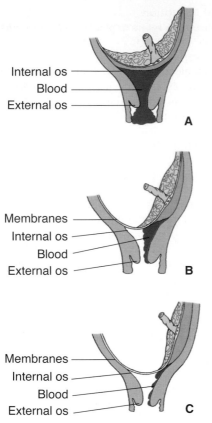

Internal os
Blood
External os
A

Membranes
Internal os
Blood
External os
B

Membranes
Internal os
Blood
External os
C

FIGURE 2-2: Placenta previa.

- **Risk factors:** tobacco use, history of cesarean delivery, history of placenta previa, history of uterine instrumentation such as curettage, increased maternal age, increased parity, multiple gestation
- **Management:** Obtain serial ultrasounds to examine placenta location and fetal growth. Avoid cervical examinations. Some patients with stable bleeding may be managed on an outpatient basis. Advise these patients to observe pelvic rest. Instruct the patient to call her HCP if she is having uterine contractions, loss of fluid, and vaginal bleeding. Discuss a plan of action with the patient regarding how she will come to the hospital. Ascertain whether the patient has access to transportation and someone to drive her.

If patient is not stable enough for outpatient management and needs to be hospitalized, she may need continuous external fetal monitoring in the labor and delivery unit. Large-bore IV access should be placed, and laboratory tests such as blood type and screen, coagulation studies, hemoglobin, hematocrit, platelet count, and fibrinogen level should be obtained, as per orders. Also, if patient is at less than 34 weeks' gestation, the HCP may order corticosteroid therapy for fetal lung maturity, and tocolysis may also be considered. If there is active bleeding, Rh-immune globulin (RhoGAM) needs to be administered if the mother is Rh-negative to prevent isoimmunization.

Mode of delivery depends on how much of the placenta is covering the cervical os, thus blocking the passageway for delivery. Most likely a cesarean section will be the mode chosen to deliver the infant.

TIP

If diagnosis of placenta previa is made before 24 weeks, 90% of these cases will resolve by term. As the uterus enlarges, the placenta "moves" away from the cervical os.

Placenta Accreta

Placenta accreta is abnormal placentation directly onto the uterine lining caused by a deficient decidua basalis.

- **Incidence:** 1 in 533 deliveries
- **Signs and symptoms:** painless vaginal bleeding
- Variations
  - Placenta increta, wherein the placenta's chorionic villi extend to the myometrium
  - Placenta percreta, wherein the placenta's chorionic villi penetrate through the myometrium and the peritoneum of the uterus
- **Risk factors:** placenta previa, history of previous cesarean section, increased parity, increased maternal age, and defects in the endometrial lining
- **Management:** Take steps to prevent and prepare for a possible postpartum hemorrhage and minimize complications (such as shock). A multidisciplinary approach should be taken, with surgery, urology, and anesthesia personnel all on board. IV access with two large-bore catheters, close monitoring of vital signs, immediate availability of blood products, and fluid resuscitation are recommended.

ALERT!

About two-thirds of patients with a diagnosis of placenta accreta require a cesarean hysterectomy. A hysterectomy is performed during a cesarean section after the delivery of the fetus to prevent significant maternal blood loss when manual separation of the placenta from the uterus is impossible.

Vasa Previa

Vasa previa is characterized by the velamentous insertion of the cord into the cervical os.

- **Incidence:** 1 in 2500
- **Signs and symptoms:** acute bleeding on spontaneous or artificial rupture of membrane
- **Risk factors:** in vitro fertilization, low-lying placenta, and multiple pregnancy
- **Management:** Historically, vasa previa was diagnosed on palpation of a pulsating cord through the membrane intrapartally.

The cord in a vasa previa is usually not surrounded with Wharton's jelly (which protects the cord), making it susceptible to lacerations and exsanguination. When bleeding is found on rupture of membranes and a vasa previa is diagnosed, urgent cesarean delivery is most likely indicated because of the high risk for fetal morbidity and mortality from rapid fetal blood loss.

Through advancement in ultrasonography, antenatal diagnosis of vasa previa is now possible. When diagnosed before 36 weeks' gestation, vasa previa is managed similarly to placenta previa, with serial ultrasounds, antenatal testing, corticosteroid therapy, and strict instructions regarding labor symptoms and pelvic rest.

Diabetes Mellitus

Diabetes is a chronic state of hyperglycemia. Pregestational diabetes, as the term implies, is diagnosed before pregnancy. Diabetes that is diagnosed during pregnancy is termed *gestational diabetes mellitus* (GDM).

Pregestational Diabetes
Diabetes diagnosed before pregnancy is classified into two major categories: type 1 and type 2.
- **Incidence:** 1% of all pregnancies
- **Type 1:** previously termed *insulin-dependent diabetes mellitus* (IDDM) or *juvenile-onset diabetes*
  - **Etiology:** autoimmune process causing the destruction of pancreatic beta cells
- **Type 2:** previously termed *non–insulin-dependent diabetes* or *adult-onset diabetes*
  - **Causative factor:** insulin resistance and insulin deficiency

Gestational Diabetes
GDM is glucose intolerance of any degree that is diagnosed during pregnancy whether it is treated with diet alone (class A_1) or with insulin (class A_2).
- **Incidence:** occurs in 2% to 5% of pregnant women
- **Screening:** Assessment for GDM risk should be performed at the first prenatal visit.
  - **Low risk for GDM:** Screening is not recommended by the American Diabetes Association for low-risk women who fulfill **all** of the following criteria:
    - **Age:** < 25 years
    - **Weight:** normal
    - **Medical history:** no history of abnormal glucose metabolism
    - **Obstetric history:** no poor obstetric outcome
    - **Ethnicity:** not a member of an ethnic group with a high diabetes prevalence such as African American, Asian American, Pacific Islander, or Native American
    - **Family history:** no first-degree relatives with diabetes
    - Average risk for GDM

Screening for women who do not meet all the criteria for low risk and who do not possess any high-risk characteristic (see later) should be done between 24 and 28 weeks of gestation.

High Risk for GDM

If the woman is found to be at high risk for GDM on obtaining her initial history, early screening should be undertaken as soon as possible. High-risk characteristics for GDM include the following:

- Marked obesity
- GDM in a prior pregnancy
- Family history of diabetes

If the initial screening is normal for someone at high risk for GDM, testing should be repeated at 24 to 28 weeks.

Diagnosing GDM

Diagnosis is confirmed by means of a fasting blood glucose level >126 mg/dL or a random plasma glucose level >200 mg/dL with hyperglycemia symptoms to be confirmed the next day with repeat testing. If repeat testing is normal, proceed to either one- or two-step approach for further evaluation.

- **One-step approach:** Proceed directly to diagnostic testing with an oral glucose tolerance test (GTT).
- **Two-step approach:** The first step includes administering a 50-g oral glucose load and measuring the plasma or serum glucose concentration 1 hour later. There is no need for fasting before this test; however, patient should not eat, drink, or smoke cigarettes once the glucose solution is administered. The threshold for abnormal 1-hour glucose value is controversial. When >140 mg/dL value is used, ~80% of women are identified with GDM. If >130 mg/dL value is used, ~90% of women are identified with GDM. The American Diabetes Association leaves the choice open to the HCP. Knowing what your practice uses as a cutoff is important. If a patient has an abnormal value from the glucose challenge screening test, the patient will need to perform the 3-hour oral GTT to diagnose GDM.

⭐ **BEST PRACTICES**

Nursing responsibilities in administering the 3-hour GTT include the following:
- Instruct patient not to eat or drink after midnight.
- Obtain a fasting serum or plasma glucose.
- Administer 100-g oral glucose solution.
- Have patient remain seated while test is being performed.
- Instruct patient not to smoke once glucose solution is administered.
- Obtain serum or plasma glucose measurement every hour for 3 hours after glucose solution ingestion.
- Two or more abnormal values are required for the diagnosis of GDM. See Table 2–1 for the criteria used for diagnosing GDM.

Table 2–1 Two Different Criteria for the Glucose Tolerance Test Used for Diagnosing Gestational Diabetes

100-g ORAL GTT	CARPENTER AND COUSTAN	NDDG
	mg/dL	mg/dL
Fasting	95	105
1 hour	180	190
2 hour	155	165
3 hour	140	145

Two different criteria are used based on O'Sullivan and Mahan's research published in 1964, one by the National Diabetes Data Group (NDDG) and one by Carpenter and Coustan.

GTT, glucose tolerance test.

Management of Diabetes in Pregnancy

The nurse has an important role in educating the patient with diabetes on keeping excellent glycemic control to optimize outcome for both the mother and the baby.

Proper Nutrition

- Assess patient's eating habits and food preferences (consider cultural and/or ethnic choices).
- Collaborate with the patient to determine appropriate nutritional goals and construct a nutritional plan specific to the patient. Research has shown that nutrition education is key in improving glycemic control.
- Refer to a nutritionist/registered dietitian for meal planning to achieve caloric goals and nutritional needs in pregnancy.
- Caloric requirement of approximately 300 kcal higher than nonpregnancy needs is the same for pregnant women with and without diabetes.
- Tailor a dietary plan that is composed of complex, high-fiber carbohydrates from whole grains, legumes, fruits and vegetables, protein from lean meats, poultry, and tofu. Limit saturated fat intake to < 7% of total calories.
- Recommended calorie distribution: breakfast 10% to 20%, lunch 20% to 30%, dinner 30% to 40%, and snack 30%.
- Recommend consuming an evening snack as important to curb nocturnal hypoglycemia.

> **TIP**
>
> In pregnancy, diabetes is classified according to age of onset, duration of disease, organ involvement, and whether the disease was diagnosed in pregnancy or before. Refer to Table 2–2 for the White classification of diabetes in pregnancy.

> **TIP**
>
> According to the U.S. Food and Drug Administration, moderate consumption of artificial sweeteners such as aspartame is safe in pregnancy.

Table 2–2	White Classification of Diabetes in Pregnant Woman	
CATEGORY	**DESCRIPTION**	
	GESTATIONAL DIABETES	
A_1	Diet controlled	
A_2	Insulin requiring	
	PREGESTATIONAL DIABETES	
B	Onset >20 years of age, lasting <10 years, with no vascular involvement, requiring insulin	
C	Onset between 10 and 19 years of age or had the disease for 10 to 19 years, with no vascular involvement, requiring insulin	
D	Onset before age 10 years or duration of disease ≥20 years or with retinopathy, requiring insulin	
F	Irrelevant of onset or length of disease, but development of nephropathy, requiring insulin	
R	Irrelevant of onset or length of disease, development of retinopathy, requiring insulin	
T	Renal transplantation, irrelevant of onset or length of disease	
H	History of myocardial ischemia, irrelevant of onset or length of disease	

Physical Activity

Educate patient on importance of physical activity, and stress that it has been proved to improve glycemic control, reduce the risk for cardiovascular disease, improve control of blood pressure, and provide psychological benefits of stress reduction and lower incidence of depression. Physical activity regimens should be closely monitored by an HCP because insulin needs may be altered by different forms and duration of activity.

Monitoring

- **Blood glucose monitoring:** Educate and/or review with the patient how to monitor blood glucose levels at home. If the patient is admitted to the hospital, obtain blood glucose levels as per prescriber's orders. A fasting glucose level measurement 1 or 2 hours before and after meals and at bedtime may be ordered by the HCP. Blood glucose goals are listed in Table 2–3.
- **Ketones and glucose in urine:** At each prenatal visit, perform a urine dip analysis for ketones and glucose. At home, patients should check their urine for ketones if their blood glucose level exceeds 200 mg/dL, and they need to be instructed to report abnormal results to their HCP immediately.

Table 2–3 **Blood Glucose Goals in Diabetes During Pregnancy**	
On awakening	≤95 mg/dL
Before meal	≤100 mg/dL
1 hour after meal	≤140 mg/dL
2 hours after meal	≤120 mg/dL

- Monitor for symptoms of hyperglycemia such as increased thirst, urination, and lethargy.
- Monitor for hypoglycemia symptoms such as confusion, visual disturbances, anxiety, tremor, sweating, and increased hunger. Although uncommon, seizures and loss of consciousness may also occur.

Medication

If diet and exercise are not enough, medication such as insulin may be prescribed. Some patients are candidates for oral medication.

Healthy Coping

- Being diagnosed with diabetes may cause an individual stress. Intervention may be needed to optimize coping and to improve the patient's quality of life. Intervention may include cognitive-behavioral treatment of depression and support groups. Assess family/significant other support and involve them when diabetes education is provided for the patient.
- Refer to a nutritionist, ophthalmologist, pediatrician, diabetes specialist, and/or a primary care physician (for postpartum follow-up), diabetes educator, and financial counselor.
- **Maternal-fetal surveillance:** Women with pregestational diabetes may need to come for prenatal care every 1 to 2 weeks in the first two trimesters and weekly in the third trimester.

Maternal Morbidity in Poorly Controlled Pregestational Diabetes Mellitus

- Retinopathy
  - Nephropathy

EVIDENCE-BASED PRACTICE

The safety and efficacy in pregnancy of all oral hypoglycemic agents has not been well studied. However, glyburide, which does not cross the placenta, has been shown to be comparable with insulin's effectiveness in a study of 404 women between 11 and 33 weeks of gestation. The research also did not find any evidence of adverse maternal and fetal effects. Glyburide is now being used to treat GDM in some patients.

- Chronic hypertension
- Coronary artery disease
- Diabetic ketoacidosis

Perinatal Morbidity and Mortality in Poorly Controlled Pregestational Diabetes Mellitus

Perinatal morbidity and mortality in poorly controlled pregestational DM are associated with the following conditions:
- Congenital anomalies
- Spontaneous abortions
- Complex cardiac defects
- Anencephaly
- Spina bifida
- Sacral agenesis

There is an increased risk in poorly controlled GDM for the following:
- Intrauterine fetal death
- Macrosomia
- Shoulder dystocia

Possible neonatal effects in poorly controlled GDM include the following:
- Hypoglycemia
- Respiratory distress syndrome
- Polycythemia
- Organomegaly
- Hyperbilirubinemia

Obstetric complications more common in poorly controlled GDM include the following:
- Preterm labor
- Polyhydramnios
- Pre-eclampsia
- Intrauterine growth restriction (IUGR)
- Primary cesarean delivery

Maternal and Fetal Complications in Poorly Controlled Gestational Diabetes Mellitus

Maternal and fetal complications in poorly controlled GDM include the following:
- Hypertensive disorders
- Macrosomia
- Hyperbilirubinemia
- Shoulder dystocia
- Operative delivery
- Birth trauma

WHY IS IT IMPORTANT TO KNOW ABOUT DIABETIC KETOACIDOSIS?

Diabetic ketoacidosis (DKA) is an emergency that is life-threatening for both mother and fetus. It is most commonly seen in women with type I pregestational DM. Risk factors include infection, unrecognized new-onset diabetes, poorly controlled DM, insulin pump malfunction, use of antenatal corticosteroids, and beta-mimetic medications used for tocolysis. A woman with DKA typically presents with nausea, vomiting (in 25% of patients, coffee-ground emesis is seen), abdominal pain, fruit-scented breath, confusion, dehydration, hypotension, and hyperventilation. Laboratory findings in a woman with DKA include plasma glucose level >250 mg/dL, positive urine and serum ketones, anion gap elevation to ≥10, serum bicarbonate level <15, and arterial pH <7.25.

Management of DKA in pregnancy should include the following:

- Laboratory assessment: Obtain baseline laboratory results every 1 to 2 hours for glucose, ketones, and electrolyte levels.
- Insulin: Typically given intravenously.
- Fluid hydration: Typically, IV fluid resuscitation is warranted.

Continued

WHY IS IT IMPORTANT TO KNOW ABOUT DIABETIC KETOACIDOSIS?—cont'd

- Glucose: When plasma glucose level declines to <250 mg/dL, patient should be given 5% dextrose in normal saline intravenously to prevent further ketosis.
- Electrolyte replacement

Antepartum Fetal Assessment for Women With Diabetes

Because of the increased morbidity and mortality associated with diabetes in pregnancy, starting at 32 to 34 weeks of gestation, the following assessments are typically recommended for women with diabetes to monitor the well-being of the fetus.

- **Fetal kick counts:** assessed daily by the mother
- **Nonstress test:** performed twice weekly
- **Ultrasounds:** to monitor fetal growth about every 3 to 4 weeks and measure the amniotic fluid volume usually twice weekly
- **Umbilical artery Doppler velocimetry:** obtained if fetal growth is poor

Hypertensive Disorders

Gestational Hypertension

Formerly called "pregnancy-induced hypertension," the condition of having high blood pressure diagnosed and isolated in pregnancy is now referred to as "gestational hypertension" by the National High Blood Pressure Education Program Working Group.

OFFERING SUPPORT

To find a diabetes teacher (nurse, dietitian, or other health professional) near you, call the American Association of Diabetes Educators toll-free at 1-800-TEAMUP4 (1-800-832-6874), or go online to www.diabeteseducator.org and click on the link "Find a Diabetes Educator."

- **Diagnosis:** blood pressure >140/90 mm Hg found after 20 weeks' gestation in a pregnant woman who previously was normotensive and with the absence of proteinuria. This increased blood pressure needs to be present on two occasions, measured 4 hours apart.
  - Gestational hypertension may very well be chronic hypertension that was undiagnosed until the patient's pregnancy.

QSEN Application

Patient-centered care includes knowledge such as the following:
- Integrating understanding of multiple dimensions of patient-centered care
  - Patient/family/community preferences, values
  - Coordination and integration of care
  - Information, communication, and education
  - Physical comfort and emotional support
  - Involvement of family and friends
  - Transition and continuity

- Counsel the patient to follow up with a primary care physician after delivery to determine whether the patient's blood pressure continues to be elevated and requires further management.
- Persistent high blood pressure past the 12th week postpartum may likely be because of chronic hypertension.

Gestational hypertension may lead to pre-eclampsia; there is an increased likelihood for pre-eclampsia if onset of increased blood pressure happens at ≥35 weeks' gestation.

- **Management:** At each prenatal visit:
  - Obtain the patient's vital signs.
  - Dip a urine sample for protein.
  - Assess the patient for signs and symptoms of worsening disease.

Pre-eclampsia

Pre-eclampsia is a condition defined by high blood pressure with accompanying proteinuria.

- **Incidence:** 5% to 8% of all pregnancies
- Risk factors
  - First pregnancy
  - African American
  - ≥35 years of age
  - Family history of pre-eclampsia
  - Obesity
  - Multifetal gestation
  - Pre-eclampsia in previous pregnancy
  - **Poor outcome in previous pregnancy:** IUGR, placental abruption, fetal demise
  - **Pre-existing medical and genetic conditions:** chronic hypertension, renal disease, type 1 DM, thrombophilias
  - Factor V Leiden
- **Diagnosis:** blood pressure >140/90 mm Hg found after 20 weeks' gestation in a pregnant woman who previously had normal blood pressure with the presence of protein in the urine ≥0.3 g in a 24-hour urine specimen

- Signs and symptoms
  - Visual disturbances
  - Headache
  - Epigastric pain
  - Edema
  - Hyper-reflexia
  - Oliguria
- Laboratory findings
  - Elevated liver enzymes
  - Elevated uric acid
  - Low platelet count
  - Proteinuria ≥0.3 g in a 24-hour urine specimen
- Fetal and placental effects

Because of a compromised uteroplacental blood flow, changes in the fetus and placenta may occur. A nonreassuring fetal heart tracing may be seen on fetal assessment together with IUGR, oligohydramnios, and placental abruption.

Mild pre-eclampsia may worsen, turning into severe pre-eclampsia. See Box 2-1 for the diagnostic criteria for severe pre-eclampsia.

- Management
  - Antihypertensives, such as labetalol or hydralazine, may be ordered by the HCP.
  - Magnesium sulfate given intravenously for seizure prophylaxis may be ordered by the HCP (see Box 2-2).
  - Careful surveillance of the patient's vital signs and fluid intake and output should be performed.

> **TIP**
>
> A finding of 0.3 g of urine correlates with ≥1+ protein on a urine dipstick.

Box 2-1 Diagnostic Criteria for Severe Pre-eclampsia

A diagnosis of severe pre-eclampsia can be made if one or more of the following criteria are met:

1. Blood pressure: systolic ≥160 mm Hg or diastolic ≥110 mm Hg taken on two separate occasions at least 6 hours apart
2. Proteinuria: ≥5 g in a 24-hour urine specimen or ≥3+ on two urine samples collected at least 4 hours apart
3. Oliguria: <500 mL in a 24-hour period
4. Visual disturbances
5. Pulmonary edema
6. Epigastric or right upper quadrant pain
7. Impaired liver function
8. Thrombocytopenia
9. Fetal growth restriction

Box 2–2 **Medication Highlight: MAGNESIUM SULFATE**

magnesium sulfate (IV, parenteral) (9.9% Mg; 8.1 mEq Mg/g) (mag-**nee**-zee-um sul-fate)

CLASSIFICATION

- Therapeutic: mineral and electrolyte replacements/supplements
- Pharmacological: minerals/electrolytes

PREGNANCY CATEGORY A

Indications

Treatment/prevention of hypomagnesemia. Treatment of hypertension. Anticonvulsant associated with severe eclampsia, pre-eclampsia, or acute nephritis. **Unlabeled Use:** Preterm labor. Treatment of torsade de pointes. Adjunctive treatment for bronchodilation in moderate to severe acute asthma.

Action

Essential for the activity of many enzymes. Plays an important role in neuro-transmission and muscular excitability. **Therapeutic Effects:** Replacement in deficiency states. Resolution of eclampsia.

Pharmacokinetics

- **Absorption:** IV administration results in complete bioavailability; well absorbed from IM sites
- **Distribution:** widely distributed; crosses the placenta and is present in breast milk
- **Metabolism and Excretion:** excreted primarily by the kidneys
- **Half-life:** Unknown

TIME/ACTION PROFILE (ANTICONVULSANT EFFECT)

ROUTE	ONSET	PEAK	DURATION
IM	60 min	Unknown	3–4 hr
IV	Immediate	Unknown	30 min

CONTRAINDICATIONS/PRECAUTIONS

- **Contraindicated in** hypermagnesemia, hypocalcemia, anuria, heart block. OB: Unless used for preterm labor, avoid continuous use during active labor or within 2 hours of delivery because of potential for magnesium toxicity in newborn.
- **Use cautiously in** any degree of renal insufficiency.
- **Adverse Reactions/Side Effects** (CAPITALS indicate life-threatening; underlines indicate most frequent.)
- **Central nervous system:** drowsiness. **Respiratory:** ↓ respiratory rate. **Cardiovascular:** arrhythmias, bradycardia, hypotension. **Gastrointestinal:** diarrhea. **Musculoskeletal:** muscle weakness. **Dermal:** flushing, sweating. **Metabolic:** hypothermia.

INTERACTIONS

- **Drug–drug:** May potentiate **calcium channel blockers** and **neuromuscular blocking agents.**

Continued

Box 2–2 **Medication Highlight: MAGNESIUM SULFATE—cont'd**

ROUTE/DOSAGE

Treatment of Deficiency (expressed as milligrams of magnesium)

- **IM, IV (adults):** *Severe deficiency*—8–12 g/day in divided doses; *mild deficiency*—1 g q6h for 4 doses or 250 mg/kg over 4 hours
- **IM, IV (children >1 month):** 25–50 mg/kg/dose q4–6h for 3–4 doses; maximum single dose: 2 g
- **IV (neonates):** 25–50 mg/kg/dose q8–12h for 2–3 doses

Seizures/Hypertension

- **IM, IV (adults):** 1 g q6h for 4 doses as needed
- **IM, IV (children):** 20–100 mg/kg/dose q4–6h as needed, may use up to 200 mg/kg/dose in severe cases

Torsade de Pointes

- **IV (infants and children):** 25–50 mg/kg/dose; maximum dose: 2 g

Bronchodilation

- **IV (adults):** 2 g single dose
- **IV (children):** 25 mg/kg/dose, maximum dose: 2 g

Eclampsia/Pre-eclampsia

- **IV, IM (adults):** 4–5 g by IV infusion, concurrently with up to 5 g IM in each buttock; then 4–5 g IM q4h *or* 4 g by IV infusion followed by 1–2 g/hr continuous infusion (not to exceed 40 g/day or 20 g/48 hr in the presence of severe renal insufficiency)

Part of Parenteral Nutrition

- **IV (adults):** 4–24 mEq/day
- **IV (children):** 0.25–0.5 mEq/kg/day

Availability (generic available)

- **Injection:** 500 mg/mL (50%). **Premixed infusion:** 1 g/100 mL, 2 g/100 mL, 4 g/50 mL, 4 g/100 mL, 20 g/500 mL, 40 g/1000 mL

NURSING IMPLICATIONS

ASSESSMENT

- **Hypomagnesemia/Anticonvulsant:** Monitor pulse, blood pressure, respirations, and electrocardiogram frequently throughout administration of parenteral magnesium sulfate. Respirations should be at least 16 per minute before each dose.
- Monitor neurological status before and throughout therapy. Institute seizure precautions. Patellar reflex (knee jerk) should be tested before each parenteral dose of magnesium sulfate. If response is absent, no additional doses should be administered until positive response is obtained.
- Monitor newborn for hypotension, hyporeflexia, and respiratory depression if mother has received magnesium sulfate.
- Monitor intake and output ratios. Urine output should be maintained at a level of at least 100 mL/4 hr.

Continued

Box 2–2 **Medication Highlight: MAGNESIUM SULFATE—cont'd**

- *Laboratory test considerations:* Monitor serum magnesium levels and renal function periodically throughout administration of parenteral magnesium sulfate.

POTENTIAL NURSING DIAGNOSES

- Risk for injury (indications, side effects)

IMPLEMENTATION

- *High Alert:* Accidental overdosage of IV magnesium has resulted in serious patient harm and death. Have second practitioner independently double-check original order, dose calculations, and infusion pump settings. Do not confuse milligram (mg), gram (g), or milliequivalent (mEq) dosages.
- IM: Administer deep IM into gluteal sides. Administer subsequent injections in alternate sides. Dilute to a concentration of 200 mg/mL before injection.

INTRAVENOUS ADMINISTRATION

- Direct IV: *Diluent:* 50% solution must be diluted in 0.9% NaCl or 5% dextrose in water (D5W) to a concentration ≤20% before administration. *Concentration:* ≤20%. *Rate:* Administer at a rate not to exceed 150 mg/min.
- Continuous infusion: *Diluent:* Dilute in D5W, 0.9% NaCl, or lactated Ringer's (LR). *Concentration:* 0.5 mEq/mL (60 mg/mL) (may use maximum concentration of 1.6 mEq/mL [200 mg/mL] in fluid-restricted patients). *Rate:* Infuse over 2–4 hr. Do not exceed a rate of 1 mEq/kg/hr (125 mg/kg/hr). When rapid infusions are needed (severe asthma or torsade de pointes), may infuse over 10–20 min.
- Y-site compatibility: acyclovir, aldesleukin, alfentanil, amifostine, amikacin, argatroban, ascorbic acid, atracurium, atropine, aztreonam, benztropine, bivalirudin, bleomycin, bumetanide, buprenorphine, butorphanol, calcium gluconate, carboplatin, carmustine, caspofungin, cefazolin, cefotaxime, cefoxitin, ceftazidime, ceftizoxime, chloramphenicol, chlorpromazine, cisatracurium, cisplatin, clindamycin, clonidine, cyanocobalamin, cyclophosphamide, cytarabine, dactinomycin, daptomycin, dexmedetomidine, digoxin, diltiazem, diphenhydramine, dobutamine, docetaxel, dopamine, doripenem, doxacurium, doxorubicin liposome, doxycycline, enalaprilat, epinephrine, epoetin alfa, eptifibatide, ertapenem, esmolol, etoposide, etoposide phosphate, famotidine, fenoldopam, fentanyl, fluconazole, fludarabine, fluorouracil, folic acid, gemcitabine, gentamicin, glycopyrrolate, granisetron, heparin, hetastarch, hydromorphone, idarubicin, ifosfamide, imipenem/cilastatin, insulin, irinotecan, isoproterenol, kanamycin, ketamine, ketorolac, labetalol, lidocaine, linezolid, lorazepam, mannitol, mechlorethamine, metaraminol, methotrexate, methyldopate, metoclopramide, metoprolol, metronidazole, micafungin, midazolam, milrinone, mitoxantrone, morphine, multivitamins, mycophenolate, nafcillin, nalbuphine, nesiritide, nicardipine, nitroglycerin, nitroprusside, norepinephrine,

Continued

Box 2–2 **Medication Highlight: MAGNESIUM SULFATE—cont'd**

octreotide, ondansetron, oxaliplatin, oxytocin, paclitaxel, palonosetron, pamidronate, pancuronium, pantoprazole, papaverine, penicillin G potassium, pentobarbital, phenobarbital, phentolamine, phenylephrine, piperacillin/tazobactam, potassium acetate, potassium chloride, procainamide, prochlorperazine, promethazine, propofol, propranolol, protamine, pyridoxine, quinupristin/dalfopristin, ranitidine, remifentanil, rituximab, rocuronium, sargramostim, sodium acetate, sodium bicarbonate, streptokinase, succinylcholine, sufentanil, tacrolimus, telavancin, teniposide, theophylline, thiamine, thiotepa, ticarcillin/clavulanate, tigecycline, tirofiban, tobramycin, tolazoline, trastuzumab, trimetaphan, urokinase, vancomycin, vasopressin, vecuronium, verapamil, vincristine, vinorelbine, vitamin B complex with C, voriconazole, zoledronic acid

- **Y-site incompatibility:** aminophylline, amphotericin B cholesteryl sulfate, amphotericin B lipid complex, amphotericin B liposome, anidulafungin, azathioprine, calcium chloride, cefepime, ceftriaxone, cefuroxime, ciprofloxacin, dantrolene, dexamethasone sodium phosphate, diazepam, doxorubicin hydrochloride, drotrecogin, epirubicin, haloperidol, inamrinone, indomethacin, methylprednisolone sodium succinate, pentamidine, phenytoin, phytonadione

PATIENT/FAMILY TEACHING

- Explain purpose of medication to patient and family.

EVALUATION/DESIRED OUTCOMES

- Normal serum magnesium concentrations
- Control of seizures associated with toxemias of pregnancy

Data from Davis's Drug Guide for Nurses. 12th ed. Philadelphia, PA: FA Davis Company; 2011.

Eclampsia

Eclampsia is characterized by seizures isolated in pregnancy and the postpartum period.

- **Incidence:** 1 in 2000 to 3448 pregnancies
- **Diagnosis:** occurrence of new-onset grand mal seizures in a woman who most likely has hypertension, proteinuria, and generalized edema
- **Associated signs and symptoms:** wide spectrum of signs that range from minimal hypertension, no proteinuria, and no edema to severe high blood pressure, severe proteinuria, and generalized edema. Clinical symptoms, such as headaches, blurred vision, photophobia, right upper quadrant pain, and altered mental status, may aid in the diagnosis of eclampsia. Hyperreflexia and oliguria may also be seen.
- **Timing:** An estimated 91% of all cases of eclampsia occur after the 28th week of gestation, during the antepartum and intrapartum periods. In the postpartum period, eclampsia likely occurs within 48 hours but may happen up to 4 weeks after delivery.

- Complications
  - Maternal death
  - Placental abruption
  - Disseminated intravascular coagulation

HELLP Syndrome

HELLP syndrome is a serious obstetric complication associated with patients with pre-eclampsia and/or eclampsia characterized by the *presence of these laboratory findings:* hemolytic anemia, elevated liver enzymes, and low platelet count.

- **Diagnosis:** laboratory findings aid in the diagnosis of HELLP syndrome
- **Incidence:** occurs in 4% to 12% of patients with pre-eclampsia
- Associated signs and symptoms
  - Right upper quadrant pain
  - Nausea
  - Vomiting
  - Headache
  - Visual changes
  - Malaise
- **Therapeutic intrapartum management may include:**
  - Bed rest
  - IV fluids

EVIDENCE-BASED PRACTICE

The range of signs for eclampsia is wide. As many as 54% of patients may have severe hypertension, and in 16% of the cases, patients may be normotensive. A study done of 399 patients with eclampsia showed that 48% of the women had severe proteinuria and 14% had no proteinuria. Generalized edema also has a wide range of severity; however, weight gain of ≥2 lb per week in the last trimester may be one of the first signs before an eclamptic seizure.

BEST PRACTICES

MANAGEMENT OF AN ECLAMPTIC SEIZURE

- Prevent injury during a convulsive episode.
  - Establish airway patency.
  - Ensure maternal oxygenation by administering oxygen via face mask.
  - Elevate padded bed rails.
  - Minimize risk for aspiration by placing the patient on her side.
- Prevent recurrent convulsions.

The drug of choice to treat and prevent further eclamptic episodes is magnesium sulfate given intravenously.

- Use of antithrombotic agents
- Steroids
- Fresh frozen plasma infusion
- Dialysis
- **Postpartum management:** For at least the first 48 hours, careful surveillance of the patient's vital signs, fluid intake and output, pulse oximetry, and laboratory values (as ordered by the HCP) should be performed.

Chronic Hypertension

Chronic hypertension is the presence of a systolic blood pressure ≥140 mm Hg, a diastolic blood pressure ≥90 mm Hg, or both, before pregnancy or before the 20th week of gestation. See Table 2–4 for criteria for mild and severe hypertension.

- **Incidence:** occurs in up to 5% of pregnant women
- Diagnosis
  - Blood pressure criteria as listed earlier
  - Use of antihypertensives before pregnancy
  - Onset of high blood pressure before the 20th week of pregnancy
  - Persistence of increased blood pressure past the 12-week postpartum period
- Implications of chronic hypertension in pregnancy
  - IUGR
  - Placental abruption
  - Development of pre-eclampsia
  - Fetal death
  - Delivery before term
- Management
  - As per the orders of an HCP, baseline laboratory work should be obtained and repeated to identify worsening disease. Liver function tests, hemoglobin/hematocrit level, platelet count, and a 24-hour urine evaluation are clinically useful.
  - For mild hypertension, antihypertensives generally are not prescribed because they have not been proved to improve perinatal outcome.
  - For severe hypertension, antihypertensives may be initiated by the HCP.
  - At each prenatal visit, obtain the patient's vital signs, dip a urine sample for protein, and assess the patient for signs and

Table 2–4 Mild Versus Severe Hypertension in Pregnancy

	MILD	SEVERE
Systolic blood pressure	≥140 mm Hg	≥180 mm Hg
Diastolic blood pressure	≥90 mm Hg	≥110 mm Hg

symptoms of worsening disease, such as headache, visual changes, and abdominal pain.

Congenital Infection (TORCHeS Syndrome)

TORCHeS syndrome refers to a set of perinatal infections that are transferred from the mother to the fetus. The TORCHeS acronym stands for the following congenital infections: **t**oxoplasmosis, **o**ther infections (parvovirus and varicella), **r**ubella, **c**ytomegalovirus, **he**rpes, and **s**yphilis.

Toxoplasmosis

Toxoplasmosis infection (*Toxoplasma gondii*) occurs primarily by the ingestion of poorly cooked infected meat or contaminated food.
- **Incidence:** 1 in 8000 pregnancies
- Maternal signs and symptoms
  - May be asymptomatic
  - May appear to have a presentation similar to mononucleosis such as fever, sore throat, fatigue, and swollen lymph glands
- **Effects on fetus/infant:** may be asymptomatic at birth but may suffer intellectual disabilities and/or blindness later in life
- **Diagnosis:** presence of IgM-specific antibody and a very high IgG antibody titer

---

★ BEST PRACTICES

Cats are the only host for this protozoan; *T. gondii* lives in the cat's intestines and is then excreted in the cat's feces. Handling of cat feces and subsequent contamination of food by improper handling and cooking, improper washing of produce, or lack of proper hand sanitation may spread the *T. gondii* oocyst to humans. Another route of infection is as follows: a cow ingests the *T. gondii* oocyst, cysts form in its muscles, and then a human eats the undercooked contaminated meat.

QSEN Application

Integration of evidence-based practice includes the following:
- Demonstrating knowledge of basic scientific methods and processes
- Differentiating clinical opinion from research and evidence summaries
- Describing reliable sources for locating evidence reports and clinical practice guidelines
- Describing how the strength and relevance of available evidence influences the choice of interventions in provision of patient-centered care

In this chapter, together with information about care of pregnant women and newborns, Quality and Safety Education for Nurses (QSEN) competencies assure delivery of the best nursing care.

http://qsen.org/competencies/pre-licensure-ksas/#patient-centered_care

- **Treatment:** An HCP may prescribe spiramycin (available only through the U.S. Food and Drug Administration), pyrimethamine (after the first trimester), or sulfonamides to prevent the risk for fetal transmission. The goal in management of toxoplasmosis is **prevention** of an acute infection, especially in pregnancy. Education must be provided regarding the following:
  - Avoidance of direct contact with cat feces/litter
  - Proper hand washing
  - Safe handling of food
  - Thorough washing of fresh fruits and vegetables
  - Avoidance of eating raw or rare meat
  - Thorough cooking of meat

Other Infections: Parvovirus and Varicella

Parvovirus B19

Transmission occurs through respiratory secretions and close infectious contact, especially via hand to mouth.

- **Cause:** single-stranded DNA named parvovirus B19
- **Diagnosis:** positive for parvovirus B19–specific IgM indicates recent infection; positive IgG without IgM is indicative of a past infection and immunity
- Maternal signs and symptoms
  - Mostly asymptomatic
  - In immunocompromised adults, onset of a rash may be seen.
- Effects on fetus/infant
  - If a mother is infected at less than 20 weeks of gestation, severe effects may occur such as anemia and myocarditis resulting in hydrops fetalis.
  - Risk for stillbirth within 1 to 11 weeks of maternal infection
- **Treatment:** Currently, there are no effective vaccinations or treatment modalities that are found to be efficacious against maternal or fetal parvovirus B19 infection. Women who are pregnant are advised to avoid potential exposure to individuals infected with parvovirus. **Routine testing in pregnancy for parvovirus is not recommended.**

Varicella

Transmission of varicella occurs through respiratory droplets and close contact.

- **Cause:** varicella zoster virus (VZV), a DNA herpes virus that causes chickenpox
- **Incidence:** 0.4 to 0.7 in 1000 pregnancies
- **Diagnosis:** positive serologies for IgM and IgG
- Maternal effects
  - Primary infection manifests as chickenpox
  - Fever
  - Malaise
  - Maculopapular pruritic rash

- VZV remains dormant in the sensory ganglion after the primary infection; VZV may become reactivated and cause herpes zoster, an erythematous vesicular skin rash
  - Encephalitis
  - Pneumonia
  - Death
- Effects on fetus/infant
  - Microcephaly
  - Skin scarring
  - Chorioretinitis
  - Limb hypoplasia
- **Neonatal VZV infection:** associated with an increased risk for death when maternal infection occurs between 5 days before delivery and 48 hours postpartum
- Treatment
  - Within 72 hours of exposure to varicella, the pregnant patient may be given varicella zoster immune globulin (VZIG), which may decrease the severity of maternal infection.
  - Oral acyclovir may be given to a pregnant patient within 24 hours of development of a rash characteristic of varicella infection. Acyclovir therapy may decrease the symptoms and duration of maternal disease.

Rubella (German Measles)

Spread of the rubella virus occurs through respiratory droplets and close personal contact.

- **Cause:** single-stranded RNA virus
- Maternal signs and symptoms
  - Nonpruritic rash
  - Malaise
  - Fever
  - Conjunctivitis
  - Lymphadenopathy
- Effects on fetus/infant
  - IUGR
  - Increased risk for miscarriage
  - Increased risk for congenital rubella syndrome (CRS)
- Congenital Rubella Syndrome

CRS is associated with sensorineural hearing loss, cataracts, glaucoma, retinitis, patent ductus arteriosus, and cardiac lesions. CRS findings are most likely to be found in infants infected within the first trimester.

- **Diagnosis:** Serology positive for IgM specific for rubella indicates exposure or infection.

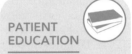

PATIENT EDUCATION

Educate your patient about the varicella vaccine.

- The varicella vaccine contains live attenuated virus and should be avoided in pregnancy.
- If you are not immune to varicella, the vaccine will be offered to you during your postpartum stay at the hospital before discharge.
- You will need to avoid pregnancy for a month after the administration of the vaccine.

- **Treatment:** Typically, rubella infection is self-limited. No current treatment modalities have been found to be efficacious in preventing rubella congenital infection. Encourage patients who are not immune to rubella to avoid possible exposure to the virus.

Cytomegalovirus

Cytomegalovirus is a virus transmitted primarily via urine or saliva, but also through blood, breast milk, cervical secretions, and semen.
- **Cause:** double-stranded DNA herpes virus
- Maternal signs and symptoms
  - May be asymptomatic
  - May appear to have a presentation similar to mononucleosis: malaise, myalgia, fever, chills, and lymphadenopathy
- Effects on fetus/infant
  - IUGR
  - Microcephaly
  - Low platelets
  - Enlarged liver and spleen
  - Jaundice
  - Later in life, sensorineural hearing loss may become evident, along with developmental delays and seizures.
- **Diagnosis:** Diagnosis includes presence of CMV-specific IgM and a fourfold increase in IgG titers in maternal serology.
- **Fetal diagnosis:** Diagnosis of fetal CMV infection can be made by the detection of CMV in amniotic fluid or fetal blood; however, this does not predict the severity of the disease. Ultrasound can also aid in the diagnosis of CMV. Findings on ultrasound may include:
  - IUGR
  - Hydrocephalus
  - Microcephaly
  - Periventricular calcifications
- **Treatment:** Currently, no vaccinations or treatment modalities have been found to be efficacious against maternal or fetal CMV infection. Women who are pregnant are advised to avoid potential exposure to CMV.

⭐ BEST PRACTICES

The goal of rubella infection management is the **prevention** of maternal infection, which, in turn, will prevent congenital rubella infection. A rubella vaccine is available for women to receive before pregnancy and in the postpartum period. The vaccine is contraindicated in pregnancy because it contains live, attenuated virus. Instruct the patient to avoid pregnancy for 4 weeks after the vaccine is given. Breastfeeding is not a contraindication to receiving the rubella vaccine.

Herpes/Syphilis

Refer to Chapter Eight "Sexually Transmitted Infections" for information about herpes and syphilis infections.

Multiple Gestation

Because of assisted reproductive technology and agents to induce ovulation, there has been a 65% increase in the frequency of twins and a 500% increase in triplets and high-order births in the United States since 1980. Some of the greatest implications for carrying multiple fetuses include an increased risk for premature labor and delivery, placental abruption, and postpartum hemorrhage. Antepartal surveillance may be recommended, as discussed in the following section.

- **Incidence:** In the United States, multiple gestations account for 3% of all live births.
- Risks
  - Perinatal morbidity is increased threefold to fourfold in multifetal pregnancies in comparison with singleton pregnancies.
  - Preterm labor
  - Preterm delivery
  - IUGR
  - Pre-eclampsia
  - GDM
  - Placental abruption
  - PROM
  - Pyelonephritis
  - Postpartum hemorrhage
  - Congenital anomalies
  - Cerebral palsy
  - Increased cost and length of stay for mother
  - Neonatal intensive care unit admission

> **TIP**
>
> On average, singleton pregnancies are delivered at 40 weeks, whereas twins, triplets, and quadruplets are delivered at 37, 33, and 29 weeks, respectively.

Death of One Fetus

There is an increased risk for death of one or more fetuses in multifetal pregnancies. There is no consensus on a protocol for fetal monitoring when a fetal demise has occurred. For an otherwise healthy surviving fetus(es), immediate delivery is likely not beneficial.

The clinician may opt to monitor fibrin and fibrinogen levels for the theoretical risk for disseminated intravascular coagulopathy, which is a complex disorder resulting in intravascular coagulation and hemorrhage.

Antepartum Surveillance

- Because of the increased risk for stillbirth in multiple gestations, clinicians may initiate antepartal surveillance using simultaneous nonstress tests or performing a biophysical profile on each fetus. However, there is no evidence to support when routine antepartal testing should be initiated.

- At each prenatal visit, vital signs including weight are obtained; urine is evaluated for protein; and each fetus's heart rate is independently identified.
- Starting at the 30th to 32nd week of gestation, educate the patient on fetal kick counts.
- Preterm labor and delivery are risks associated with multifetal gestation. Research has not been able to prove that placing a mother on routine bed rest, placing a prophylactic cerclage, using home uterine monitoring devices, or prescribing prophylactic tocolytic medication improves perinatal outcome.

Preterm Labor

Preterm labor is defined as contractions with cervical change occurring before 37 weeks of gestation.
- **Incidence:** unclear
- **Causes:** unclear
- Intervention
  - **Nonpharmacological:** Effectiveness of these modalities is uncertain.
    - Bed rest
    - Pelvic rest (including abstinence from sexual intercourse)
    - Hydration (orally and intravenously)
  - **Pharmacological:** These drugs work by inhibiting uterine muscle contractions and may prolong a pregnancy for about 2 to 7 days.
    - Indomethacin
    - Magnesium sulfate
    - Nifedipine
    - Ritodrine
    - Terbutaline
  - **Corticosteroid therapy:** Although this intervention is not intended to manage preterm labor, administration of corticosteroids has been found beneficial to an infant whose mother is in true preterm labor between 24 and 34 weeks of gestation. Two courses of corticosteroids are available:
    - Betamethasone, 12 mg intramuscularly (IM) × 2 doses, given 24 hours apart
    - Dexamethasone, 6 mg IM × 4 doses, given 6 hours apart
  - **Group beta streptococcus (GBS) prophylaxis:** Once a preterm labor diagnosis is established, antibiotic prophylaxis may be considered by the HCP for women whose GBS status is positive or unknown with risk factors such as prematurity.

Rho(D) Isoimmunization

Isoimmunization is the formation of maternal antibodies (in a mother who is Rh [D]–negative) that cross the placenta and destroy red cells in the fetal circulation (in a fetus who is Rh [D]–positive). Theoretically, there is supposed to be no mixing of blood between the maternal and fetal circulations; however, in reality, some degree of fetomaternal bleeding occurs (see Fig. 2–3). As little as 0.1 mL of Rh (D)–positive fetal blood can result in isoimmunization.

- Events associated with fetomaternal bleeding include the following:
  - Delivery of the fetus (most common cause)
  - Ectopic pregnancy
  - Abortion
  - Abdominal trauma
  - Chorionic villus sampling (CVS)
  - Multifetal pregnancy
  - Bleeding with placenta previa and placental abruption
  - External cephalic version
  - Amniocentesis
  - Delivery of placenta
- **Prevention:** Prevention of isoimmunization is recommended by the administration of Rho(D) immune globulin (RhoGAM) to pregnant Rh(D)–negative women who are not sensitized. Blood type and antibody screen testing is performed at the initial prenatal visit. If the woman is not isoimmunized, 300 mcg of RhoGAM should be administered IM at 28 weeks' gestational age and within 72 hours postpartum. RhoGAM administration should also be considered in other events associated with fetomaternal bleeding.
- **Management:** Women who are already isoimmunized are monitored for fetal anemia using ultrasound to assess for fetal hydrops, amniotic fluid bilirubin assessment, and middle cerebral artery (MCA) Doppler ultrasound.

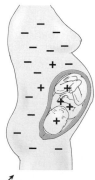
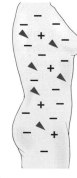
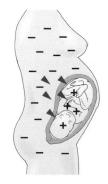

⊕ Rh⁺ father   ♀ Rh⁻ mother   ◢ Anti-Rh(O) antibodies

FIGURE 2-3: Rh isoimmunization.

Thyroid Disease

Thyroid disease is a disorder that occurs when the thyroid gland does not produce the appropriate amounts of thyroid hormones. Pregnancy-related hormones, such as estrogen and hCG, affect the level of thyroid hormones in the body. Maintenance of normal thyroid levels is essential for the proper development of the fetal brain and nervous system.

Hyperthyroidism

Hyperthyroidism is the result of a hyperfunctioning thyroid gland.

- Causes
  - Graves disease
  - Hyperemesis gravidarum
  - Molar disease
  - Nodular thyroid disease
  - Subacute thyroiditis
  - Iatrogenic
- Signs and symptoms
  - Tachycardia
  - Palpitations
  - Nervousness
  - Tremors
  - Heat intolerance
  - Insomnia
  - Goiter
  - Palpitations
- **Diagnosis:** thyroid function tests
- Maternal implications related to uncontrolled hyperthyroidism
  - Severe pre-eclampsia
  - Preterm delivery
  - Heart failure
- Fetal and neonatal effects
  - Low birth weight
  - Fetal loss
  - Development of hypothyroidism/ hyperthyroidism in neonate
- **Treatment:** drugs of choice in pregnancy are propylthiouracil (PTU) and methimazole

Hypothyroidism

Hypothyroidism is an illness caused by the underproduction of thyroid hormone.

- Signs and symptoms
  - Cold intolerance

- Hair loss
- Dry skin
- Constipation
- Fatigue
- Muscle cramps
- Untreated hypothyroidism may cause the following complications:
  - Myxedema
  - Myxedema coma
  - Pre-eclampsia
- Fetal and neonatal effects
  - Low birth weight
  - Preterm delivery
  - Congenital cretinism (if hypothyroidism is caused by iodine deficiency)
  - Congenital hypothyroidism
- **Diagnosis:** thyroid function test
- **Treatment:** drug of choice is the same for pregnant and nonpregnant women: levothyroxine (Synthroid)

Premature Rupture of Membranes

PROM involves the rupture of membranes before the onset of labor. If PROM happens before 37 weeks' gestation, this is termed *preterm PROM*.
- **Incidence:** 8% of all term pregnancies
- Causative factors
  - In a term pregnancy, weakening of membranes leading to PROM may be because of uterine contractions.
  - In preterm PROM, intra-amniotic infections are a commonly associated cause.
- Risk factors associated with PROM
  - Previous preterm birth
  - Short cervical length
  - Preterm labor
- Risk factors associated with preterm PROM
  - Uterine overdistention (such as in multifetal pregnancies)
  - Maternal cigarette smoking
  - Cervical cerclage
  - Amniocentesis
- Maternal implications of PROM
  - Intrauterine infection
- Fetal implications of PROM
  - Umbilical cord compression
  - Infection
- Maternal implications of preterm PROM
  - Intrauterine and postpartum infection

- Fetal implications of preterm PROM
  - Complications because of prematurity such as intraventricular hemorrhage and necrotizing enterocolitis
  - Placental abruption
  - Fetal malpresentation
- Diagnosis of PROM
  - Diagnosis of PROM may be based on both history and physical examination.
  - Some patients may give a good history of a gush or a trickle of fluid from the vagina.
  - Visualization of amniotic fluid leakage into the cervical canal may be seen.
  - The fluid obtained may be tested for pH levels to help differentiate amniotic fluid from vaginal secretions. Amniotic fluid has a pH 7.1 to 7.3, as opposed to vaginal pH 4.5 to 6.0.
  - Allowing the fluid sample to dry on a slide and finding a fern-like pattern under microscopy suggests that this is amniotic fluid and helps with the diagnosis of membrane rupture.
  - While performing the sterile speculum examination, careful inspection for possible umbilical cord prolapse and/or for a presenting fetal part (such as a limb) through the cervical os should also be done.
- Management of PROM
  - Determine correct gestational age, fetal well-being, and fetal presentation.
  - Assess for the presence of intrauterine infection by physical examination and obtaining *Neisseria gonorrhoeae* and *Chlamydia trachomatis* cultures (refer to institutional policy if this may be obtained by the nurse at your site), if indicated.
  - Use electronic fetal monitoring to assess for well-being. One must remember, however, that fetuses less than 32 weeks' gestation may not have a reactive fetal heart tracing because of immaturity despite being healthy.
- Management of term PROM
  - Without intervention, half of women with PROM will deliver within 5 hours and 95% within 28 hours.
  - Certified Nurse-Midwife (CNM) or MD may suggest induction of labor.
- Management of preterm PROM
  - **34 to 36 weeks:** same as term
  - 32 to 33 weeks
    - Expectant management
    - GBS prophylaxis is recommended, as indicated.
    - Some HCPs may order a course of corticosteroids for lung maturity.
    - Antibiotics may be given to possibly treat or prevent an infection for the prolongation of the pregnancy.

- 24 to 31 weeks
  - Same as 32 to 33 weeks except that there is a consensus that corticosteroid therapy is recommended for this gestational age group.
  - Some CNMs or MDs may order tocolytics, such as magnesium sulfate, to prolong the duration of pregnancy.

3 Intrapartum

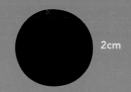

2cm

CHAPTER 3

Intrapartum

Labor

Onset of labor usually occurs between 38 and 42 weeks of gestation and is characterized by regular contractions and cervical dilation.

Initial Assessment

Maternal Signs of Approaching Labor

- **Lightening** is reported by the mother, around the 38th week of gestation, as a change in the shape of her gravid abdomen as the fetus settles, or "drops," into the pelvis.
- **Bloody show** is the passage of the cervical mucus that acted as a protective plug for the uterus during the pregnancy. Cervical dilation and effacement may cause the rupture of small cervical vessels, causing the mucus to be blood tinged.
- **Rupture of membranes**, also referred to as "breaking water," occurs for some women before the onset of labor. The fluid-filled amniotic sac that surrounds the fetus either spontaneously breaks or is artificially ruptured by her health-care provider.
- **Uterine contractions** are the tightening and relaxing of the uterine muscle. The purpose of the contractions is to thin and dilate the cervix and to move the fetus down the birth canal for delivery.

BRAXTON HICKS R_x

Braxton Hicks contractions are irregular contractions that are often felt by the mother who is nearing or at full-term gestation.

Determining True Versus False Labor

Distinguishing between true and false labor is an essential nursing assessment skill. True labor involves contractions that lead to cervical effacement and dilation. False labor is associated with irregular contractions that may decrease in intensity, with rest, or with change of position. Review Table 3–1 for the differences between true and false labor.

Table 3–1 Determining True Versus False Labor	
TRUE LABOR	**FALSE LABOR**
Contractions occur at regular intervals that increase in intensity, duration, and frequency.	Braxton Hicks contractions, which are irregular and decrease in intensity with rest or change of position
Cervical effacement and dilation occurs	No cervical change

The Three Ps of Labor and Delivery

Power

Power refers to the forces that expel the fetus from the womb. Types of power are as follows:

- **Primary power** describes involuntary uterine muscle contractions.
- **Secondary power** describes the voluntary maternal efforts to push out the fetus.

Characteristics of Uterine Contractions

Uterine contraction may be determined by palpation, external monitoring, and internal monitoring.

- **Intensity** of a contraction may be palpated as mild, moderate, or strong. External fetal monitoring is not a good indicator of contraction intensity because of factors such as maternal habitus and positioning of the tocodynamometer. Internal measurement of contractions is in millimeters of mercury (mm Hg) but is often reserved for high-risk pregnancies because of the increased risk for infection associated with this invasive procedure.
- **Frequency** of a contraction is timed from the beginning of one contraction to the start of the next.
- **Duration** of a contraction is measured from the beginning to the end of the same contraction.

Cervical Effacement and Dilation

- **Effacement** is the shortening of the cervix from about 2 cm in length (0% effaced) to completely thinned out (100% effaced).
- **Dilation** is the opening of the cervix measured in centimeters from 0 (closed cervix) to 10 (complete/fully dilated cervix; Fig. 3–1).

Passenger

The passenger is the fetus.

- **Fetal attitude** refers to the relationship of the fetal head to the spine.
  - **Complete flexion:** when the chin of the fetus is flexed and touches the sternum
  - **Moderate flexion:** also called the "military position," when the fetal chin is not touching the chest but is in an alert position
  - **Deflexion or extension:** when the back is arched and head is extended (Fig. 3–2)

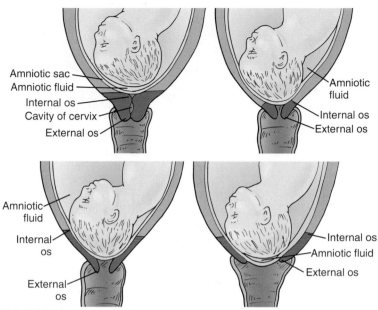

FIGURE 3-1: Cervical effacement and dilation.

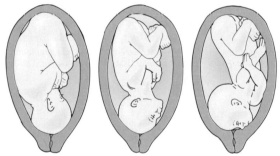

FIGURE 3-2: Fetal attitude.

- **Fetal lie** refers to the relationship of the long axis of the fetus to the long axis of the mother.
  - **Longitudinal lie:** when the long axis of the fetus is parallel to the long axis of the mother
  - **Transverse lie:** when the long axis of the fetus is perpendicular to the long axis of the mother
  - **Oblique lie:** when the fetal lie is at an angle between the transverse and longitudinal lie
- **Fetal position** refers to the relationship of the presenting fetal part to the maternal pelvis (Fig. 3–3).

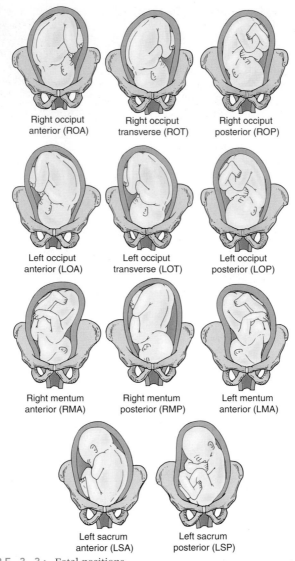

Right occiput
anterior (ROA)

Right occiput
transverse (ROT)

Right occiput
posterior (ROP)

Left occiput
anterior (LOA)

Left occiput
transverse (LOT)

Left occiput
posterior (LOP)

Right mentum
anterior (RMA)

Right mentum
posterior (RMP)

Left mentum
anterior (LMA)

Left sacrum
anterior (LSA)

Left sacrum
posterior (LSP)

FIGURE 3-3: Fetal positions.

- **Fetal presentation** refers to the part of the fetus that is first to enter the pelvic inlet.
  - **Cephalic:** the fetus is positioned with the head as the presenting part.
  - **Breech:** the fetus is positioned with the buttocks as the presenting part.
  - **Shoulder:** the fetus is positioned with the shoulder as the presenting part.

- **Fetal size** is estimated through palpation or ultrasound.
- **Fetal station** is the measurement in centimeters of the fetal head in relation to the level of the maternal ischial spines.
  - Measurement ranges from −5 to +5
  - 0 station refers to the fetal head being at the level of the ischial spines (Fig. 3–4)

Passage

Passage refers to the shape and measurement of the maternal bony pelvis through which the fetus must travel during delivery. The four basic pelvic classifications are gynecoid, android, anthropoid, and platypelloid (Fig. 3–5).

Stages of Labor

First Stage

The first stage of labor starts at the onset of labor and lasts to full dilation.

- **Latent phase** begins at the onset of regular contractions every 3 to 30 minutes lasting 30 to 40 seconds.
  - **Cervical dilation:** 0 to 3 cm
  - Duration
    - **Nullipara:** 7.3 to 8.6 hours
    - **Multipara:** 4.1 to 5.3 hours

Nursing Role During Latent Phase

Often, at this stage, the mother is still at home. If the mother is admitted to the hospital at this time, an initial assessment of the mother and her

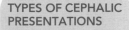

TYPES OF CEPHALIC PRESENTATIONS

- Occiput or vertex: presentation refers to the head completely flexed
- Chin or mentum
- Brow

TIPS

- Frank breech: the fetus is flexed at the hip with the legs pointing straight up in front of the fetal body
- Complete: the legs are flexed at the knee
- Footling: one or both fetal feet are in the maternal pelvic inlet

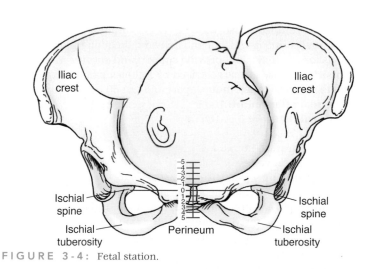

Iliac crest

Iliac crest

Ischial spine

Ischial spine

Ischial tuberosity

Perineum

Ischial tuberosity

F I G U R E 3 - 4 : Fetal station.

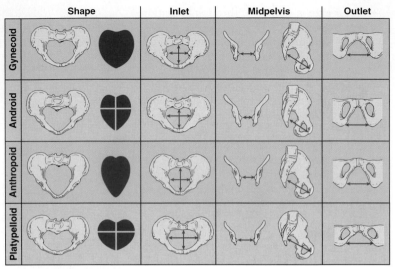

	Shape	Inlet	Midpelvis	Outlet
Gynecoid				
Android				
Anthropoid				
Platypelloid				

FIGURE 3-5: Pelvic types.

fetus is performed; the nurse should orient the mother and her support person to the room, equipment, and procedures. Encourage ambulation.

- **Active phase** is characterized by intensifying contractions that are at 2 to 5 minutes apart and last 40 to 60 seconds.
  - **Cervical effacement:** ≥80%
  - **Cervical dilation:** 4 to 7 cm
  - Duration
    - **Nullipara:** 4.6 hours
    - **Multipara:** 2.4 hours

Nursing Role During Active Phase

When a mother presents in active labor, she will likely be admitted to the hospital by the Certified Nurse-Midwife (CNM) or physician. Discuss different maternal positions for labor and delivery, breathing and relaxation, and options for pain relief and provide support and encouragement.

- **Transition phase** is characterized by intense, painful contractions that are 1.5 to 2 minutes apart and last 60 to 90 seconds.
  - **Cervical effacement:** 100%
  - **Cervical dilation:** 8 to 10 cm
  - Duration
    - **Nullipara:** 3.6 hours
    - **Multipara:** varies

Nursing Role During Transition Phase

Offer emotional support and encouragement, especially for the mother who is feeling tired, agitated, panicked, and anxious during this phase. Encourage patient to rest between contractions, relax, and breathe deeply. Offer nonpharmacological pain relief such as massage, and provide pain medication as prescribed by the CNM or physician.

Second Stage

The second stage of labor is the period from full cervical dilation (10 cm) to the delivery of the newborn.

- Contractions are about 2 to 3 minutes apart lasting 40 to 60 seconds.
- Duration
  - **Primigravida:** up to 3 hours
  - **Multigravida:** 0 to 30 minutes

Effective Pushing by the Mother

Varying techniques for pushing are used in labor. Two methods of pushing are generally used during the second stage.

1. **Closed glottis:** Using this approach, the mother is directed to take a deep breath and hold it for at least 10 seconds while she bears down three to four times during each contraction.
2. **Open glottis:** This technique involves involuntary pushing by the mother wherein she instinctively holds her breath for about 6 seconds while bearing down, followed by taking several breaths between urges to bear down. The woman is more in control with her labor as she responds to her own body.

Maternal Positions in Labor

Women may choose different positions during labor and delivery; these include sitting, kneeling, squatting, on all fours, or lying down supine or on her side.

ALERT!

The Association of Women's Health, Obstetric, and Neonatal Nurses (AWHONN) states that sustained use of the closed-glottis type of pushing should be avoided. This pushing technique may lead to decreased uteroplacental blood flow, hypoxemia, academia, and lower Apgar scores. AWHONN encourages the use of the open-glottis, involuntary technique, because this has been shown to avoid fetal stress and results in a shorter second stage of labor.

Nursing Role During the Second Stage of Labor

Assist and support with maternal pushing efforts in different laboring positions that are most comfortable to the mother and optimal for uteroplacental flow. If the mother has opted for anesthesia, such as an epidural, she may have less feeling in her lower extremities and will need help changing positions. Inform the woman ahead of time that she may feel intense burning pressure when the head descends to the vaginal introitus, also known as crowning. As per institution policy and CNM and/or physician orders, provide ice chips if patient is not placed on an NPO (nothing by mouth) status. Uphold the woman's privacy throughout the labor and delivery process (Fig. 3–6).

Third Stage

The third stage of labor lasts from the delivery of the infant up to the delivery of the placenta. The duration of this stage may be 5 to 10 minutes but could be up to half an hour.

Nursing Role During the Third Stage of Labor

The focus of the third stage of labor is providing immediate newborn care (review the "Newborn Assessment" section of Chapter Six "Newborn"),

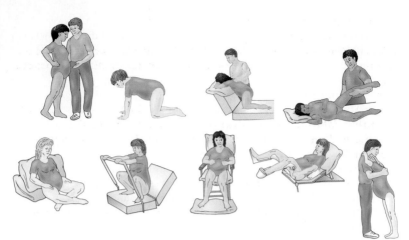

FIGURE 3-6: Labor positions: different maternal positions for labor and delivery.

QSEN Application

Teamwork and collaboration include skills such as the following:
- Functioning competently within own scope of practice as a member of the health-care team
- Assuming role of team member or leader based on the situation
- Initiating requests for help when appropriate to situation
- Clarifying roles and accountabilities under conditions of potential overlap in team member functioning
- Integrating the contributions of others who play a role in helping patient/family achieve health goals

In this chapter, together with information about care of pregnant women and newborns, Quality and Safety Education for Nurses (QSEN) competencies assure delivery of the best nursing care.

http://qsen.org/competencies/pre-licensure-ksas/#patient-centered_care

---

assisting with the expulsion of the placenta, close monitoring of the mother, and facilitating bonding and attachment between the couplet. Per institution protocol and the CNM and/or physician orders, oxytocin is administered intramuscularly or intravenously to stimulate uterine contractions and decrease bleeding. When the placenta is delivered, careful examination is needed to ensure that it is intact. (Retained placenta is associated with infection and postpartum hemorrhage.)

Fourth Stage

The fourth stage of labor is the postpartum period. (Review Chapter 4 "Postpartum" for further details.)

Maternal and Fetal Assessments in Labor and Delivery

Maternal Vital Signs

Take vital signs at least every 4 hours. Interval is increased as labor progresses to the active phase and if the mother's membranes are ruptured.

Fetal Heart Rate

- In the absence of risk factors or use of oxytocin, obtain and evaluate fetal heart rate (FHR) every 30 minutes during the active phase of the first stage of labor, increasing interval to every 15 minutes once the second stage begins.
- In the presence of risk factors and/or use of oxytocin, continuous electronic fetal monitoring is recommended. Evaluate FHR every 15 minutes during the active phase of the first stage of labor, increasing interval to every 5 minutes once second stage begins.

Uterine Contractions

Assess each time the FHR is checked.

Amniotic Fluid

Assess clarity, color, and odor of amniotic fluid.

Pain

Assess level and source of maternal pain and discomfort, knowledge of pain relief measures, and effectiveness of current pain relief modalities. It is imperative that the nurse follow the protocols of the hospital/birth center regarding how often assessments are performed for each phase and stage of labor.

Intrapartum Fetal Heart Rate Monitoring

Uterine Activity

- **Normal:** ≤5 in 10 minutes, averaged over 30 minutes of monitoring
- **Tachysystole:** >5 contractions in 10 minutes, averaged over 30 minutes of monitoring

Electronic Fetal Monitoring Terminology

- **Baseline** is the average FHR in a 10-minute segment of fetal monitoring, rounded to the nearest five beats.
  - **Normal:** between 110 and 160 bpm
  - **Tachycardia:** >160 bpm
  - **Bradycardia:** <110 bpm
- **Baseline variability** is the fluctuation in the baseline FHR.
  - **Absent:** undetectable amplitude
  - **Minimal:** amplitude range ≤5 bpm
  - **Moderate:** amplitude range 6 to 25 bpm
  - **Marked:** amplitude ≥25 bpm
- *Acceleration*
  - **≥32 weeks:** accelerations have a peak of ≥15 bpm above the baseline lasting ≥15 seconds, but less than 2 minutes from beginning to end of the acceleration

- **≤32 weeks:** accelerations have a peak of ≥10 bpm above the baseline lasting ≥10 seconds, but less than 2 minutes from beginning to end of the acceleration
  - Prolonged acceleration ≥2 minutes but less than 10 minutes
- **Early deceleration** is a gradual decrease in FHR ≥30 seconds with the nadir (lowest point) of the deceleration occurring at the same time as the peak of the uterine contraction (Fig. 3–7).
- **Late deceleration** is a gradual decrease in FHR ≥30 seconds with the nadir (lowest point) of the deceleration occurring after the peak of the contraction (Fig. 3–8).
- **Variable deceleration** is an abrupt decrease in FHR with the onset to the nadir of the deceleration being less than 30 seconds. The decrease in FHR from the baseline is ≥15 bpm lasting ≥15 seconds but less than 2 minutes (Fig. 3–9).
- **Prolonged deceleration** is a decrease in FHR from the baseline that is ≥15 bpm, lasting between 2 and 10 minutes.

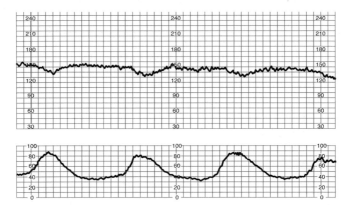

FIGURE 3-7: Early decelerations.

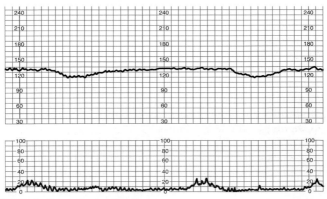

FIGURE 3-8: Late decelerations.

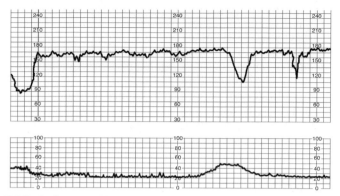

FIGURE 3-9: Variable decelerations.

- **Sinusoidal pattern** is characterized by 3 to 5 cycles per minute of sine wave–like FHR pattern lasting ≥20 minutes.

Fetal Heart Rate Tracings Classification

According to the 2008 National Institute of Child Health and Human Development Workshop, fetal heart tracings are categorized as follows:

- **Category I** tracings are considered normal and are strongly associated with normal fetal acid-base status.
  - Normal baseline
  - Moderate FHR variability
  - Absent late or variable decelerations
  - Present or absent early decelerations
  - Present or absent accelerations
- **Category II** tracings are considered indeterminate and not predictive of fetal acid-base status requiring continued evaluation and close monitoring.
  - Baseline rate of either bradycardia (without an absent baseline variability) or tachycardia
  - Baseline FHR variability that is either minimal, absent with no recurrent decelerations, or marked
  - No accelerations despite fetal stimulation
  - Periodic recurrent variable decelerations with minimal or moderate baseline variability, prolonged decelerations between 2 and 10 minutes, recurrent late decelerations with moderate baseline variability, or variable decelerations that have overshoots or shoulders
- **Category III** tracings are considered abnormal and are associated with abnormal fetal acid-base status. They are characterized by absent baseline FHR variability and any of the following:
  - Bradycardia
  - Recurrent variable decelerations
  - Recurrent late decelerations
  - Sinusoidal FHR pattern

Pain Management in Labor

Nonpharmacological Pain Management

- **Localized pressure on lower back:** to relieve back labor
- **Massage:** to relieve muscle tension, provide distraction, and stimulate local release of endorphins
- **Therapeutic touch:** performed by trained individuals who lay their hands on the patient's energy fields to ease the pain
- **Heat and cold:** some cultures prefer one over the other at certain periods during childbirth; heat generally eases muscle tension; a cold washcloth over the forehead or the back of the neck may relieve a woman's feeling of warmth during the active and transitional phases of labor.
- **Hydrotherapy:** use of water to relieve pain and provide comfort, typically by showering or getting into a tub filled with warm water
- **Relaxation:** a skill that should be introduced in childbirth classes and used throughout the labor process; relaxation conserves the energy the mother needs during labor and delivery and may prevent maternal exhaustion
- **Imagery:** used to keep the mother relaxed and focused on getting through the childbirth process by imagining calming scenarios and pleasant experiences
- **Patterned breathing:** used in labor as a form of distraction and relaxation; initially taught in childbirth classes
- **Music:** to relax and distract the mother from the painful contractions of labor
- **Acupuncture:** performed by certified acupuncturists by placing needles into specific points on the body to relieve pain
- **Hypnosis:** patient may use to alter her behavior pattern in response to pain during labor
- **Effleurage:** use of light, gentle touch, such as rhythmically stroking the abdomen during a contraction

ALERT!

Naloxone (Narcan), an opioid antagonist, reverses the effects of opioids such as respiratory repression, hypotension, and sedation. For rapid effects, give intravenously. May also be given intramuscularly or subcutaneously, but reversal effects are less rapid.

Pharmacological Management of Pain
Parenteral Anesthesia

- **Systemic analgesia** such as morphine, nalbuphine (Nubain), and meperidine (Demerol) administered intramuscularly or intravenously
  - **Maternal adverse effects:** nausea and vomiting, respiratory depression
  - **Neonatal adverse effects:** may affect neonate depending on dose and timing of administration in relation to birth
  - **Nursing consideration:** monitor closely for maternal respiratory depression; if being given as an intravenous (IV) push, administer at the beginning of a contraction to decrease fetal effects

Regional Anesthesia

Regional anesthesia is provided by the CNM or physician.

- Local anesthesia is provided during the second stage of labor by injecting an anesthetic, such as chloroprocaine hydrochloride, into the perineum to numb the perineal area before episiotomy and for the repair of perineal lacerations.
- Pudendal block is provided during the second stage of labor by injecting an anesthetic, such as lidocaine hydrochloride, through the lateral vaginal walls into the pudendal nerve to numb the lower vagina, vulva, and perineum for temporary relief of pain during an operative vaginal delivery using forceps or vacuum.

Regional Anesthesia Provided by an Anesthesiologist or a Certified Registered Nurse Anesthetist

- Epidural block is a type of regional anesthesia provided during the first stage of labor by placing a catheter into the epidural space between the fourth and fifth vertebrae. It provides anesthetic effects to the uterus, cervix, vagina, and perineum within 5 to 20 minutes. Epidural block may be used for both vaginal and cesarean deliveries.
- Combined spinal-epidural is a type of regional anesthesia that provides immediate pain relief affecting the uterus, cervix, vagina, and perineum. It may be used for vaginal and cesarean deliveries.
- Spinal anesthesia has an immediate onset and may be used in both vaginal and cesarean births depending on the dose and placement of the single-shot medication in the dural sac.

Adverse Effects of Regional Anesthesia

- **Maternal:** hypotension, fever, pruritus, lower extremity weakness, loss of uterine contraction sensation, post–dural puncture headache, dizziness, sedation, longer second stage of labor, fetal malposition (occiput posterior), increased rate of forceps- or vacuum-assisted delivery, higher rate of using oxytocin for augmentation
- **Fetal:** bradycardia and late decelerations

ALERT! !

Post-dural puncture headache (PDPH), commonly referred to as a "spinal headache," typically occurs within the first 48 hours after spinal or combined spinal-epidural anesthesia. The cause of PDPH is theorized to be leakage of cerebrospinal fluid into the dura mater. The obstetrician/CNM and the anesthesiologist will need to be alerted if a postpartum patient complains of a headache to rule out a PDPH, among other causes.

⭐ **BEST PRACTICES**

NURSING CONSIDERATION

Monitor for complications such as hematoma, infection, hypotension, seizures, and cardiac arrhythmias if medication is injected into a vein.

General Anesthesia

General anesthesia is provided by the anesthesiologist or Certified Registered Nurse Anesthetist (CRNA) for emergent cesarean sections or when epidural or spinal anesthesia is contraindicated. This type of anesthesia may be given intravenously or may be inhaled and results in maternal loss of consciousness; airway maintenance and management by the anesthesiologist or CRNA will be required. Risks include aspiration, hypoxia, hemorrhage (because of uterine relaxant effects), and fetal depression.

Induction and Augmentation of Labor

Labor induction is the process of artificially stimulating uterine contractions before labor begins on its own. **Labor augmentation** is the process of stimulating a labor that has already started and may have slowed or stalled.

Indications

Indications for the induction or augmentation of labor include the following:

- Maternal medical conditions such as uncontrolled hypertension or diabetes
- Post-term pregnancy (>42 weeks' gestation)
- Compromised fetus such as in severe intrauterine growth restriction
- Fetal death
- Chorioamnionitis

Procedure

- Use of cervical ripening agents such as misoprostol and prostaglandin E_2
- IV infusion of oxytocin (see Box 3–1)

Risks

The following risks are associated with the induction or augmentation of labor:

- Hypertonic uterus
- Uterine rupture
- Increased bleeding postpartum

NURSING CONSIDERATIONS

- Secure an IV line and infuse fluids as per orders.
- Administer oral antacid before procedure, time permitting.
- Administer IV antacids such as ranitidine hydrochloride (Zantac) or cimetidine (Tagamet) as per orders.

QSEN Application

Patient-centered care includes knowledge such as the following:

- Demonstrating comprehensive understanding of the concepts of pain and suffering, including physiological models of pain and comfort
- Discussing principles of effective communication

In this chapter, together with information about care of pregnant women and newborns, Quality and Safety Education for Nurses (QSEN) competencies assure delivery of the best nursing care.

http://qsen.org/competencies/pre-licensure-ksas/#patient-centered_care

Box 3–1 Medication Highlight: OXYTOCIN

oxytocin (ox-i-**toe**-sin)
Pitocin

CLASSIFICATION

Therapeutic: hormones
Pharmacological: oxytocics

PREGNANCY CATEGORY X

Indications

- **IV:** Induction of labor at term
- **IV:** Facilitation of threatened abortion
- **IV, IM:** Postpartum control of bleeding after expulsion of the placenta

Action

Stimulates uterine smooth muscle, producing uterine contractions similar to those in spontaneous labor. Has vasopressor and antidiuretic effects.
Therapeutic Effects: Induction of labor. Control of postpartum bleeding.

Pharmacokinetics

- **Absorption:** IV administration results in 100% bioavailability.
- **Distribution:** widely distributed in extracellular fluid; small amounts reach fetal circulation
- **Metabolism and excretion:** rapidly metabolized by liver and kidneys
- **Half-life:** 3 to 9 minutes

Continued

Box 3–1 **Medication Highlight: OXYTOCIN—cont'd**

TIME/ACTION PROFILE (REDUCTION IN UTERINE CONTRACTIONS)

ROUTE	ONSET	PEAK	DURATION
IV	Immediate	Unknown	1 hr
IM	3–5 min	Unknown	30–60 min

CONTRAINDICATIONS/PRECAUTIONS

- **Contraindicated in** hypersensitivity, anticipated nonvaginal delivery
- **Use cautiously in** first and second stages of labor; slow infusion over 24 hours has caused water intoxication with seizure and coma or maternal death because of oxytocin's antidiuretic effect
- **Adverse reactions/side effects** (CAPITAL LETTERS indicate life-threatening; <u>underlines</u> indicate most frequent.) **Maternal adverse reactions are noted for IV use only.**
- **Central nervous system—maternal:** COMA, SEIZURES; **fetal:** INTRACRANIAL HEMORRHAGE. **Respiratory—fetal:** ASPHYXIA, hypoxia. **Cardiovascular—maternal:** hypotension; **fetal:** arrhythmias. **F and E maternal:** hypochloremia, hyponatremia, water intoxication. **Miscellaneous—maternal:** ↑ <u>uterine motility, painful contractions</u>, abruptio placentae, ↓ uterine blood flow, hypersensitivity

INTERACTIONS

- **Drug–drug:** Severe hypertension may occur if oxytocin follows administration of **vasopressors.** Concurrent use with **cyclopropane** anesthesia may result in excessive hypotension.

ROUTE/DOSAGE

Induction/Stimulation of Labor

- **IV (adults):** 0.5–2 milliunits/min; ↑ by 1–2 milliunits/min q15–60 min until pattern established (usually 5–6 milliunits/min; maximum: 20 milliunits/min), then ↓ dose

Postpartum Hemorrhage

- **IV (adults):** 10 units infused at 20–40 milliunits/min
- **IM (adults):** 10 units after delivery of placenta

Incomplete/Inevitable Abortion

- **IV (adults):** 10 units at a rate of 20–40 milliunits/min

Availability (generic available)

- **Solution for injection:** 10 units/mL

NURSING IMPLICATIONS

ASSESSMENT

- Assess fetal maturity, presentation, and pelvic adequacy before administration of oxytocin for induction of labor.
- Assess character, frequency, and duration of uterine contractions; resting uterine tone; and FHR frequently throughout administration. If contractions

Continued

Box 3–1 **Medication Highlight: OXYTOCIN—cont'd**

occur less than 2 min apart and are more than 50 to 65 mm Hg on monitor, if they last 60 to 90 seconds or longer, or if a significant change in FHR develops, stop infusion and turn patient on her left side to prevent fetal anoxia. Notify health-care professional immediately.

- Monitor maternal blood pressure and pulse frequently and FHR continuously throughout administration.
- This drug occasionally causes water intoxication. Monitor patient for signs and symptoms (drowsiness, listlessness, confusion, headache, anuria), and notify physician or other health-care professional if they occur.
- *Laboratory test considerations:* Monitor maternal electrolytes. Water retention may result in hypochloremia or hyponatremia.

POTENTIAL NURSING DIAGNOSES

- Deficient knowledge, related to medication regimen (patient/family teaching)

IMPLEMENTATION

- **Do not confuse Pitocin (oxytocin) with Pitressin (vasopressin).**
- Do not administer oxytocin simultaneously by more than one route.

IV ADMINISTRATION

- **Continuous infusion:** Rotate infusion container to ensure thorough mixing. Store solution in refrigerator, but do not freeze.
- Infuse via infusion pump for accurate dose. Oxytocin should be connected via Y-site injection to an IV of 0.9% NaCl for use during adverse reactions.
- Magnesium sulfate should be available if needed for relaxation of the myometrium.
- **Induction of labor—***Diluent:* Dilute 1 mL (10 units) in 1 L of compatible infusion fluid (0.9% NaCl, 5% dextrose in water [D5W], or lactated Ringer's [LR]). *Concentration:* 10 milliunits/mL. *Rate:* Begin infusion at 0.5–2 milliunits/min (0.05–0.2 mL); increase in increments of 1–2 milliunits/min at 15- to 30-min intervals until contractions simulate normal labor.
- **Postpartum bleeding—***Diluent:* For control of postpartum bleeding, dilute 1–4 mL (10–40 units) in 1 L of compatible infusion fluid. *Concentration:* 10–40 milliunits/mL. *Rate:* Begin infusion at a rate of 20–40 milliunits/min to control uterine atony. Adjust rate as indicated.
- **Incomplete or inevitable abortion—***Diluent:* For incomplete or inevitable abortion, dilute 1 mL (10 units) in 500 mL of 0.9% NaCl or D5W. *Concentration:* 20 milliunits/mL.
Rate: Infuse at a rate of 20–40 milliunits/min.
- **Y-site compatibility—**heparin, hydrocortisone sodium succinate, insulin, meperidine, morphine, potassium chloride, vitamin B complex with C, warfarin, zidovudine
- **Solution compatibility—**dextrose/Ringer's or LR combinations, dextrose/saline combinations, Ringer's or LR injection, D5W, D10W, 0.45% NaCl, 0.9% NaCl

Continued

Data from Davis's Drug Guide for Nurses. 12th ed. Philadelphia, PA: FA Davis Company; 2011.

Cesarean Delivery

A cesarean delivery or cesarean section is the delivery of the fetus through a surgical incision into the abdomen and the wall of the uterus.

Indications

There are maternal and fetal indications for having a cesarean delivery. Sometimes the surgery is planned ahead of time because of certain circumstances such as prior cesarean births or medical conditions such as a tumor obstructing the birth canal. Other times the surgery is unplanned when situations arise during the labor process and the decision is made at that time by the obstetrician.

Maternal
- Medical issues such as certain cardiac and respiratory diseases
- Multiple pregnancy, particularly triplets, or a higher-order pregnancy
- Obstruction of the passageway by fibroids or tumors
- Maternal infection such as an active herpetic lesion on vulva/perineum
- Failure of labor to progress

Fetal
- Malpresentation such as breech or transverse lie
- Nonreassuring fetal status

Maternal-Fetal
- Placenta previa
- Placental abruption
- Cephalopelvic disproportion

Procedure

Preparation

For a planned cesarean delivery, the patient is typically scheduled in advance for a specific time and date to come to the labor and delivery unit for the surgery. Patients are usually advised not to eat or drink anything after midnight the day before the surgery. When the patient comes in for her surgery, the nurse brings her to her room to change into a patient gown and reviews with the patient and her support person the series of events that will take place before, during, and immediately after the surgery.

- An IV catheter is placed in a vein, typically in the arm, to administer fluids and medications for the surgery and afterward.
- A Foley catheter is placed to continuously empty the bladder during the surgery and in the immediate postpartum period.
- The abdomen is shaved and cleansed with a solution such as Betadine. (Refer to your institution's policy.)
- Anesthesia such as an epidural or spinal block is then given by the anesthesiologist and/or CRNA. (Refer to section on pharmacological management of pain for the different types of anesthesia available for surgery.)

Delivery

- An incision is made by the surgeon into the abdomen. The three most common incision types are midline, Maylard, and Pfannenstiel. The Pfannenstiel incision is the most common and is a horizontal incision made just above the symphysis pubis.
- An incision is then created into the anterior wall of the uterus. In about 90% of cesarean sections, a low transverse incision is made. This type of incision results in less bleeding and allows for the woman to have a subsequent trial of labor. In other cases, such as in the delivery of an extremely premature baby in a breech position, a vertical incision is used.
- After the baby is delivered through the incisions, the umbilical cord is cut and the placenta removed or spontaneously expulsed; the incisions are repaired and closed with dissolvable sutures.

Possible Complications

Intraoperative
- Maternal mortality (ranges from 6 to 22 per 100,000)
- Injury to surrounding organs such as the ureters, bladder, and bowel
- Hemorrhage

Postoperative
- Endometritis
- Wound infection
- Deep venous thrombosis
- Septic pelvic thrombophlebitis

Vaginal Birth or Trial of Labor After a Cesarean Section

It was once thought that a woman who had had a cesarean section could no longer have a vaginal delivery. Many women who have had one previous low-transverse cesarean section in the past, however, can be candidates for a trial of labor after a cesarean section (TOLAC) and vaginal birth after a cesarean section (VBAC). The main risk of a TOLAC is a

1% chance for uterine rupture with a history of a low-transverse cesarean delivery.

Reasons to Consider Trial of Labor After a Cesarean Section Instead of a Repeat Cesarean Delivery

First and foremost, a woman who has a successful TOLAC or VBAC will avoid having an abdominal surgery and its risks, such as the following:

- Longer period of recovery
- Increased risk for infection
- Greater blood loss and risk for hemorrhage
- Injury to surrounding pelvic organs
- Increased possibility of placenta accreta with succeeding pregnancies

Criteria for Identifying Candidates for a VBAC

According to the American College of Obstetrics and Gynecology (ACOG), criteria for identifying candidates for a VBAC include the following:

- One prior low-transverse cesarean section
- No history of uterine rupture
- No other uterine surgery
- Facility with physician immediately available and capable of performing an emergency cesarean section

Operative Vaginal Delivery

Forceps or vacuum extraction is sometimes used when women in labor are experiencing a prolonged second stage and/or the FHR tracing is nonreassuring. For a forceps or vacuum extractor to be applied, the following criteria need to be met:

- Membranes ruptured
- Cervix completely dilated
- Fetus vertex and engaged
- Adequate maternal pelvis size

The well-trained physician also needs to explain the procedure and its risks to the patient and obtain an informed consent. Maternal analgesia should be offered and provided.

Risks

Maternal

Operative vaginal delivery has the following maternal risks:

- Perineal trauma
- Urinary and fecal incontinence

Fetal

Operative vaginal delivery has the following fetal risks:

- Cephalohematoma
- Intracranial hemorrhage
- Facial trauma

4 Postpartum

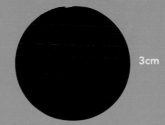

3cm

CHAPTER 4

Postpartum

The postpartum period, or puerperium, is the first 6 to 8 weeks after childbirth wherein the new mother's body returns to a non-pregnant state. This is a dynamic time where she learns how to care for herself and her newborn baby. The following sections cover the thorough assessment of a postpartum patient.

Maternal Assessment

Vital Signs

Refer to hospital policy for the frequency of monitoring vital signs and performing a postpartum assessment. Typically, vital signs are obtained in the following intervals:

- Vaginal delivery
  - **First hour:** every 15 minutes
  - **Second hour:** every 30 minutes
  - **Third hour:** one time
  - Thereafter, every 8 hours of the hospital stay until discharge
- Cesarean section
  - **First hour:** every 15 minutes
  - **Second to fifth hours:** every 30 minutes
  - **Sixth to eighth hours:** once each hour
  - Thereafter, every 4 to 8 hours of the hospital stay until discharge
- Temperature
  Normal: < 100.4°F
- Pulse
  Normal: 60 to 100 bpm
- Respiration
  Normal: 12 to 20/min
- Blood pressure
  - Normal range
    - **Systolic:** 90 to 120 mm Hg
    - **Diastolic:** 60 to 80 mm Hg

ALERT!

Elevated temperature in the first 24 hours postpartum may be caused by dehydration and physical exertion during labor and delivery. After the first 24 hours, an elevated temperature may be indicative of an infection.

ALERT!

Tachypnea may be caused by blood loss, pain, or anxiety. When adventitious lung sounds are auscultated and are accompanied with chest pain and/or shortness of breath, suspicion of pulmonary emboli should be reported to the health-care practitioner (HCP) immediately.

According to the American Autonomic Society and the American Academy of Neurology, orthostatic hypotension is defined as a systolic blood pressure decrease of at least 20 mm Hg or a diastolic blood pressure decrease of at least 10 mm Hg from a supine to a sitting or standing position. May be accompanied with symptoms such as dizziness, lightheadedness, blurred vision, palpitations, nausea, and impaired cognition. Orthostatic hypotension may indicate excess bleeding.

The Postpartum Assessment: BUBBLE PLEB

The mnemonic BUBBLE PLEB is used to assist with the assessment of a postpartum patient:

B—Breasts and chest
U—Uterus and abdomen
B—Bladder
B—Bowels
L—Lochia
E—Episiotomy/Lacerations
P—Pain
L—Lower and upper extremities
E—Emotional status
B—Bonding and attachment

1. Gather supplies before going into the patient's room:
   - Stethoscope
   - Blood pressure machine
   - Thermometer
   - Gloves
   - Mini-flashlight
2. Wash hands or use a hand sanitizer before approaching the patient.

Breasts and Chest

- Assess method of infant feeding.
  - If breastfeeding:
    - Affirm that breastfeeding is beneficial to the infant and the mother.
    - For first-time breastfeeders, reassure them that although they do not see copious amounts of milk in the first 2 to 3 days postpartum, they are making colostrum, which is rich in nutrients and immunoglobulins (IgG), to boost the infant's immunity.
    - Determine the amount and frequency of feedings: Record the last feeding in the infant's flow chart.
    - Encourage the mother to breastfeed every 2 to 3 hours for 10 to 20 minutes or for as long as the infant wants. This will help establish and maintain milk production.
  - If bottle feeding:
    - Instruct patient not to stimulate her breasts because this may cause her body to think that she needs to make milk for her baby.
    - Advise patient to turn her back to the shower when bathing to avoid any type of nipple stimulation. Encourage her to wear a well-supporting bra such as a sports bra.
    - Record and update the feeding(s) in the infant's flow chart. Write the type of formula, amount of formula taken, and at what time.
    - Encourage the mother to bottle-feed every 3 to 4 hours.

For a multipara, ask about previous experience.

RN: Did you breastfeed your older child/children?

Patient: Yes, I breastfed my older son for 12 months.

Ask about the current feedings:

RN: How are the feedings going?

Patient: I think they are going well. The baby latches on well.

RN: That is wonderful! So, you are able to see the baby get your nipple and the areola, the most darkened area surrounding your nipple, into his mouth?

Patient: Yes, he latches and sucks well. I do not feel any pain. But I'm concerned he is not getting adequate milk.

RN: Is he making wet diapers and stools?

Patient: Yes! He's made about four wet diapers and he had passed meconium stool today.

RN: That's a wonderful sign that the baby is getting sufficient amounts of milk from breastfeeding, along with the fact that I see on his chart that he feeds for 15 minutes on each side and is feeding every 2 hours.

Patient: Yes, he feeds well.

RN: You are doing a great job. Breastfeeding definitely takes patience and hard work. I am available to further assist you and answer any questions you may have.

- If feeding via breast and bottle:
  - Discuss with patient the physiology of supply and demand.
  - Encourage to place infant on breast and empty breasts of milk before supplementing with formula.

Assess Breasts

- **Inspect:** Visually assess breasts for symmetry, fullness/engorgement, and/or erythema. Assess for flat, retracted nipples and for signs of trauma from breastfeeding such as redness, blisters, and fissures.
- **Palpate:** Assess for engorgement, tenderness, and plugged ducts.
- **Expected findings:** Breasts may be initially soft during the first 24 to 48 hours after delivery. Colostrum production also occurs during this time. During days 2 to 4, the breasts may feel fuller with milk and warmer to the touch because of vasocongestion. Small nodules because of a plugged duct may be present.
- **Abnormal findings:** If a nodule persists despite proper milk transfer, further evaluation is needed to rule out fibrocystic changes or malignant disease. Cracked and bleeding nipples may be indicative of an improper latch. Refer to Chapter Five "Breastfeeding" to learn more about assisting mothers with proper positioning and latch.
- **Patient education:** Encourage use of a well-supporting and properly fitted bra for lactation suppression in mothers who choose not to breastfeed. For breastfeeding mothers, instruct on use of a

cotton nursing garment with flaps that open for breastfeeding. Refer to Chapter Five "Breastfeeding" for further information.

Assess Chest

- **Auscultate:** Listen to heart and lungs.
- **Expected findings:** Normal cardiac rate and rhythm and clear lungs. Both the respiratory and cardiovascular systems begin returning to their prepregnant states after delivery of the newborn. The heart returns to its normal position and there is more room for diaphragmatic expansion.
- **Abnormal findings:** Adventitious lung sounds need further evaluation to rule out complications such as pulmonary embolism.
- **Patient education:** After a cesarean section, it is vital that the patient is instructed to cough, turn, deep breathe, and use an incentive spirometer to prevent fluid accumulation in the alveoli (a condition called *atelectasis*). About 12 hours after surgery, and within a few hours after a vaginal delivery, the patient should be encouraged to gradually ambulate to mobilize the fluids in the lungs. The nurse should assist the patient getting out of bed for the first time and make sure she is hemodynamically stable.

REEDA

Redness
Ecchymosis
Edema
Drainage
Approximation of skin edges

TIP

The contractions may cause pain that women find comparable with severe menstrual cramps. Breastfeeding and medication to aid the uterus to involute (such as oxytocin [Pitocin]) may increase the intensity of the cramping pain. See the section on pain later in this chapter to review methods to alleviate pain.

Uterus and Abdomen

- **Inspection:** Visually inspect abdomen for any distention. If patient had a cesarean section or a postpartum tubal ligation, assess the incision for redness, ecchymosis, edema, drainage, approximation of skin edges (remember the mnemonic REEDA). Note whether staples or sutures were used to close the abdominal incision. Staples are usually removed before the patient's discharge from the hospital.
- **Auscultate:** Listen for bowel sounds in all four quadrants.
- **Palpation:** Determine the descent of the uterus in relation to the umbilicus using finger breadths as your measuring tool. For example, U-1 or U/1 means that the uterus is 1 finger breadth below the umbilicus. Assess the firmness of the uterus and its position in relation to the midline of the abdomen.
- **Percuss:** If tympany (drum-like sound) is heard, this may be an indication that the abdomen is filled with gas and causing the patient discomfort.

- **Expected findings:** The skin of the abdomen will appear loose and floppy. The cesarean section or tubal ligation incision should look clean, dry, and intact. Within the first 12 hours after surgery, bowel sounds may be hypoactive and will return to normal active sounds within 12 to 24 hours. Abdomen is soft to palpation and nontender. The uterus should be firm and not boggy, located midline of the abdomen, and appropriately descended.
- **Abnormal findings:** A distended abdomen with hypoactive bowel sounds, and no report of passing flatus 72 hours after surgery, may be an indication of a paralytic ileus and needs to be evaluated by an HCP. A displaced uterus from the midline, commonly to the right, is likely due to a distended bladder. If this is the case, assist the patient to the bathroom to empty her bladder and reassess the uterus after voiding. Uterine tenderness, foul-smelling drainage, and an erythematous, tender, dehiscing incision may be signs of an infection.

Bladder

- **Expected findings:** After a vaginal delivery, the patient will usually void within the first 6 hours postpartum. An indwelling Foley catheter is inserted before a cesarean section and usually remains after surgery to continuously empty the patient's bladder. The catheter is discontinued at 12 hours when the patient is able to ambulate.
- **Abnormal findings:** If patient is unable to void on her own, she may need to be catheterized to empty bladder of urine. Refer to your institution's protocol. If patient is experiencing pain upon urination, accompanied with urgency and frequency, these may be signs of a urinary tract infection and must be reported to the HCP.
- **Patient education:** Instruct patient to pat dry from front to back after voiding. Teach

ALERT!

If there is wound drainage from a cesarean section incision, an episiotomy, or a perineal laceration, assess Color, Odor, Consistency, Amount (remember the mnemonic COCA). Any type of drainage must be monitored closely. Copious, foul-smelling, and/or pus-like drainage may be an indication of infection, which requires further evaluation by an HCP. If there is no drainage from the incision, the wound dressing for a cesarean section or a tubal ligation should be taken off after 24 hours and left open to air to dry. This will prevent moisture from accumulating, which may cause an environment suitable for increased bacterial growth.

ALERT!

A boggy uterus feels spongy and may be a sign of uterine atony or may be due to retained placental fragments. Uterine atony, which is the loss of uterine muscle tone, is the most common cause of postpartum hemorrhage (PPH). Retained placental fragments may inhibit the uterus to adequately contract and also result in PPH. A boggy uterus that does not firm up after fundal massage needs immediate attention. Refer to the PPH section for a step-by-step guide on how to manage a PPH with the HCP.

When was the last time
you went to the bathroom
to urinate? Are you experiencing any pain upon
urinating? Are you feeling
the urge to go all the time?
Are you finding that you
are not making it to the
bathroom to urinate?

patient to perform Kegel exercise to strengthen her perineal muscle.

Bowels

- **Expected findings:** Anesthesia adminis-tered during labor and delivery may de-crease gastrointestinal motility. A patient should be able to tolerate a regular diet after a vaginal delivery. Depending on in-stitutional policy, a patient who underwent a cesarean section is advanced to a liquid, then to a regular diet at 12 to 24 hours after surgery. Bowel movement usually occurs within 2 to 3 days postpartum.

- **Abnormal findings:** If a patient is not able to tolerate the appro-priate diet and experiences nausea and vomiting, her diet may need to be changed back to a clear fluid diet or she may even need to be placed on an NPO status. If patient continues to have nausea and vomiting, with excessive bloating, and constipation, the patient needs to be evaluated to rule out a paralytic ileus.

- **Patient education:** Encourage the patient to ambulate as soon as tolerated to help with gastrointestinal motility.

Lochia

- **Inspection:** Assess amount and characteris-tics of lochia.

  - **Expected findings**
    - **Lochia rubra (days 0–3):** red, rust-colored discharge
    - **Lochia serosa (days 3–14):** pink, brownish colored discharge
    - **Lochia alba (2 weeks and beyond):** whitish yellow discharge

  - **Abnormal findings:** Foul-smelling odor may be a sign of an infection. In-creased bleeding needs to be assessed (Fig. 4–1).

TIP

The amount of lochia is
typically documented as
scant, moderate, or heavy
and is assessed in relation
to when the patient delivered. Keep in mind that
visual inspection of pads
is subjective. Weighing
pads will give a better
estimation of the amount
of blood loss. Remember,
1 g = 1 mL.

SPEAKING OUT

Are you passing gas? Have you moved your bowels yet? Are you eating food without any nausea or vomiting?

SPEAKING OUT

How is your bleeding? Are you soaking your pads every 1 to 2 hours or pass-ing clots?

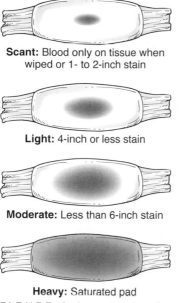

Scant: Blood only on tissue when wiped or 1- to 2-inch stain

Light: 4-inch or less stain

Moderate: Less than 6-inch stain

Heavy: Saturated pad

FIGURE 4-1: Estimation of lochia amount on a peripad.

Episiotomy and/or Laceration

- **Inspection:** Assess the patient's perineum. If she had an episiotomy or laceration, note the presence of redness, ecchymosis, edema, drainage, and approximation of skin edges (remember the mnemonic REEDA; Fig. 4–3).
- **Expected findings:** Include slight edema. Skin edges should be well approximated. Hemorrhoids may be present.
- **Abnormal findings:** Include redness, ecchymosis, drainage, skin that is not approximated, hematoma, and tenderness.
- **Patient education:** Discuss with patient that discomfort and pain at the site of the episiotomy or laceration may be present especially in the first week postpartum. See following section on pain for how to manage pain effectively. Offer ice packs for the first 24 hours to prevent further edema, then heat by using warm water in a sitz bath. Educate on topical anesthetic creams/sprays appropriate for perineal use and witch hazel pads. The patient may be hesitant to defecate in fear of pain and/or the stitches coming apart. Stool softeners may be offered as prescribed by HCP.

Pain

- Ascertain the presence and location of pain. Depending on the severity and the location, examine the site appropriately.
- Explain nonpharmacologic interventions to alleviate pain, such as massage, imagery, breathing, distraction, and hot/cold therapy.

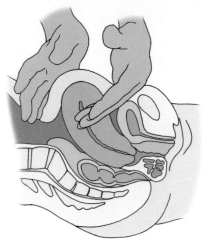

FIGURE 4-2: How to perform a fundal massage. Don procedure gloves and assist patient to a supine position. Place one hand at the top of the uterus, called the *fundus*. The fundus should feel like a hard, globular mass. Place the other hand above the pubic symphysis to stabilize the uterus. Proceed to gently but firmly massage the uterus in a circular motion. The mother may feel afterbirth pains when this procedure is performed and should be offered pain-relieving measures.

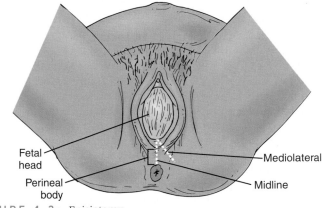

Fetal head

Perineal body

Mediolateral

Midline

FIGURE 4-3: Episiotomy.

- Discuss pharmacologic options that are prescribed by the HCP. Typical pain relievers used postpartum are: acetaminophen, ibuprofen, oxycodone, morphine, ketorolac tromethamine, and hydromorphone. Check your orders for the appropriate dosing, frequency, and route of administration. (More detailed information about these medications is available in Appendix A at the back of the book.)

What causes the cramping pain after having a baby?

Patient: Nurse, why do I feel like I am still contracting? The cramping pain is causing me discomfort.

RN: Your uterus, the baby's home inside your abdomen, is made up of muscle. The uterus was about the size of a fist before you were pregnant and it expanded in size to accommodate your growing baby. The cramping sensation you are feeling is caused by the uterus contracting back down to its prepregnancy size. This is called *uterine involution*, a normal process after delivery that may continue for up to 2 to 4 weeks—You mentioned that the cramping is causing you discomfort; what is the level of your pain at this time? Zero being no pain, and 10 being the worst pain you have ever experienced.

Patient: I am not having any at this moment.

RN: Well, that's good to hear. But I just want you to know that there are options to relieve your pain such as heat packs and medications like ibuprofen. Please let me know when you are starting to experience pain and I can provide you with these pain-relieving measures.

Patient: Ok, I will. Thank you.

- Narcotics may cause constipation. Ask HCP to prescribe stool softeners and encourage patient to drink plenty of fluids and ambulate.
- Patient's pain needs to be reevaluated 30 minutes after therapy is implemented. If no change in pain status has occurred, alert HCP.

Legs and Extremities

- **Inspection and palpation:** Assess extremities for signs and symptoms of thrombophlebitis such as erythema, warmth, and tenderness in the affected area and unilateral swelling of an extremity. Palpate pedal pulses. Do not forget to inspect intravenous (IV) site(s) for symptoms of infiltration such as swelling, tenderness, or cool skin, and for symptoms of phlebitis such as tenderness, warmth, and erythema.
- **Expected findings:** Include extremities free of signs and symptoms of thrombophlebitis, and IV sites free of signs and symptoms of infiltration or phlebitis. If there is no calf pain elicited when

QSEN Application

Patient-centered care includes skills such as:

- Assessing presence and extent of pain and suffering
- Assessing levels of physical and emotional comfort
- Eliciting expectations of patient and family for relief of pain, discomfort, or suffering
- Initiating effective treatments to relieve pain and suffering in light of patient values, preferences, and expressed needs

In this chapter, together with information about care of pregnant women and newborns, Quality and Safety Education for Nurses (QSEN) competencies assure delivery of the best nursing care.

http://qsen.org/competencies/pre-licensure-ksas/#patient-centered_care

dorsiflexing the foot, Homans' sign is considered negative. This does not rule out deep vein thrombosis.

- **Abnormal findings:** If calf pain is elicited, this is a positive Homans' sign and may be indicative of a deep vein thrombosis along with warm, erythematous, and tender extremities.

Emotional Status

- **General assessment:** There is a wide spectrum of emotions during childbirth. The mother may experience excitement and joy together with anxiety, fear, and stress.
- Assess appropriateness of patient's emotions according to the situation. For example, a woman whose infant is diagnosed with an unexpected illness may become sad or even depressed. It is important to assess for family support.
- If patient states or you observe that she is in a depressed state, the patient needs to be further assessed using a tool such as the Edinburgh postpartum depression tool. If the woman screens positive for depression, the HCP needs to be alerted. Ask the HCP whether he or she can place a social services and/or psychiatry consultation for further evaluation, management, treatment, and follow-up.

Bonding and Attachment

- **Bonding** is the process of a *unidirectional* affection and regard from parent to neonate. It is the instant affection a mother feels. It is important that during the first 30 to 60 minutes after birth, the "sensitive period," the mother is given the time and privacy to initiate this bond with her infant. Perhaps delay procedures such as vitamin K administration, if it is possible.
- **Attachment** is the *interaction* between parent and neonate that is mutually satisfying. This is enhanced by positive feedback from the infant. The mother strokes the baby's cheeks and in response (perhaps the rooting reflex) the neonate moves his mouth a certain way and the mother perceives it as a smile. The mother feels good and continues to stroke and touch the neonate to reciprocate the perceived happiness. Attachment is the beginning of a lifelong bond between mother and her child.

Self and Newborn Care Education

Also refer to the patient education sections of the BUBBLE PLEB assessment.

EVIDENCE-BASED PRACTICE

Postpartum blues is experienced by 70% to 80% of postpartum women within 2 to 4 days after delivery. On the other hand, postpartum depression happens in about 10% of women about 2 weeks to a year after childbirth. Postpartum psychosis is rare and may happen 2 to 3 days postpartum. See Table 4–1 for the categories of postpartum mood disorders.

Table 4-1 Categories of Postpartum Mood Disorders

	POSTPARTUM BLUES	POSTPARTUM DEPRESSION	POSTPARTUM PSYCHOSIS
Incidence (%)	70–80	≥10	0.1–0.2
Average time	2–4 days postpartum	2 weeks to 12 months postpartum	2–3 days postpartum
Average duration	2–3 days, resolution within 10 days	3–14 months	Variable
Symptoms	Mild insomnia, tearfulness, irritability, poor concentration, depressed affect	Irritability, labile mood, difficulty falling asleep, phobias, anxiety, symptoms worsen in the evening	Similar to organic brain syndrome: confusion, attention deficit, distractibility, clouded sensorium
Treatment	None; self-limited	Antidepressant pharmacotherapy; psychotherapy	Antipsychotic pharmacotherapy, antidepressant pharmacotherapy (50% of patients also meet depression criteria)

Infant Feeding

Breastfeeding

Please refer to Chapter 5 "Breastfeeding."

Formula Feeding

If a mother chooses to formula-feed her infant, provide the following information regarding safe practices, proper formula preparation, and lactation suppression.

- Wash hands before preparation of formula and feeding the infant.
- Use hot, soapy water to clean bottles and nipples.

SPEAKING OUT

KEGEL EXERCISE

Named after Dr. Kegel who developed this exercise to strengthen the pelvic floor muscles that support the uterus, bladder, and bowels.

How to perform Kegel exercises: Contract your pelvic muscles (as though you are stopping the flow of urine) and hold it for 10 seconds. Relax for another 10 seconds. Repeat for 15 minutes, four times a day.

Continued

SEXUAL ACTIVITY AND PELVIC REST

Avoid sexual intercourse and maintain pelvic rest (this means not placing anything inside the vagina such as tampons) for 4 to 6 weeks to allow for adequate healing of the pelvic organs. It may be wise to wait for the HCP to examine you at your follow-up visit before resuming sexual intercourse.

FAMILY PLANNING

Refer to Chapter Seven "Contraceptive Counseling" for more information.

NUTRITION

- Eat a well-balanced diet. Drink to satisfy thirst.
- For a nonlactating mother: Return to your diet before pregnancy using the Recommended Daily Allowances to guide you with your nutritional requirements.
- For a lactating mother: While lactating, you will need to increase caloric intake by 500 calories more than the recommended amount for you before pregnancy. Typically, this is 2300 to 2500 Kcal/day for most women who are moderately active. Continue taking your prenatal vitamins, as recommended by your HCP. Another goal for you is to ingest 1000 mg calcium a day through diet and supplementation.

RETURN OF MENSTRUATION

For a nonlactating mother: Your periods will likely return within 4 to 8 weeks postpartum.

For a lactating mother: Your periods may not return for months or until you have weaned your infant.

Do not rely on the return of menses as a form of birth control. There is a chance of pregnancy if you engage in sexual intercourse before the onset of your menses without using contraception. Remember that your ovaries will have to release an egg prior to you having your first period after childbirth.

WEIGHT LOSS

Losing weight gained in pregnancy is a common concern for most postpartum women. The recommended weight loss for most women is 4.5 lbs/mo. You should not let your calorie intake fall below 1800 kcal/day, because this may contribute to postpartum fatigue and decreased bone mineral density.

EXERCISE

The amount, intensity level, and initiation of exercise are highly dependent on your level of fitness, medical history, whether there were any complications during pregnancy, labor, and delivery, and your postpartum recovery. We recommend that you resume exercise gradually and consult your HCP.

FOLLOW-UP VISIT

We recommend that you schedule a postpartum follow-up visit with your HCP within 6 weeks after delivery.

- Many different types of nipples and bottles are available on the market, and choosing which type usually depends on your preference.
- Read the instructions on how to prepare, properly store, and reconstitute the formula you choose to give your baby.
- Follow any instructions for mixing formula on the packaging. Overdilution of formula may cause water intoxication, and the use of too much formula in ratio to water may cause hypernatremia in an infant.
- It is safe to give formula at room temperature. If warm formula is preferred, the bottle may be placed in hot (not boiling) water. Advise parents to test the temperature of the formula by shaking the bottle and placing a few drops on the inside of the preparer's wrist. The formula should feel warm, not hot.
- Formula should never be microwaved because of inconsistent heating of the liquid, which may burn the infant.
- Even if you do not choose to breastfeed, you may start lactating and may find colostrum leaking out of your breasts. You may suppress lactation by wearing a well-supporting bra and avoiding nipple stimulation.
- If engorgement occurs and you are uncomfortable, place warm packs on the breast and manually express breast milk, only to the point that you feel comfortable and your breasts soften. Do not overly stimulate the breasts, because this may cause further breast milk production. Immediately place ice packs on the breasts to prevent further lactation.

Complications in the Postpartum Period

Complications in the postpartum period may fall into three main categories: postpartum hemorrhage (PPH), which is the excessive bleeding experienced after delivery, perineal trauma, and perineal infections.

Postpartum Hemorrhage

PPH is ≥500 mL for a vaginal delivery and ≥1000 ml for a cesarean section.

- **Incidence:** 4% of all deliveries
- **Types**
  - **Immediate:** Occurs within the first 24 hours after childbirth. Caused by uterine atony, genital laceration, retained products of conception, placenta accreta/increta/percreta, uterine rupture, uterine inversion, and coagulopathy.
  - **Delayed:** Occurs after the first 24-hour period after childbirth and until 6 weeks postpartum. Caused by subinvolution of the uterus, retained products of conception, infection, and coagulopathy.

Causes

Following are common causes of PPH.

Uterine Atony

Atony is the failure of the myometrium to effectively contract and control the bleeding at the placental site. With relaxed muscles, blood flows out rapidly and causes a hemorrhage.

- **Incidence:** 1 in 20 deliveries
- Risk factors
  - Grand multiparity
  - Multiple gestation

SPEAKING OUT

If your labor and delivery and postpartum units do not have a PPH kit, suggest to your Nurse Manager that this is a necessity in your unit. It is a kit that can be grabbed quickly when there is a PPH, much like a crash cart for a code. The kit contains the essential equipment necessary when caring for a woman experiencing a PPH.

- Supplies to start an IV: tourniquet, alcohol swab, 18-gauge catheter, heparin lock, clear tape, 2×2 gauze, transparent dressing, IV flush with sterile saline
- Blood draw supplies: tourniquet, butterfly, venipuncture, tubes to draw labs for complete blood cell count (CBC) and coagulopathy studies (prothrombin time [PT]/partial thromboplastin time [PTT]/fibrinogen), bandage, 2×2 gauze, clear tape
- Needle and syringe for medicine administration
- Ring forceps
- 4×4 gauze
- Vaginal speculums in different sizes
- Flashlight
- Sterile gloves, if possible, long gloves
- Nonsterile gloves
- Goggles
- Medications (expiration dates will need to be checked routinely): morphine, Pitocin, 15-methyl prostaglandin (Hemabate), methylergonovine (Methergine); see Appendix A.
- IV bag of normal sterile saline and IV tubing

- Polyhydramnios
- Fetal macrosomia
- Chorioamnionitis
- Placenta previa
- Precipitous delivery
- Prolonged labor
- Management
  - Bimanual massage by the HCP
  - **Administration of uterotonic therapy:** intramuscular (IM) methylergonovine (Methergine), oxytocin (Pitocin) diluted in IV infusion, per vagina/rectum misoprostol (Cytotec), PO Hemabate. See Table 4–2.
  - Make sure pain medication is administered as soon as possible in order for patient to tolerate procedures well.
  - IV resuscitation with fluids and/or blood
  - HCP may consider prescribing antibiotics to prevent infection.
  - If other measures fail, the obstetrician may consider medical/surgical interventions such as uterine ligation, embolization, or hysterectomy.

Perineal Trauma

Trauma to the cervix, vulva, perineum, and/or vagina is the second most common cause of PPH regardless of whether a woman had a vaginal or caesarean delivery.

- Risk factors
  - Operative vaginal delivery
  - Fetal macrosomia
  - Fetal malpresentation
  - Precipitous delivery
- Suspect perineal trauma if you notice:
  - Bright red bleeding (compared with the dark red color of lochia)
  - Decreasing hemoglobin values
  - Hypotension
  - Tachycardia
  - Continuation of bleeding despite a firm uterus at the appropriate location
- Types of trauma
  - Laceration
    - **First degree:** involves the perineal skin and the vaginal mucous membrane
    - **Second degree:** includes muscles of the perineum
    - **Third degree:** not only includes the skin, mucous membranes, and the muscles of the perineum, but also the anal sphincter
    - **Fourth degree:** extends all the way through the mucosa of the rectum
  - Hematoma
    - **Vulvar hematoma:** Usually caused by injury to the superficial fascia wherein the collection of blood protrudes to the skin.

Table 4–2 Medication Index for PPH

AGENT	DOSE	ROUTE	DOSING FREQUENCY	SIDE EFFECTS	CONTRA-INDICATIONS
Oxytocin (Pitocin)	10 – 80 units in 1,000 ml of crystalloid solution	1st line: IV 2nd line: IM or IU	Continuous	Nausea, emesis, water intoxication	None
Methylergonovine (Methergine)	0.2 mg	1st line: IM 2nd line: IU or PO	Q 2 – 4 h	HTN, hypotension, nausea, emesis	HTN, preeclampsia
15-Methyl Prostaglandin F2∞ (Hemabate)	0.25 mg	1st line: IM 2nd line: IU	Q 15 – 90 min (max is 8 doses)	Nausea, emesis, diarrhea, flushing, chills	Active cardiac, pulmonary, renal or hepatic disease
Prostaglandin E2 (Dinoprostone)	20 mg	PR	Q 2 h	Nausea, emesis, diarrhea, flushing, chills, HA	Hypotension
Misoprostol (Cytotec)	600 – 1000 mcg	1st line: PR 2nd line: PO	Single dose	Tachycardia, fever	None

From Gabbe SG, Niebyl JR, Simpson JL, et al., eds. *Obstetrics: Normal and Problem Pregnancies.* 5th ed. Philadelphia, PA: Churchill Livingstone; 2007:138.

NURSING ACTION DURING A PPH

If you feel a boggy uterus and you note excessive uterine bleeding and/or passage of clots, *do not leave your patient's bedside. You* are the director and you should avoid leaving the set. Call for assistance instead. Direct a nurse for each task:

- Call the HCP.
- Obtain uterotonics (likely IM or IV Pitocin, IM Methergine, IM Hemabate).
- Obtain pain medications (likely IM or IV morphine sulfate).
- Get the PPH kit.
- Start a large-bore IV, if no IV present.

Direct nursing assistant(s) to:

- Take the patient's vital signs.
- Bring the baby to the nursery to allow more room for staff to work.
- If visitors are in room, guide the visitors to the waiting area.

When the HCP arrives, *you* are the one who will be expected to give the quick rundown of the patient's history:

- Patient name
- Gravida and para
- Type of delivery
- Degree of laceration and/or type of episiotomy
- Asthma history (avoid giving asthmatics Hemabate)
- Hypertension history (avoid giving methylergonovine [Methergine] to patients with hypertension)
- Medical/Surgical history

Nursing actions:

- Provide support and ensure patient experiences as little pain and discomfort as possible.
- Assist the HCP while he or she manages the PPH. The HCP may need to perform a bimanual massage of the uterus and manual extraction of clots.
- Once the patient is stable and comfortable, assist cleaning the patient while she is in bed, using a warm, damp wash cloth. Help change the patient's soiled bed linens and gown.
- Place the call bell near the patient and remind her to call for assistance the first time she wants to get out of bed.
- The HCP will likely order follow-up blood work such as a CBC, PT/PTT, and fibrinogen.
- Uterotonic therapy may also be prescribed by the HCP for 24 to 48 hours after the PPH.
- Assess the patient's vital signs, bleeding, pain level, and check for signs and symptoms of hemodynamic instability as per your institution's protocol.

- Management
  - HCP may incise skin to evacuate the hematoma of trapped blood. Pressure dressing is then applied to this area to prevent further bleeding
  - Ask HCP whether a Foley catheter should be placed to empty patient's bladder until swelling around the area has subsided.
- **Vaginal hematoma:** Results from vaginal delivery or use of forceps. The accumulation of blood in this type of hematoma happens above the pelvic diaphragm.
- Management
  - Similar to management for vulvar hematoma, the HCP will place an incision at the site to drain the blood. Often, a vaginal packing is placed to put pressure at the site.
- **Retroperitoneal hematoma:** Occurs at the time of a cesarean section wherein the uterine arteries continue to bleed or resulting from uterine scar rupture during labor. This type of hematoma is not visibly obvious and may be suspected if patient becomes hemodynamically unstable.
- Management
  - Surgery to look for and drain the hematoma
  - Arterial ligation

Retained Products of Conception

Retained products of conception are leftover placental fragments and amniotic membranes that may prevent the uterus from contracting to its normal size, thus resulting in excessive bleeding.
- **Incidence:** 1 in 100 to 200 deliveries
- **Management:** Removal of products of conception using manual extraction or uterine curettage performed by the HCP

Uterine Rupture

Uterine rupture is the spontaneous dehiscence or opening of the uterine wall. This may cause massive bleeding and the fetus and placenta may extrude into the abdomen.
- **Incidence:** 1 in 2000 deliveries
- Risk factors
  - Prior caesarean delivery
  - Induction of labor
- Clinical manifestations
  - **Fetal heart tracing findings:** late decelerations and bradycardia
  - **Maternal findings:** tachycardia, hypotension, change in uterine shape, abdominal pain, uterine tenderness, cessation of contractions
- Management
  - After HCP delivers fetus and placenta, the site of rupture will be sutured close.
  - Hysterectomy may be a possibility if the site of rupture cannot be closed and/or the mother's status starts to deteriorate because of the blood loss.

Uterine Inversion

Uterine inversion happens when the top of the uterus collapses into the inner cavity possibly because of excessive traction on the umbilical cord or application of too much fundal pressure.

- **Incidence:** 1 in 2500 deliveries
- Clinical manifestations
  - Inability to palpate the fundus
  - Maternal hypotension and tachycardia
- Management
  - IV fluid resuscitation through a large-bore IV catheter
  - HCP manually or surgically replaces uterine fundus

Postpartum Infection

A puerperal infection is a fever of a 100.4°F (38°C) occurring after the first 24 hours postpartum.

Types of Postpartum Infections

Mastitis

- **Incidence:** 5% of lactating women
- **Onset:** 2 to 3 weeks postpartum
- **Causative organism:** usually *Staphylococcus aureus*
- Risk factors
  - Stasis of milk likely because of infrequent, inconsistent breastfeeding
  - Nipple trauma
- Signs and symptoms
  - Fever, tachycardia, chills, malaise, headache
  - Often unilateral breast tenderness that may have localized area of inflammation and redness
  - Enlarged axillary lymph nodes on the side of the affected breast
- Management
  - Notify HCP of patient status.
  - Administer antibiotics and antipyretics as prescribed by HCP.
  - It is usually acceptable for patient to continue to breastfeed infant unless an abscess is present and/or HCP advises to discard breast milk.
  - Encourage breastfeeding on unaffected side first to facilitate letdown and softening of the infected breast, thus allowing for a more comfortable feeding when the affected breast is offered to the infant.
  - Encourage breastfeeding every 2 to 3 hours exclusively and avoid supplementing with formula, which will likely decrease the infant's interest to breastfeed.
  - Place warm compress to increase circulation and massage breasts to decrease breast engorgement and soften them before a feeding.
  - If patient is advised to discard breast milk until infection/abscess is treated, and patient wishes to maintain lactation,

patient may manually express milk and/or use a breast pump until it is safe to resume breastfeeding.

- Offer ice packs between feedings for comfort and to reduce edema. Ice packs may also be used to suppress further milk production if patient decides to switch feeding method to formula.
- Complication
  - **Breast abscess:** Needle-point surgical drainage and hospitalization may be necessary, along with IV antibiotics and antipyretics.

Endometritis

An infection of the lining of the uterus, also called the *endometrium*.

- Incidence
  - **Vaginal delivery:** 1% to 3%
  - **Cesarean section:** 15% to 20%
- **Causative organisms:** group beta streptococcus (GBS), enterococcus, *Escherichia coli*, *Klebsiella pneumoniae*, *Proteus*, *Bacteroides*, *Prevotella*
- **Onset:** 2 to 4 days postpartum
- Risk factors
  - Operative procedure such as a cesarean section and forceps-assisted vaginal delivery
  - Multiple cervical examinations during labor
  - Prolonged rupture of membranes (≥18 hours)
  - Manual extraction of placenta
- Signs and symptoms
  - Fever
  - Tachycardia
  - Chills
  - Malaise
  - Abdominal or uterine tenderness
  - Foul-smelling lochia
- Management
  - Notify HCP of patient status.
  - Administer antibiotics and antipyretics as ordered.
  - Instruct patient on proper perineal care.
  - Place patient in Fowler's position to help drainage of lochia.
  - Discuss with the patient and her family the possibility of a longer hospital stay but that improvement of symptoms usually occurs within 48 to 72 hours after initiation of antibiotics.
  - Facilitate continued mother–infant bonding and attachment.
  - If patient is breastfeeding, discuss with HCP that patient will need antibiotics that are compatible with lactation.
  - Provide comfort measures such as cool compresses, warm packs, and pain medication.

- Complications
  - Salpingitis
  - Oophoritis
  - May result in sterility

Wound Infection

A postpartum woman may experience development of a wound infection at two likely sites: the abdominal incision from a cesarean section or the episiotomy/laceration from a vaginal delivery.

- Risk factors
  - Chorioamnionitis
  - Obesity
  - Diabetes
  - Advanced maternal age
  - Malnutrition
- **Onset:** Early onset is a wound infection that occurs within the first 2 days. Late onset occurs between days 2 and 7.
- Signs and symptoms
  - Erythematous, tender incision with purulent discharge
  - Low-grade temperature with fever spikes
- Management
  - Antibiotic therapy as prescribed by the HCP
  - Offer both nonpharmacologic and prescribed pharmacologic pain management modalities

Cesarean incision

- Assist the HCP with the irrigation, débridement, and packing of the wound.
- Change the dressing regularly and dispose of soiled dressings properly, as per institutional protocol.
- Teach the family how to care for the patient's wound in the event that the patient is discharged from the hospital with a wound dressing that needs to be changed on a regular basis.

Episiotomy/Laceration

- Instruct patient on sitz bath use to cleanse the affected site and to increase the circulation to the perineal area.
- Encourage the patient to wipe from front to back and to use the peri bottle to clean after each time she voids or moves her bowels.
- Offer stool softeners, as prescribed, in order for the patient not to have to strain with moving her bowels.
- **Complications from cesarean or episiotomy/laceration infection:** sepsis and necrotizing fasciitis

Urinary Tract Infection

- **Incidence:** 2% to 4%
- **Onset:** can occur at any time during antepartum and postpartum periods
- **Causative organism:** *E. coli*, GBS, *Klebsiella, Enterobacter, Proteus, S. aureus*

- Risk factors
  - Catheterizations
  - Multiple vaginal examinations
  - Diabetes
  - Cesarean section
  - Asymptomatic bacteriuria in pregnancy
- Signs and symptoms
  - Fever
  - Dysuria
  - Frequency
  - Urgency
  - Hematuria
  - Costovertebral angle tenderness
- Management
  - Notify HCP of patient status.
  - Administer antibiotics and antipyretics as prescribed.
  - If uncomplicated UTI, patient may not need to prolong her hospital stay. HCP may choose to initiate PO antibiotic therapy in the hospital and have the patient complete therapy at home as long as she is afebrile and pain is well-controlled.
  - Instruct patient on proper perineal care, and encourage her to pat dry from front to back.
  - Advise the patient to increase fluid intake.
  - Encourage the patient to rest.
- **Complications:** pyelonephritis, an infection of the kidneys; treated with antibiotics and antipyretics and may necessitate hospitalization

5 Breastfeeding

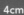

4cm

CHAPTER 5

Breastfeeding

B reast milk is the best food for infants. It is naturally and perfectly tailored to the needs of the newborn. Breast milk contains the right amount of nutrients to satisfy and nourish the infant. Breast milk also contains vital antibodies that are passed from the mother that help protect the infant against certain infections. Promoting breastfeeding needs to be a priority of all health-care staff caring for both the mother and the infant.

Benefits of Breastfeeding for the Infant

- Decreases incidence/severity of infections including bacterial meningitis, otitis media, necrotizing enterocolitis, and urinary tract infection
- Reduces postneonatal infant mortality rate by approximately 21%
- Decreases rate of sudden infant death syndrome
- Decreases incidence of insulin-dependent (type 1) diabetes mellitus, non–insulin-dependent (type 2) diabetes mellitus, leukemia, obesity, and asthma
- Enhances performance on cognitive development tests
- Provides pain relief when infant is breastfed during a procedure such as a heel stick when drawing blood

EVIDENCE-BASED PRACTICE

One of the goals of *Healthy People 2010* is to: "Increase the percentage of live births that occur in facilities that provide recommended care for lactating mothers and their babies." Research has proved that women who deliver in facilities that provide adequate support and guidance for lactating mothers breastfeed longer and more exclusively.

U.S. Department of Health and Human Services, Office of Disease Prevention and Health Promotion: *Healthy People 2010*. Retrieved November 11, 2010, from www.health.gov/healthypeople.

Benefits of Breastfeeding for the Mother

- The release of oxytocin during letdown causes the uterus to contract, thus potentiating uterine involution back to prepregnancy state and decreasing bleeding in the postpartum period
- Enhances feelings of attachment and relaxation because of oxytocin and prolactin release
- It is a convenient method of feeding: no need to bring bottles and formula when traveling; no need for washing and cleaning bottles and nipples after feeding
- May lower the risk for osteoporosis
- Associated with decreased risk for development of ovarian and breast cancer
- More cost-effective than formula feeding

Women Who Should Not Breastfeed

Despite the countless benefits of breastfeeding, some women should not breastfeed because their current health status may cause harm to the infant. Women who should be discouraged from breastfeeding include those who:

- Test positive for HIV
- Have untreated tuberculosis or varicella
- Currently have an active herpes lesion on breast
- Take street drugs
- Abuse alcohol
- Are currently being treated for breast cancer
- Take antineoplastic, thyrotoxic, and immunosuppressive medications
- Have an infant with galactosemia

Initiating Breastfeeding

- Babies are born with the natural ability to breastfeed; however, both the infant and the mother need continued practice to develop the skill of breastfeeding.

QSEN Application

Ensuring safety includes skills such as:
- Demonstrating effective use of strategies to reduce risk for harm to self or others
- Using national patient safety resources for own professional development and to focus attention on safety in care settings

In this chapter, together with information about care of pregnant women and newborns, Quality and Safety Education for Nurses (QSEN) competencies assure delivery of the best nursing care.

http://qsen.org/competencies/pre-licensure-ksas/#patient-centered_care

- Before labor and delivery, ascertain the mother's plans regarding breastfeeding.
- Initiate breastfeeding as soon as possible after the birth of the infant; this is the period wherein the infant is aroused and alert, and it is an optimum time for breastfeeding.
- Assist the mother in finding a comfortable position for breastfeeding. Make sure her back and arms are well-supported, which will allow for her to comfortably hold her baby (see Figs. 5–1 through 5–4 for the different breastfeeding positions; see page 112 for more on common breastfeeding positions).
- Instruct the mother to cup her breast with one hand and stroke the baby's lower lip with her nipple to encourage the baby to open wide.
- Have the mother hug the infant closer while centering her nipple into the baby's mouth to properly latch the infant.
- The infant should never be latched to the nipple only. He should have a good amount of the mother's areola (the dark

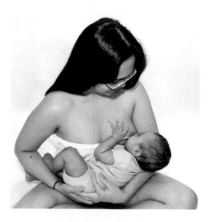

FIGURE 5-1: Cradle hold.

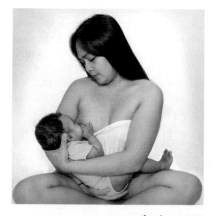

FIGURE 5-2: Cross-cradle or transitional hold.

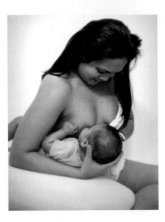

FIGURE 5-3: Football or clutch hold.

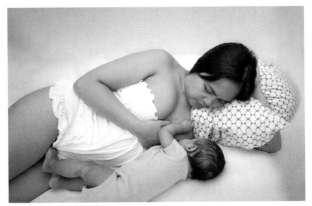

FIGURE 5-4: Side-lying position.

area surrounding the nipple) in his mouth with both lips turned out and relaxed, and with the tongue cupped under her breast.

- If the mother reports that she is experiencing breast pain from feeding, the infant is likely not latched on properly. Teach the mother to slide her clean finger between her breast and the infant's gums. This breaks the suction and she will hear a faint pop. She can then proceed to pull her nipple out of the infant's mouth and reposition for a better latch.
- Encourage the mother to room-in with her infant so that she will get used to learning her own baby's feeding cues. The infant may start rooting, sucking, putting his hand in his mouth, and nuzzling into the mother's chest as a sign that he is ready to breastfeed. Crying is often a late sign of hunger.

UNICEF-WHO BABY-FRIENDLY HOSPITAL INITIATIVE

TEN STEPS TO SUCCESSFUL BREASTFEEDING

Offering Support

Every facility that provides maternity services and care for newborn infants should:

1. Have a written breastfeeding policy that is routinely communicated to all health-care staff.
2. Train all health-care staff in skills necessary to implement this policy.
3. Inform all pregnant women about the benefits and management of breastfeeding.
4. Help mothers initiate breastfeeding within half an hour of birth.
5. Show mothers how to breastfeed and how to maintain lactation even if they should be separated from their infants.
6. Give newborn infants no food or drink other than breast milk, unless medically indicated.
7. Practice rooming-in: allow mothers and infants to remain together 24 hours a day.
8. Encourage breastfeeding on demand.
9. Give no artificial teats or pacifiers (dummies or soothers) to breastfeeding infants.
10. Foster the establishment of breastfeeding support groups and refer mothers to them on discharge from the hospital or clinic.

United Nations Children's Fund. (1991). Baby-Friendly Hospital Initiative. Retrieved November 11, 2010, from www.unicef.org/programme/breastfeeding/baby.htm#10.

QSEN Application

Utilization of evidence-based practice includes knowledge such as:
- Differentiating clinical opinion from research and evidence summaries
- Describing reliable sources for locating evidence reports and clinical practice guidelines
- Explaining the role of evidence in determining best clinical practice
- Describing how the strength and relevance of available evidence influences the choice of interventions in provision of patient-centered care
- Discriminating between valid and invalid reasons for modifying evidence-based clinical practice based on clinical expertise or patient/family preferences

In this chapter, together with information about care of pregnant women and newborns, Quality and Safety Education for Nurses (QSEN) competencies assure delivery of the best nursing care.

http://qsen.org/competencies/pre-licensure-ksas/#patient-centered_care

Common Breastfeeding Positions

- **Cradle hold:** While sitting straight up, have the mother cradle the infant in her arm with the infant's head resting comfortably in the bend of her elbow. The infant's whole body is facing the mother's. This hold is the most commonly used and most comfortable for the majority of mothers (see Fig. 5–1).
- **Cross-cradle or transitional hold:** While sitting straight up, the mother cradles the infant along the opposite arm from the breast she is using. The infant's head is supported with the palm of her hand at the base of his head. This allows for more control of the infant's head during the latching-on process. This hold is ideal for infants who are premature and more likely hypotonic (see Fig. 5–2).
- **Clutch or football hold:** While sitting up straight, instruct the mother to hold her infant at her side (like tucking a football under the arm). The baby should be at the mother's waist level and the infant's head at the level of the nipple. The infant's head is supported by the mother's palm placed at the base of the head. This hold is good for mothers who had a cesarean section, have large breasts, or have inverted nipples (see Fig. 5–3).
- **Side-lying position:** Assist the mother to lie on her side with the baby positioned parallel to her body and facing her. The mother is able to either hold her breast to guide her nipple into the baby's mouth or use her hand to guide the baby's head to her breast. This hold is good for mothers who had a cesarean section because it keeps the baby's weight off the incision (see Fig. 5–4).

> **TIPS**
>
> - Instruct the mother to bring the baby to her breast and not her body to the baby.
> - Use pillows to support the mother and the infant.
> - The more comfortable both the mother and the newborn are, the easier it will be for the mother to breastfeed, maintain proper latch, and continue breastfeeding.

Assessment of the Infant's Latch

An infant needs to properly latch on to the mother's breast to be able to effectively breastfeed, get enough milk, and prevent nipple soreness. The LATCH Evaluation Tool may be used to objectively assess an infant's latch by assigning numeric points to key characteristics necessary for an effective latch (see Table 5–1).

EVIDENCE-BASED PRACTICE

Research has shown that infants who are placed skin-to-skin with their mothers within 30 minutes of birth while at the delivery room cried less, stayed warmer, initiated interaction with their mother, and were more likely to breastfeed and for a longer duration.

Table 5-1 LATCH Evaluation Tool

	0	1	2
L—Latch	Too sleepy or reluctant No sustained latch or suck achieved	Repeated attempts for sustained latch or suck Hold nipple in mouth Stimulate suck	Grasps breasts Tongue down Lips flanged Rhythmical sucking
A—Audible swallowing	None	A few with stimulation	Spontaneous intermittent <24 hours old Spontaneous and frequent >24 hours old
T—Type of nipple	Inverted	Flat	Everted (after stimulation)
C—Comfort (breast/nipple)	Engorged Cracked, bleeding, large blisters, or bruises Severe discomfort	Filling Reddened/small blisters or bruises Mild/moderate discomfort	Soft Tender
H—Hold (positioning)	Full assist (staff holds infant at breast)	Minimal assist (i.e., elevate head of bed; place pillows for support) Teach one side; mother does the other Staff holds and then mother takes over	No assist from staff Mother able to position/hold infant

From Jensen D, Wallace S, Kelsay P. LATCH: a breastfeeding assessment and documentation tool. *J Obstet Gynecol Neonat Nurs.* 23(1):27–32, 1994.

QSEN Application

Patient-centered care includes knowledge such as:
- Eliciting patient values, preferences, and expressed needs as part of clinical interview, implementation of care plan, and evaluation of care
- Communicating patient values, preferences, and expressed needs to other members of health-care team
- Providing patient-centered care with sensitivity and respect for the diversity of human experience
- Assessing own level of communication skill in encounters with patients and families
- Participating in building consensus or resolving conflict in the context of patient care
- Communicating care provided and needed at each transition in care

In this chapter, together with information about care of pregnant women and newborns, Quality and Safety Education for Nurses (QSEN) competencies assure delivery of the best nursing care.

http://qsen.org/competencies/pre-licensure-ksas/#patient-centered_care

Frequency and Duration of Breastfeeding

During the first weeks:
- 8 to 12 feedings at the breast per 24 hours
- Offer both breasts for at least 10 to 15 minutes each and allow for infant to stay on the breasts for as long as desired by the newborn.
- A newborn may need rousing to be fed every 4 hours from the beginning of the last feeding.

Once breastfeeding is well-established:
- Frequency of feeding may go down to about 8 times every 24 hours.
- Frequency may sporadically increase to accommodate infant growth spurts and/or an increase in milk volume demand.

Appearance and Amount of Breast Milk

Both the appearance and amount of breast milk changes from the small amounts of colostrum on the first day of lactation to copious amounts of bluish white breast milk once breast milk production is established (see Table 5–2).

Reassurance That Newborn Is Getting Adequate Amount of Breast Milk

Because breast milk that is directly transferred from the breast into the infant's mouth cannot be measured, some parents need further reassurance that their infant is receiving an adequate amount of milk. The following are signs that can be observed in the infant that the nurse can discuss with the mother to give her further reassurance:
- Audible swallowing sounds while breastfeeding
- Adequate weight gain of ≥4 to 7 oz/wk after the fourth day of life

Table 5–2 **Appearance and Amount of Breast Milk**	
	APPEARANCE AND AMOUNT
Birth	Colostrum is produced. The color is yellow or golden. Drops: 1 teaspoon in amount at each feeding.
Days 1–2	Colostrum is produced. The color is yellow or golden. About 1 teaspoon at each feeding.
Days 2–5	Mature milk comes in. May continue to be yellow or golden but transitioning to bluish white. Mother feels breasts becoming full and may start leaking.
First 4–6 weeks	Milk may now appear to be watery and have a bluish white color at the beginning of each feeding (foremilk) and creamy white toward the end of the feeding (hind milk).

From The National Women's Health Information Center, U.S. Department of Health and Human Services, Office of Women's Health: Learning to Breastfeed. Retrieved November 11, 2010, from www.womenshealth.gov/breastfeeding/learning-to-breastfeed.

- Adequate amount of wet diapers (Table 5–3)
- Stools that transition from dark, tarry (meconium) to greenish yellow to soft, seedy, yellow-mustard stools by the fifth day of life
- Normal skin turgor

See Table 5–3 for elimination patterns in the first week of life.

Routine Pediatric Follow-up After Discharge

- First follow-up visit with a pediatrician at 3 to 5 days of age
- Next routine follow-up is at 2 to 3 weeks of age

Length of Breastfeeding

The American Academy of Pediatrics recommends:
- Breastfeeding exclusively for the first 6 months of life
- Continued breastfeeding for at least the first year of life along with the gradual introduction of iron-enriched foods into the infant's diet starting at 6 months of age
- Continued breastfeeding for as long as both the mother and infant desire to do so

Using a Breast Pump

Mothers may need to use a breast pump in the hospital for several different reasons. Commonly, it is because her infant is presently not able to take in anything orally because of prematurity and the mother would like to initiate lactation. The mother will need assistance to use the

Table 5–3 **Elimination Patterns in the First Week of Life**		
BABY'S AGE	**WET DIAPERS**	**DIRTY DIAPERS**
Day 1 (birth)	1	Thick, tarry and black stool (meconium)
Day 2	2	Thick, tarry and black stool (meconium)
Day 3	3	Greenish yellow
Days 4–7	5–6	Transition to seedy, watery mustard color

From the National Women's Health Information Center, U.S. Department of Health and Human Services, Office of Women's Health: Learning to Breastfeed. Retrieved November 11, 2010, from www.womenshealth.gov/breastfeeding/learning-to-breastfeed.

breast pump and to store pumped breast milk. Most hospitals have a separate refrigerator for milk storage. Instruct the mother to label the container of breast milk with her name and the date the milk was pumped.

Because many breast pumps are available in the market today, the mother will need to read and follow the instructions for the specific breast pump she has purchased for use at home or for when she goes back to work.

Safe Preparation and Storage of Expressed Breast Milk

See Table 5–4 for guidelines on proper storage of expressed breast milk. Instruct the mother to:

- Wash hands before expressing and handling breast milk.
- Collect and store milk in clean containers that can be tightly closed.
- Remember to label her breast milk and to use the oldest milk first.
- Not add fresh milk to milk that already has been frozen.
- Not save milk from a used bottle for use at another feeding.

Table 5–4 Milk Storage Guidelines

LOCATION	TEMPERATURE	DURATION	COMMENTS
Countertop	Room temperature (up to 77°F or 25°C)	6–8 hours	Container should be covered and kept as cool as possible.
Insulated cooler bag	5–39°F or −15°C to 4°C	24 hours	Keep ice packs in contact with milk at all times. Limit opening the cooler bag.
Refrigerator	39°F or 4°C	5 days	Store milk in the back main body of the refrigerator and not in the shelves of the door.
Freezer compartment of refrigerator	5°F or −15°C	2 weeks	Place the breast milk container toward the back of the freezer where the temperature is most consistent.
	0°F or −18°C	3–6 months	
Chest or upright deep freezer	−4° F or −20° C	6–12 months	

Data from The Academy of Breastfeeding Medicine: *Clinical Protocol #8: Human Milk Storage Information for Home Use for Healthy Full Term Infants*. Princeton Junction, NJ: Academy of Breastfeeding Medicine, 2004.

Safely Thawing Breast Milk

Counsel the mother to:

- Avoid using the microwave because liquids do not heat evenly and excess heat can destroy the nutrient quality of the breast milk
- Place the container of frozen breast milk in a bowl of warm (not hot) water
- Not refreeze thawed breast milk

Common Problems Encountered With Breastfeeding

- **Nipple soreness:** Sore nipples are a common complaint by mothers who are initiating breastfeeding. Usual causes of nipple soreness are incorrect latch and improper position that results in ineffective sucking. Instruct the mother to break the suction properly, reposition the infant, and attempt latching the baby on again. After breastfeeding, the mother may rub breast milk or ultra-purified lanolin on her nipples to soothe them. Encourage the mother to air-dry her nipples after feeding, change nursing pads often, and avoid wearing bras that are too tight.
- **Engorgement:** Between the second and sixth day after delivery, the mother will start making larger quantities of milk. Naturally, her breasts will feel full, larger, heavier, and maybe even slightly tender. This fullness may turn into engorgement when the breasts become hard, painful, warm, and throbbing with flattening of the nipples. Engorgement occurs if milk builds up because of irregular and incomplete emptying of the breasts as a result of poor latching and incorrect positioning, infrequent feedings, supplementation, nipple damage, or fatigue. To minimize engorgement, avoid supplementing (unless prescribed by a pediatrician) and overusing pacifiers. Instruct the mother on how to hand express milk to soften the breasts before feeding to allow for the infant to have a better latch. Assist the mother on how to properly latch and position infant.
- **Plugged duct:** Breast engorgement may lead to plugged ducts, which are sore, tender lumps that are usually unilateral. This is not an infectious state as the mother remains without a fever. To relieve the plugged duct, teach the mother to massage the lump before and during feeding. Breastfeed on the unaffected side first and ensure complete emptying.
- **Mastitis:** See "Types of Postpartum Infections" in Chapter Four "Postpartum."

Breastfeeding Resources

- **Academy of Breastfeeding Medicine:** www.bfmed.org
- **American Academy of Pediatrics:** www.aap.org/breastfeeding

- **Centers for Disease Control and Prevention:** www.cdc.gov/breastfeeding
- **La Leche League:** www.llli.org
- **U.S. Department of Health and Human Services:** www.womenshealth.gov/breastfeeding
- **National Women's Health Information Center (NWHIC) Breastfeeding Helpline:** 1-800-994-9662, www.womenshealth.gov
- **World Health Organization:** www.who.int/topics/breastfeeding
- **Association of Women's Health, Obstetric and Neonatal Nurses:** www.awhonn.org
- **LactMed, United States National Library of Medicine's web-based database of drugs and other chemicals to which breastfeeding mothers may be exposed:** lactmed.nlm.nih.gov/ (LactMed also has a smartphone application for easy access to the database.)

6 Newborn

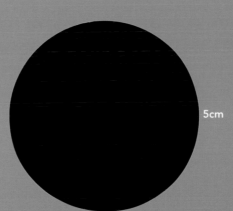

5cm

CHAPTER 6

Newborn

The newborn period, also referred to as the neonatal period, begins the moment the infant is born up to the first 28 days of life.

Physiological Adaptation of the Newborn

Transition to extrauterine life begins when the umbilical cord is cut. The placenta no longer works as lungs. The lungs begin to exchange gases. The first breath causes the lungs to inflate and blood to circulate through the heart, lungs, and the rest of the body.

- Transition period can last 6 to 12 hours.
- Typical timing for assessing a healthy newborn
    1. Assess immediately after birth.
    2. Assess within 1 to 4 hours after birth.
    3. Assess within first 24 hours or before discharge.
- Three phases of transition
    1. Phase one: "Period of reactivity" lasts 1 to 2 hours.
    2. Phase two: "Sleep period" occurs 1 to 4 hours after birth.
    3. Phase three: "Second period of reactivity" is the next 2 to 8 hours.

For the transition to extrauterine life to be successful, physiological changes must occur in the following systems:

- Respiratory system
    - Alveoli inflate with the help of surfactant.
    - The lungs expand after the newborn takes his or her first breath.
    - There is marked increase in blood flow through the pulmonary circulation.
    - Mixing of oxygen-rich and oxygen-poor blood through the ductus arteriosus stops.
    - Catecholamines trigger breathing movements.
    - Breathing increases oxygenation.
    - The lungs clear of fluid.

- Cardiovascular system
  - Pulmonary vascular resistance decreases.
  - Blood flow improves through the pulmonary artery to the lungs.
  - Circulation includes the lungs.
- Neurological system and sensory functioning
  - Newborn reflexes have a role in a successful transition to extrauterine life. For example, the rooting and suck reflex aid in latching on and feeding.
- Hematological system
  - Fetal hemoglobin (Hb) has a high affinity for oxygen to promote good oxygenation while the infant begins to produce his or her own new Hb postnatally.
- Gastrointestinal/Hepatic system
  - Conjugation of bilirubin begins.
  - Digestive enzymes are excreted for infant feedings.
  - Peristalsis increases for bowel motility.
  - The fetus is dependent on the mother for a supply of glucose in utero, but after birth, the newborn must produce his or her own energy source. Glycogen is synthesized in the liver and muscle.
- Urinary system
  - Blood perfuses the newborn kidney to stimulate urine production.
  - The immature newborn kidney does not have the sophisticated ability to concentrate urine or dilute it as necessary.
- Immune system
  - The newborn is protected from certain infections, in part because of maternal antibodies circulating in his or her system until about 4 to 6 months of age.
  - Immunoglobulin G (IgG) crosses the placenta to the fetus while in utero.
  - Infants who are breastfed receive antibodies from the breast milk, including IgE, IgA, IgM, and IgG.
  - Healthy infants begin to produce their own antibodies, starting at 2 to 3 months of age.

QSEN Application

Integration of evidence-based practice includes knowledge such as:
- Demonstrating knowledge of basic scientific methods and processes
- Differentiating clinical opinion from research and evidence summaries
- Describing reliable sources for locating evidence reports and clinical practice guidelines
- Describing how the strength and relevance of available evidence influences the choice of interventions in provision of patient-centered care

In this chapter, together with information about care of pregnant women and newborns, QSEN competencies assure delivery of the best nursing care.

http://qsen.org/competencies/pre-licensure-ksas/#patient-centered_care

Newborn Assessment

Newborns are sensitive to touch; therefore, the newborn examination should be done in an opportunistic manner from least invasive to most invasive to avoid arousing the baby from a quiet state to an agitated one. It is difficult to conduct a meaningful assessment for a crying infant.

Head-to-Toe Examination

Performing the head-to-toe examination is a systematic approach to assessing the newborn to ensure that all important systems are carefully inspected.

Vital Signs

A baseline set of vital signs need to be obtained while the infant is as calm and comfortable as possible.

Heart

Auscultate the heart and obtain the apical pulse while the newborn is at rest using an infant stethoscope for better accuracy.

- Point of maximal impulse should be noted in the left midclavicular line at the fifth intercostal space.
- A normal resting apical heart rate is between 120 and 160 bpm (may range from as low as 100 during sleep to as high as 180 bpm when crying; see Fig. 6–1).
- Murmurs are common during the first few hours as the foramen ovale is closing.

⭐ **BEST PRACTICES**

Begin your assessment by observing first, then auscultating without disturbing the infant, and palpating after finishing the rest of the examination. Percussion is rarely performed in newborns.

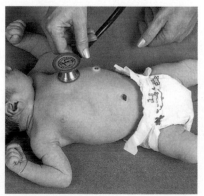

FIGURE 6-1: Auscultating the heart.

Respirations

- Assess respirations by observing the rise and fall of the neonate's chest for 1 full minute. Auscultate lung sounds using an appropriate-sized stethoscope.
- Normal rate is 30 to 60 bpm, shallow and irregular, with apneic periods of 5 to 10 seconds.
- During the first hour after birth, crackles may be auscultated while fluid is still being expelled or absorbed.
- Acrocyanosis is likely to be present and is not related to respiratory function. This is a normal circulatory finding that occurs during the transition to extrauterine life.

Temperature

- A normothermic infant should have an axillary temperature between 36.4°C and 37.2°C (97.5°F and 99.0°F).
- Place thermometer under the newborn's axilla and place his arm over his chest to keep the thermometer in place and provide comfort to the newborn (see Fig. 6–2).

Anthropometrics (Body Measurements)

- Birth weight is an important measure of health and well-being. Weights are most commonly recorded using the metric system (see Fig. 6–3). For converting pounds and ounces to kilograms and grams, refer to Table 6–1, a metric conversion table.
- Term infants (between 37 and 41 weeks) normally weigh 2500 to 4000 g (5 lb 8 oz to 8 lb 13 oz).

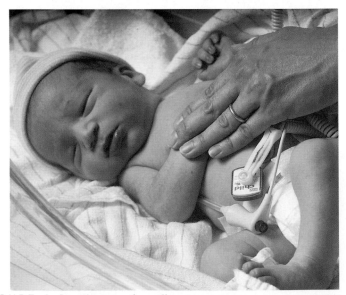

FIGURE 6-2: Obtaining the axillary temperature.

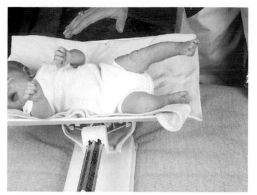

FIGURE 6-3: Weigh infant and record weight in grams.

Table 6–1 Metric Conversions

	POUNDS							
OUNCES	2	3	4	5	6	7	8	9
0	907	1361	1814	2268	2722	3175	3629	4082
1	936	1389	1843	2296	2750	3203	3657	4111
2	964	1417	1871	2325	2778	3232	3685	4139
3	992	1446	1899	2353	2807	3260	3714	4167
4	1021	1474	1928	2381	2835	3289	3742	4196
5	1049	1503	1956	2410	2863	3317	3770	4224
6	1077	1531	1984	2438	2892	3345	3799	4252
7	1106	1559	2013	2466	2920	3374	3827	4281
8	1134	1588	2041	2495	2948	3402	3856	4309
9	1162	1616	2070	2523	2977	3430	3884	4337
10	1191	1644	2098	2551	3005	3459	3912	4366
11	1219	1673	2126	2580	3033	3487	3941	4394
12	1247	1701	2155	2608	3062	3515	3969	4423
13	1276	1729	2183	2637	3090	3544	3997	4451
14	1304	1758	2211	2665	3118	3572	4026	4479
15	1332	1786	2240	2693	3147	3600	4054	4508

Note: 1 lb = 453.59237 g; 1 oz = 28.349523 g; 1000 g = 1 kg.

- Initial weight loss of 5% to 10% of birth weight occurs in the first 3 to 5 days of life.
- Length is the measurement from the top of the head to the heel, which is 46 to 56 cm (18–22 in.), on average (see Fig. 6–4).
- Head circumference is the distance around the infant's head. A general rule of thumb is normally about half the baby's body length plus 10 cm. Expected head circumference for a term infant is between 32 and 37 cm (12.5–14.5 in.; see Fig. 6–5).
- Abdominal circumference is the girth measured at one fingerbreadth above the umbilicus around the abdomen.
- Chest circumference is the distance around the chest, measured just below the nipple line. Most term infants have a chest girth averaging 32 cm (12.5 in.; see Fig. 6–6).
- Resting posture is an important part of the neurological examination and gestational age assessment. It is best to observe the infant's positioning and tone (flexion) before handling the infant.

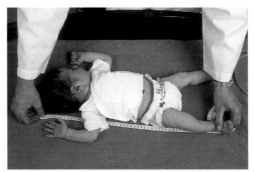

FIGURE 6-4: Measure the infant from the top of the head to the bottom of the heel.

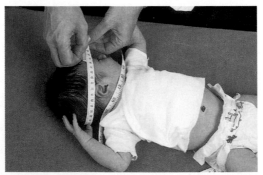

FIGURE 6-5: Measure the head circumference by placing the tape measure above ears and brow.

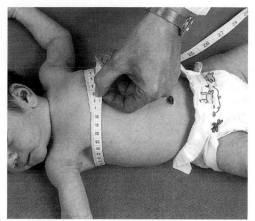

FIGURE 6-6: Chest circumference is measured just below the nipple line.

Skin
- Color should be pink and well perfused.
- **Acrocyanosis** is a bluish discoloration of the *hands and feet*, commonly present in the first 6 to 8 hours after birth until the cardiopulmonary changes have stabilized and fully oxygenated blood has circulated to the extremities. This condition occurs during the transition to extrauterine life.
- **Mottling** is a marbling of the skin. This occurs in newborns as a result of temperature instability. In the first few weeks of life in the term infant (or longer in preterm infants), mottling is also a sign of overstimulation to the autonomic nervous system. For example, mottling is a type of avoidance behavior in the newborn, which means he or she is trying shut out stimulation.
- **Harlequin sign** is a unilateral color change where one side of the newborn's body is ruddy, whereas the other side appears pale. The Harlequin sign is characterized by a transient color change, usually lasting 10 to 20 minutes. It is a vasomotor disturbance where the blood vessels on the reddish side dilate, whereas the vessels on the pale side constrict.
- **Jaundice** is yellowing of the skin that is most visible after blanching. Jaundice appears first and progresses in a head-to-toe pattern—most noticeable on the head and face, and lightens in the trunk area. Jaundice is often seen in the sclera as well. Physiological jaundice can simply be the result of mild dehydration or breastfeeding.

ALERT!

Jaundice also results from excess bilirubin occurring from excess bruising (by-product of red blood cell [RBC] breakdown), blood incompatibility, immature liver function, or disease involving the liver. Jaundice can be a sign of sepsis.

- Perfusion is best assessed by capillary refill, which should be 2 seconds or less in the newborn.
- Good skin turgor is assessed when the skin springs back readily when pinched. Moist mucous membranes also show the infant is well hydrated.
- Texture should be dry, soft, and smooth in term, well-hydrated infants. Postmature infants' (>41 weeks' gestation) skin will be dry with cracking of the feet and hands. If the infant is more than 42 weeks' gestation, the skin on the back and extremities will also be dry and peeling.
- **Lanugo** is a fine, downy hair covering most areas of the neonate's body. Lanugo is most abundant at 28 through 32 weeks' gestational age and gradually decreases with fetal maturity. The first place lanugo disappears is the face and lastly the extremities.
- **Milia** are exposed sebaceous glands that look like whiteheads on the infant's face, especially across the nose. They spontaneously disappear in the first month of life.
- **Vernix caseosa** is a waxy, cheesy substance covering the fetal and newborn skin. It protects the skin by keeping it from drying out with the astringent effect of amniotic fluid. Vernix gradually disappears the closer the infant is to term. Most post-term infants have little vernix, which can be found in the skin creases, particularly the neck and groin folds (see Fig. 6–7).
- **Erythema toxicum** is a rash often making its first appearance in the first few days of life. Also known as newborn rash, yellow or

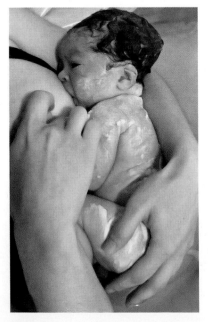

FIGURE 6-7: Vernix caseosa.

white papules erupt abruptly on a reddened base. The size of papules varies from 1 to 3 mm. Lesions do not appear on palmar surfaces. No treatment is recommended. Lotions often irritate an erythema toxicum rash. The cause of erythema toxicum is unknown, although thought to be related to an "awakened" immune system. A smear of aspirated cells shows eosinophils with no microbial source.

ALERT!

Café au lait spots can be the earliest manifestation of a serious neurocutaneous syndrome, called *neurofi-bromatosis*. These macules can also indicate other conditions, such as tuberous sclerosis, Fanconi anemia, Gaucher disease, or McCune–Albright syndrome. Newborns with six or more café au lait spots larger than 1 cm in diameter require further investigation.

- Birthmarks
  - **Café au lait spots** are hyperpigmented lesions (macules) that are typically irregularly shaped and light brown; hence, the name "coffee with milk." When small or few, the lesions are likely to be benign.
  - **Mongolian spot** is a bluish gray pigmentation in the lower back and buttocks region but also common to the shoulders or hips and legs. Although this flat birthmark resembles a bruise, it is actually a collection of melanocytes. It is common among dark-skinned infants. Most spots gradually fade over time (see Fig. 6–8).
  - **Port wine stain (nevus flammeus)** is a capillary hemangioma that extends deep into the epidermis. It is flat, sharply demarcated, and red to deep purple. It does not grow in size, nor does it fade on its own over time. This birthmark can be associated with a neurological disease called *Sturge–Weber* (involving the fifth cranial nerve) that involves seizures.
  - **Strawberry hemangioma (nevus vasculosus)** is a red, raised, capillary nevus. It usually increases in size for the first few months of life but gradually disappears by age 10 years. Any

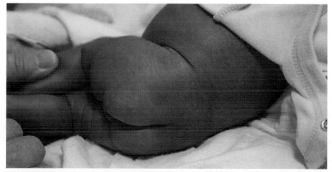

FIGURE 6-8: Mongolian spots.

capillary hemangioma occurring near the eye and interfering with vision should be removed.

- Moles, also known as *congenital pigmented nevi*, are not usually a cause for concern, even when hair is noted within the moles. Moles are worrisome if bleeding; very large; or prone to changes in shape, size, color, or texture. Giant congenital nevi are associated with melanoma, even within the first few years of life.

- **Stork bite**, also known as *telangiectatic nevus* or *nevus simplex*, is a pale pink or even reddish discoloration of the skin at the nape of the neck or lower occipital bone, eyelids, and above the nasal bridge. This type of discoloration is more prominent in fair-skinned, especially light-haired, infants. This is a superficial, vascular nevus that is more noticeable with crying. These typically fade by the second birthday, although they can persist into adulthood, particularly those at the nape of the neck.

Head

- Head size should be approximately one-fourth the total body length but should be consistent with other growth parameters (length and weight). Head size in the newborn is approximately the size of or slightly larger than the chest diameter. An excessively large head might indicate hydrocephalus (excessive cerebrospinal fluid within the brain cavity) or early intrauterine growth retardation. Conversely, if the head is undergrown, the infant may have microcephaly.

- **Fontanels** are cartilaginous "soft spots" at the juncture of the cranial sutures. The anterior fontanel, located at the top of the skull, is nearly diamond shaped, 3 to 4 cm long by 2 to 3 cm wide. It closes within 18 months of age. The posterior fontanel at the base of the skull is smaller and triangular. It is 0.5 by 1 cm and closes within 8 to 12 weeks after birth.

- **Sutures** are the cartilaginous growth plates of the skull that allow for brain growth without compression and pressure. The sutures should be palpable and unjoined. When sutures are overlapping, the head is said to be molded (cone shaped); this commonly occurs with head compression during the birthing process. The degree of molding varies with the length of labor. Within the first week of life, molding typically diminishes.

- **Cephalohematoma** is a collection of blood under the periosteum, caused by external pressure during labor and delivery. It feels boggy and edematous in areas, most commonly on the right side, although it can also be bilateral. The distinguishing feature of bilateral cephalohematomas is that they do not cross the suture line. This condition spontaneously resolves within 2 to 6 weeks, depending on its extent. Large cephalohematomas can lead to increased bilirubin levels (jaundice; see Fig. 6–9).

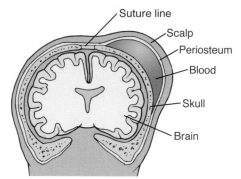

FIGURE 6-9: Cephalohematoma.

- **Caput succedaneum** is localized swelling of the soft tissues of the scalp, caused by pressure on the head during labor and delivery. It is a normal finding and tends to spontaneously resolve within a few hours or a couple days of life. The fluid may be fluctuant and cross the suture line (see Fig. 6–10).

Face
- Symmetry of the face is expected.
- Facial features should also be symmetric in size and shape (see Fig. 6–11).

Eyes
- Size and shape should be symmetric.
- Sclera is a white or bluish white color.
- Color of the iris is usually blue or gray for light-skinned and brown for darker-skinned newborns. Permanent eye color is not established until later.

ALERT!

Facial paralysis is evident when the mouth is asymmetric with crying—that is, one side moves readily, but the other side is immobile. This can occur from pressure on the facial nerve caused by pressure of the maternal pelvis or forceps during delivery. Facial paralysis usually resolves on its own within the first few days to weeks but can be permanent in some cases.

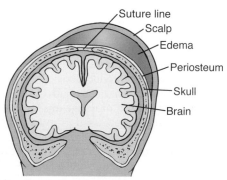

FIGURE 6-10: Caput succedaneum.

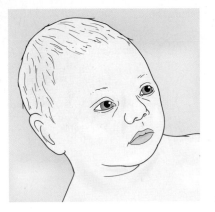

FIGURE 6-11: Symmetrical facial features.

- Lacrimal tear ducts are immature, and tear production does not usually begin until 2 months of age. "Tearless crying" is seen in the newborn. Later, these ducts may become clogged but often respond to manual pressure on the side of the nasal bridge.
- Blink reflex can be elicited by bright light, a tap on the glabella, or lightly brushing the eyelids.
- Pupils should be equal and reactive to light stimuli.
- The retina should be checked with the ophthalmoscope for a positive *red light reflex.* This is the orange–red color seen in light-skinned infants and paler for those with darker skin color.
- Opacified lens (cloudy white) should be referred for evaluation of congenital cataracts.
- Eyelids are edematous in the first few days of life because of pressure of the face through the vaginal canal during the birth process. Excess fluid is evident until normal diuresis begins.
- Subconjunctival hemorrhages appear in about 10% of newborns as a result of intravaginal pressure during birth. The ruptured, superficial blood cells within the sclera resolve within a few weeks and have no pathological significance to the eye or vision.
- Purulent drainage can indicate congenital eye infection, such as chlamydia, gonorrhea, or staphylococcus.
- Chemical conjunctivitis might occur with instillation of routine eye medication. Redness and drainage are far less common with ophthalmic ointment now used in routine newborn treatment.
- Transient strabismus, or crossed eyes, occurs in the first few months of life when the oculomotor muscles are not yet strengthened and coordinated.

- Visual acuity is reportedly best at 8 to 15 inches, which is the same distance from the infant at breast and mother's face. Newborns' vision allows for preference of human faces, due, in part, to the portion of the brain dedicated to allowing for facial recognition.

TIP

Color vision occurs after the first 3 months. This is the reason newborns tend to have the most attraction to contrasts of dark and light rather than brightly colored objects.

Nose

- Newborns are *obligate nose breathers* in the first few months of life.
- Passageways are narrow and can easily become obstructed with mucous or amniotic fluid.
- Sneezing is a reflex to aid in the clearing of nasal passageways. It can also be an avoidance behavior that occurs with overstimulation of the autonomic nervous system.
- Smell is demonstrated at birth, even in the preterm baby. This innate sense is protective in that newborns turn their heads toward milk, whether breast or formula. Newborns show preference to their own mother's milk as opposed to the milk of another woman. Shortly after birth, newborns react to noxious smells.

Mouth

- Lips and mucous membranes should be pink and moist; this indicates hydration and oxygenation status.
- Sucking blister occurs with latching.
- Saliva should not be excessive. Saliva that is draining out of the mouth can indicate swallowing dysfunction or a tracheoesophageal fistula (TEF).
- Taste buds developed before birth discriminate mother's milk and can differentiate sweet from bitter.
- Tongue should be freely movable, smooth, and pink. A protruding tongue can be a sign of trisomy 21 (Down syndrome).
- **Thrush (Candida albicans)** is white plaque that appears like milk curds on the tongue, gums, and inside of the throat and is not easily scraped off.
- **Epstein's pearls** are small, white cysts that contain keratin. They are located on the gum and feel firm to the touch. Epstein's pearls are benign and resolve spontaneously within the first weeks of life.
- **Precocious tooth** is premature eruption of a dentition through the gum, particularly in the region of the lower central incisors. These are nonfunctional for nutrition. They are almost always loose and should be removed to prevent aspiration.
- Shortened *frenulum* (tongue-tied) gives the appearance of a heart-shaped tip. Do not clip.
- The hard and soft *palate* should be intact. *Cleft* lip and/or palate should be referred for surgical intervention. There is a normal anatomical ridge in the roof of the mouth to accommodate the

nipple for a good seal that usually disappears in the first few months of life.

- Taste buds are developed before birth. Newborns demonstrate preference to their own mothers' milk and can discriminate between sweet and bitter.

Ears

- The cartilage of the pinna should be firm and well formed in the term infant. With prematurity, the cartilage is soft and pliable— the less recoil there is, the younger the gestational age is.
- Placement of the ears should be along an imaginary line from the inner canthus of the ear to the top of the pinna. Low-set or abnormally shaped ears may indicate a genetic anomaly.
- Pre-auricular cleft (dimple in front of the pinna) can be a sign of a renal disorder.
- Hearing can be assessed at birth by the infant's responsiveness to loud noise unaccompanied by vibration. A sleeping newborn should respond to sudden, noxious sound. Habituation to noise occurs when the sound level is constant. See Evidence for Practice Box 6–1 regarding the American Academy of Pediatrics' (AAP) recommendations on hearing screening.

QSEN Application

Continuous quality improvement includes knowledge such as:
- Describing strategies for learning about the outcomes of care in the setting in which one is engaged in clinical practice
- Explaining the importance of variation and measurement in assessing quality of care
- Recognizing that nursing and other health profession students are parts of systems of care and care processes that affect outcomes for patients and families

In this chapter, together with information about care of pregnant women and newborns, QSEN competencies assure delivery of the best nursing care.

http://qsen.org/competencies/pre-licensure-ksas/#patient-centered_care

EVIDENCE FOR PRACTICE BOX 6–1

The American Academy of Pediatrics (AAP) recommends universal screening as well as periodic hearing assessment for every child through adolescence. Every child with a risk factor for hearing loss (family history, intrauterine viral infection [e.g., cytomegalovirus]) should be screened at birth. Any parental concern about hearing loss should be taken seriously and followed up with screening. A failed hearing screening should always be confirmed by further, more definitive testing and appropriate referral, including audiology, genetics, and speech-language pathology. Hearing loss is the most common congenital condition in the United States. Failure to detect hearing loss in children may result in lifelong deficits in speech and language acquisition, personal-social adjustment, poor academic performance, and emotional difficulties.

Neck
- Appearance of the neck is short with skin folds. There should not be *webbing*, which is associated with trisomy 21 (Down syndrome).
- Head lag is a sign of overall tone. Head lag is associated with prematurity—the greater the lag, the more premature the infant.
- **Range of motion:** the neck should be freely mobile. Neck rigidity can indicate injury to the sternocleidomastoid muscle (congenital torticollis), which can occur during the birthing process.

Chest
- **Shape:** the chest should be somewhat barrel shaped—that is, cylindrical and symmetrical.
- Breast engorgement is normal in the first week or two of life while maternal hormone is circulating in the infant. Infrequently, breast discharge can occur from the newborn nipple—also related to maternal hormone. Nipple size is associated with gestational age; in the term infant, the firm nipple width is approximately 6 mm.
- Respirations are primarily diaphragmatic in newborns. For infants breathing normally, there are no sternal, subcostal, or supraclavicular retractions. The respiratory effort, or work of breathing, is comfortable.
- Clavicles should be smooth without separation, *crepitus*, bruising, or nodule.

Abdomen
- Shape is round and domed.
- Bowel sounds are usually heard by 1 or 2 hours of life. If abdominal sounds cannot be auscultated and the abdomen is distended, a more extensive assessment for obstruction or poor intestinal motility is needed.

ALERT!

Poor head control can indicate a neurological problem, genetic abnormality (e.g., trisomy 21), or overall illness (e.g., sepsis).

ALERT!

A pigeon-shaped chest, also known as *pectus carinatum*, which is an overgrowth of cartilage causing the sternum to protrude outward, is a sign of a genetic abnormality, such as Marfan syndrome, Noonan syndrome, or osteogenesis imperfecta.

TIP

Extra nipples, called *supernumerary nipples*, are rarely noted, found commonly in dark-skinned infants. They do not contain glandular tissue.

⭐ **BEST PRACTICES**

Closely examine large-for-gestational age (LGA) infants and those with shoulder dystocia for fractured clavicle during the birth process.

- Palpation to all four quadrants should reveal a soft, nontender abdomen with no distention. Loops of bowel should not normally be palpated.
- Liver can usually be felt 1 to 2 cm below the right costal margin in the healthy, term infant.
- Kidneys are most easily palpated in the first day of life by capturing the smooth, egg-like mass while pressing downward on the lateral, anterior abdomen and holding the posterior flank with the fingers of the other hand. Urine should be passed within 24 hours after birth.

- Spleen is rarely palpated in the lateral area of the right upper quadrant.
- Umbilical cord normally has two arteries and one vein. A thin, scrawny umbilical cord indicates poor nutrition to the fetus in utero. This can lead to an undergrown infant (small for gestational age [SGA]). The cord is odorless.
- Anus should be patent. Imperforate anus or rectal atresia is usually ruled out with the passage of meconium, although not always if meconium is below the obstruction.
- **Meconium**, a dark, sticky stool, is normally passed within the first 24 hours of life. The stools of breastfed infants are yellow and have a looser, seedy-type consistency.

Genitals
Male
- **Undescended testes**, also called *cryptorchidism*, is the failure of the testes to lower into the scrotal sac in the term infant. Testicular descent occurs during the third trimester of fetal development; therefore, the more premature the infant is, the higher the testes are.
- **Hypospadias** is when the urinary meatus is located on the ventral surface (underside) of the penile shaft. The urethral opening should be located at the tip of the penis. If it is located on the dorsal surface (top side), the condition is called *epispadias*.
- **Phimosis** is when the foreskin cannot be fully retracted.
- **Hydrocele** is a somewhat common condition where there is a collection of fluid surrounding the testes in the scrotal sac. It is benign and will reabsorb over time.
- Discoloration of the testes is suspicious for *testicular torsion*, which is twisting of the spermatic cord.
- **Crepitus** in the groin or scrotal sac indicates the presence of a hernia.

Female
- In girls, the *labia minora, majora,* and *clitoris* should be examined for size. Labia majora develop to cover the labia minora and clitoris when the infant is close to term gestation.

- Milky vaginal drainage is normal and is due to the effect of maternal hormone on the infant. Blood-tinged vaginal mucous, called *pseudomenses*, is caused by the hormones of pregnancy.
- Vaginal tag (also called *hymenal tag*) usually disappears in the first weeks of life.

Extremities

Upper

- Extra digits (fingers or toes) is called *polydactyly*. Fusing, or webbing, of the fingers or toes is *syndactyly*.
- Palmar creases should be inspected during the newborn examination. A single crease, called *simian line*, is characteristic in trisomy 21 (Down syndrome).
- The newborn should be assessed for full range of motion of the arms and shoulders. Partial or complete paralysis is a *brachial palsy*, which can occur when the arm is stretched over the head when delivering the shoulder over the maternal symphysis pubis with shoulder dystocia. Brachial plexus injury can also occur with breech presentation.
- **Erb–Duchenne paralysis** (Erb's palsy) involves injury to the brachial plexus where the arm lies limply to the side. The arm is extended with the forearm pronated. Because the newborn is unable to lift the affected arm, the Moro reflex cannot be demonstrated. Complete recovery usually occurs within a few months when the trauma is minimal.

> **WHY IS THE BRACHIAL PLEXUS IMPORTANT?**
>
> When injury to the brachial plexus is severe, recovery is not likely to occur without surgical intervention and nerve implant.

Lower

- Leg length should be equal and *gluteal creases* symmetrical.
- **Barlow and Ortolani's maneuver** indicate developmental hip dysplasia (previously known as congenital hip dislocation) in the newborn. This positional deformity can develop in utero, particularly with breech positioning. These screening tests assess hip stability by attempting to slide the hip in and out of the acetabulum, which produces a "clunk" movement. A positive finding might be treated with a Pavlik harness initially. However, casting or surgical intervention might be necessary at a later time, if severe.
- **Club foot**, also known as talipes equinovarus, is a positional deformity of the foot. In some cases, it is associated with other congenital deformities of the skeleton. Assessment involves straightening the foot to midline. Tight resistance indicates club foot. Without intervention, the calf muscle becomes underdeveloped. Club foot is commonly corrected with stretching and casting or surgery if unresponsive to more conservative measures.

Back
- Alignment should be straight and flexible without mass or lesion. Sacral curves will not be evident until the infant starts to sit.
- **Pilonidal dimple** is a cleft at the base of the sacrum. Generally, this is noncommunicating to the spinal cord and is benign.

Reflexes
- **Babinski**, also called the plantar reflex, is hyperextension of the toes when the sole is stroked from the heel upward to the ball of the foot. The fanning movement occurs from infancy to 2 years of age (see Fig. 6–12).
- **Galant reflex** is the incurvation of the trunk when stroking or tapping the spine in a prone position. The pelvis turns to the stimulated side in newborns to age 6 months.
- **Palmar grasp** reflex is elicited when an object, such as the mother's finger, is placed on the infant's palm. The infant's fingers will then close around it. When attempting to remove the object, the infant's grasp will become tighter. Sometimes this grip is firm enough the infant can almost be lifted off the surface of the bed (see Fig. 6–13).

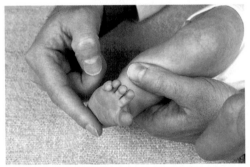

FIGURE 6-12: Babinski reflex.

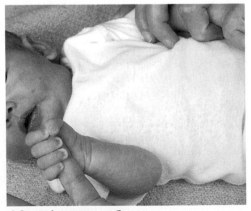

FIGURE 6-13: Palmar grasp reflex.

- **Moro** is a reflex that can be evoked by startling the infant. This can be done by striking the surface on which the infant is lying. The Moro reflex can also be tested by supporting the infant's head with your hand and then suddenly releasing it, allowing it to fall backward momentarily. Be sure to quickly support the head again without allowing it to hit the surface below it. The infant will respond by symmetrically extending the arms outward while the knees flex. Then slowly the arms return to the chest while the fingers spread to form a C. The Moro is the most sensitive assessment for an intact neurological system in a newborn. It disappears by about 3 to 4 months of age but can last as many as 6 months.

ALERT!

Absence of the Moro reflex bilaterally in an infant can suggest brain or spinal cord damage. Unilateral Moro reflex suggests the possibility of a fractured clavicle or, perhaps, a palsy of the brachial plexus. Presence of a Moro reflex in an older infant, child, or adult is abnormal and could indicate neurological injury or disease.

- **Rooting** reflex occurs when the side of the mouth or cheek is stroked or stimulated with the mother's breast, commercial nipple, or human touch. The infant turns toward that side and opens his or her lips and mouth to suck. Present at birth until 3 to 4 months, the rooting reflex is a primitive reflex to aid in latching on for nutritive feedings (see Fig. 6–14A and B).
- **Sucking** reflex occurs when anything is placed in the infant's mouth or touches the lips.
- **Startle** reflex, drawing the arms and legs inward after a loud noise, typically lasts until the infant is 6 months of age.
- **Stepping** reflex is stimulated when the sole of the foot touches a firm surface while the infant is supported in an upright position. This reflex can be somewhat tricky to elicit for the inexperienced person. Stepping typically disappears between 4 and 8 weeks.

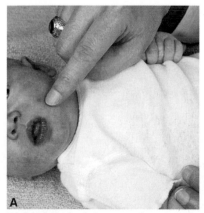
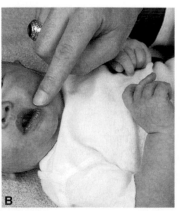

FIGURE 6-14: (A and B) Rooting reflex.

- **Tonic neck** reflex, the fencing position, is elicited when the newborn is positioned supine and his or her head is turned to the side. The extremities on the same side straighten, and those of the opposite side flex.
- **Blinking** reflex can be evoked by a light flash. The eyelids spontaneously close for a brief time.

Apgar Scoring

Apgar scoring was designed to rapidly evaluate a newborn's physical condition after delivery to determine any immediate need for support or emergency care (Table 6–2). A numeric score is assigned at 1 minute of age, again at 5 minutes after birth, and then 10 minutes later if the newborn shows any signs of possible distress or delayed transition to extrauterine life. You will assign a score on a scale of 0 to 2 for each of five key areas:

1. Appearance (skin color)
2. Activity and muscle tone
3. Pulse (heart rate)
4. Grimace response (also known as reflex irritability)
5. Respiration (breathing effort and rate)

Gestational Maturity Assessment

Physical and neuromuscular characteristics indicate gestational maturity. Muscle tone increases as the infant is closer to term; body hair decreases; breast buds increase in size; vernix disappears and skin gets drier; soles develop more creases; pinna are firmer; testes descend and scrotal rugae are more defined; labia majora become more prominent as infants advance gestational age.

The Ballard gestational age assessment tool is used to determine a neonate's gestational age between 20 and 44 weeks. A score is assigned to various parameters, and the total score corresponds to a maturity rating in weeks of gestation (see Fig. 6–15). The tool is divided into two

Table 6–2 Apgar Scoring

SIGN	SCORE		
	0	**1**	**2**
RESPIRATORY EFFORT	Absent	Slow, irregular	Good cry
HEART RATE	Absent	Slow, below 100 bpm	Above 100 bpm
MUSCLE TONE	Flaccid	Some flexion of extremities	Active motion
REFLEX ACTIVITY	None	Grimace	Vigorous cry
COLOR	Pale, blue	Body pink, blue extremities	Completely pink

Chapman L, Durham RF. *Maternal-Newborn Nursing: The Critical Components of Nursing Care.* Philadelphia, PA: FA Davis Company; 2009.

Neuromuscular Maturity

	−1	0	1	2	3	4	5
Posture							
Square Window (Wrist)	−90°	90°	60°	45°	30°	0°	
Arm Recoil		180°	140°-180°	110°-140°	90°-110°	<90°	
Popliteal Angle	180°	160°	140°	120°	100°	90°	<90°
Scarf Sign							
Heel To Ear							

Physical Maturity

	−1	0	1	2	3	4	5
Skin	sticky, friable, transparent	gelatinous, red, translucent	smooth pink, visible veins	superficial peeling or rash, few veins	cracking, pale areas, rare veins	parchment, deep cracking, no vessels	leathery, cracked, wrinkled
Lanugo	none	sparse	abundant	thinning	bald areas	mostly bald	
Plantar Surface	heel-toe 40–50 mm:-1 <40 mm:-2	>50 mm no crease	faint red marks	anterior transverse crease only	creases ant. 2/3	creases over entire sole	
Breast	imperceptible	barely perceptible	flat areola no bud	stippled areola 1–2 mm bud	raised areola 3–4 mm bud	full areola 5–10 mm bud	
Eye/ear	lids fused loosely:-1 tightly:-2	lids open, pinna flat, stays folded	sl. curved pinna; soft; slow recoil	well-curved pinna; soft but ready recoil	formed and firm, instant recoil	thick cartilage, ear stiff	
Genitals (Male)	scrotum flat, smooth	scrotum empty, faint rugae	testes in upper canal, rare rugae	testes descending, few rugae	testes down, good rugae	testes pendulous, deep rugae	
Genitals (Female)	clitoris prominent, labia flat	prominent clitoris, small labia minora	prominent clitoris, enlarging minora	majora and minora equally prominent	majora large, minora small	majora cover clitoris and minora	

Maturity Rating

Score	Weeks
−10	20
−5	22
0	24
5	26
10	28
15	30
20	32
25	34
30	36
35	38
40	40
45	42
50	44

FIGURE 6-15: Ballard gestational age assessment tool.

sections: the *Neuromuscular Maturity Assessment* and the *Physical Maturity Assessment.*

- Physical maturity
  - **Skin:** maturation of the skin, presence of vernix caseosa, thickness, cracking, and presence of veins
  - **Lanugo:** location and abundance of fine, downy hair
  - **Plantar surface:** smoothness or creasing on the surface of the sole
  - **Breast:** size of areolar bud
  - **Eye/ear:** eyelids fused or not; stiffness of the pinna (ear)
  - **Genitals (male):** smoothness of the scrotal sac (rugae) and descent of testicles
  - **Genitals (female):** prominence of the labia and clitoris
- Neuromuscular maturity
  - **Posture:** preferred body position while at rest
  - **Square window:** wrist flexibility or resistance when the examiner applies gentle pressure against the dorsum of the hand

toward the wrist. The extent of resistance is a measure of neuromuscular maturity.

- **Arm recoil:** tone of the flexors (arm) when the arms are briefly extended and released. The angle the arms spring back is an indication of neuromuscular maturity.
- **Popliteal angle:** test of resistance when the lower extremity is extended when the infant is in supine position. The knee is flexed and the thigh is gently supported to the abdomen.
- **Scarf sign:** tests flexor tone at the shoulder when the examiner supports the infant's lower extremity across the upper chest.
- **Heel-to-ear:** maneuver to assess passive flexor tone at the hip area. The examiner supports the thigh and grasps the foot, pulling it toward the ear.

WHY IS TEMPERATURE REGULATION IMPORTANT?

Temperature regulation is essential for weight gain, feeding, respiratory function, and overall normal physiological function.

Newborn Thermoregulation

Thermoregulation is the ability of the newborn to balance heat production and heat loss for stabilizing his or her own internal body temperature. Remember that a normothermic infant should have an axillary temperature between 36.4°C and 37.2°C (97.5°F and 99.0°F).

- The newborn has special requirements for temperature maintenance:
- Infants have a larger body surface area relative to body weight.
- Adipose tissue and subcutaneous fat are less in newborns.
- Newborn infants have underdeveloped sweating and shivering mechanisms.
- Blood vessels are relatively close to the skin surface, thus contributing to heat loss.
- Increased metabolic processes (nonshivering thermogenesis) produce heat beyond basal production.
- Heat production consumes a large number of calories.

QSEN Application

Continuous quality improvement includes skills such as:
- Using tools (such as flow charts, cause–effect diagrams) to make processes of care explicit
- Using quality measures to understand performance
- Using tools (such as control charts and run charts) that are helpful for understanding variation
- Identifying gaps between local and best practice

In this chapter, together with information about care of pregnant women and newborns, QSEN competencies assure delivery of the best nursing care.

http://qsen.org/competencies/pre-licensure-ksas/#patient-centered_care

- All infants are at risk for difficulty maintaining temperature, especially:
  - Term newborns, specifically during the first 12 hours of life
  - Near-term infants (34–37 weeks' gestation)
  - Preterm infants
  - SGA infants
  - Environmental causes (e.g., overheating)
  - Infection or maternal fever during labor
  - Dehydration
  - Medication effects and drug withdrawal
  - Congenital hypothyroidism
  - Infants with hypoglycemia
  - Infants with perinatal acidosis
  - Fetal distress, shown by fetal decelerations, low cord pH, or low Apgar score at 5 minutes after birth
  - Infants with endocrine, neurological, or cardiorespiratory disorder
  - Infants with congenital anomalies
- Interventions to maintain thermoregulation
  - Heat can be lost or gained by four mechanisms.
    1. Evaporation is loss of heat as surface moisture is converted to a vapor.
    2. Conduction is heat loss resulting from direct contact with a cooler surface.
    3. Convection is loss of heat from the flow of heat from the body's surface to cooler ambient air.
    4. Radiation is heat loss from the body's surface to a cooler solid that is close to the infant but not touching the infant.

> **TIP**
>
> Prewarm the radiant warmer, isolette, or blankets after birth to prevent the baby from getting cold. Pad the surface of a scale before weighing and warm your stethoscope before placing it on the newborn's chest.

⭐ **BEST PRACTICES**

To reduce evaporative heat loss, dry the newborn thoroughly with a warm, dry blanket. Bathe only one area of the baby at a time, drying thoroughly as you go.

⭐ **BEST PRACTICES**

To prevent convective heat loss, keep newborns away from air-conditioning vents. Swaddle the infant in a blanket.

Newborn Medications: Immunizations and Prophylactic

The following are common medications given to newborns before
discharge.

1. Administer 0.5% erythromycin eye ointment within an hour
   of birth to prevent transmittal of gonococcal infection from the
   mother to the newborn.
2. Inject vitamin K (phytonadione) within an hour of birth. Newborns do not have vitamin K at birth; the vitamin is necessary
   to form blood clots and prevent hemorrhage.
3. Administer hepatitis B vaccine and hepatitis B Ig within
   12 hours if the maternal hepatitis B surface antigen status is
   positive or unknown. If the maternal hepatitis B surface antigen is negative, hepatitis B Ig is not necessary. However,
   the first shot of the hepatitis B vaccine series may be offered
   before discharge. The second dose is recommended 1 to
   2 months after the first, and the third shot is given 6 months
   after the first at the pediatrician's office. A mother who is negative for hepatitis B may opt to wait and receive the hepatitis
   B vaccine series at her pediatrician's office instead of the
   hospital/birth center.

Prior to administration, the nurse needs to discuss with the infant's
parents the risks and benefits of these medications and immunizations.
The nurse may need to obtain signatures showing consent.

Blood Glucose Monitoring

The stress of delivery causes conversion of fats and glycogen to glucose
for energy. The goal for newborn blood sugar management is a glucose
level of 40 mg/dL on the first day and more than 40 to 50 mg/dL thereafter. Obtain baseline glucose at 30 minutes to 1 hour of age if infant appears to show signs of hypoglycemia and/or as hospital protocol and/or
as prescribed orders (see Table 6–3).

Screening Tests

- State-mandated metabolic screening testing (varies from state to
  state) should be completed before discharge. Newborn screening
  is best done as close as possible to the time of discharge from the
  hospital after the infant has received at least 24 hours of feeding.

Table 6–3 Procedure Highlight: Newborn Heel Stick

The heel stick is the most common way that blood is drawn from a neonate because of the rich capillary bed in the heel. The heel stick is typically used for newborn screening and determining blood glucose levels, bilirubin levels, and a complete blood count (see Fig. 6-16).

Materials:	1. Warm, moist cloth or heel-warming device 2. Alcohol wipes 3. Gauze 4. Gloves 5. Sterile 2-mm lancet 6. Blood collection tube 7. Newborn screening filter paper
Procedure:	1. Confirm the order for the blood draw and identify the infant. 2. Discuss with the neonate's parents the purpose of the blood draw and the procedure involved. 3. Swaddle the infant to provide him or her comfort, but leave the foot out of the blanket for access for the blood draw. 4. Gather your supplies. 5. Wash your hands well and put on clean gloves. 6. Apply a warm, moist cloth or heel-warming device for 3 minutes. This increases blood flow to the site. 7. Cleanse the neonate's heel with 70% isopropyl alcohol. 8. Allow the heel to air-dry. 9. Using a 2-mm lancet, perform the puncture on the plantar surface of the neonate's heel (see Fig. 6–16), making sure to avoid the bottom of the heel where the calcaneus, the heel bone, is closest to the surface. If possible, also avoid a recently punctured area. The National Committee for Clinical Laboratory Standards (NCCLS) instructs puncturing no deeper than 2.0 mm. The NCCLS also warns that puncturing deeper than 2.0 mm may cause bone damage. 10. Wipe off first drop of blood because this contains tissue fluids and may dilute the sample. 11. Apply gentle pressure with thumb on the neonate's heel and wait for droplet of blood. 12. If performing the newborn screening, gently touch the droplet of blood with the printed side of the newborn screen filter paper. Allow for the blood to soak through and fill the preprinted circle evenly. Repeat this step for the rest of the circles. Avoid having the actual filter paper touch the infant. 13. If performing the heel stick to draw blood for tests such as a bilirubin level or a complete blood count, bring the blood collection tube to the droplet of blood. Collect sufficient amount of blood in the tube as per the institution's laboratory protocol. 14. If performing the heel stick to draw blood for a glucose level, bring the glucometer to the heel and gently touch the test strip to the droplet of blood. Make note of the glucose level reading and record in the infant's chart. 15. Dispose of all the materials in proper receptacles and the sharps in biohazard containers. 16. Apply gentle pressure with a sterile gauze to the puncture site to stop the bleeding. 17. Reswaddle the infant and provide comfort measures such as a pacifier, if being used.

Continued

Table 6–3 **Procedure Highlight: Newborn Heel Stick—cont'd**

18. Document the procedure on the infant's chart, together with the type of test; puncture site location; neonatal pain response before, during, and after the procedure; and comfort measures performed.

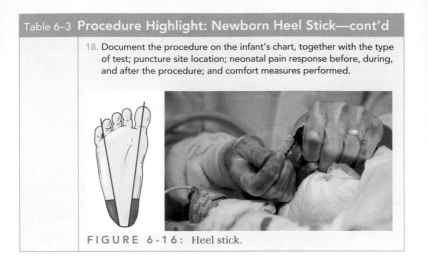

FIGURE 6-16: Heel stick.

If testing is obtained at less than 24 hours of age, repeat testing is needed before 3 weeks of age.

- Phenylketonuria is screened in all states, because when undetected, it leads to mental retardation. The condition can be prevented if it is diagnosed before symptoms develop, and the child is treated with a special diet.
- Screening is also done for hypothyroidism, which can also lead to mental retardation if not detected early and treated with supplemental thyroid hormone.
- Some states mandate testing for galactosemia and sickle cell anemia.
- Other common screening tests include cystic fibrosis, maple syrup urine disease, homocystinuria, HIV infection, and other organic or inborn errors of metabolism.
- Screening for retinopathy of prematurity per AAP guidelines for high-risk infants should be performed (or arranged as outpatient) with adequate follow-up for neonatal patients with active disease.
- Hearing screening should be completed before discharge with follow-up plans for infants requiring a full audiology assessment. If an infant is discharged without an initial screening, arrangements should be made for timely assessment as an outpatient.

Patient Education

A key role of the nurse caring for the mother and her newborn is patient education. It is crucial for the nurse to educate the mother and the family on caring for the newborn and to give anticipatory guidance as to what to expect when they bring the baby home.

Feeding
Please refer to "Infant Feeding" in Chapter Four "Postpartum."

Circumcision

Circumcision is the surgical removal of the foreskin of the penis. It is an elective procedure, typically based on cultural, religious, and personal factors. Contraindications to circumcision include abnormalities of the penis or the positioning of the urethra (epispadias, hypospadias), or a sickly infant. Post-procedure care for circumcision includes:

- Monitoring for bleeding
  - Assessing and recording first void after circumcision
  - Providing analgesia to the infant, as per pediatrician orders

Swaddling

Swaddling not only provides warmth to the newborn whose temperature-regulating system is immature at birth, but also provides security to the infant who has been in a flexed position in a tight environment in utero. The technique will help to keep newborns from awakening from their own startle reflex. Swaddling is a good way to calm infants and reduce extraneous stimulation in their surroundings. By 1 month of age, most infants will not want to be bundled up (see Table 6–4).

When providing anticipatory guidance to parents learning to care for their newborns, explain what developmental milestones they can expect and when it is appropriate to call a primary care provider. See Table 6–5.

OFFERING SUPPORT

Educate parent on newborn circumcision. Explain the procedure: *A circumcision is a surgical procedure to remove the foreskin of the penis.*

- Calm fears: The pediatrician will provide local anesthesia (confirm with agency protocols) before the procedure.
- With each diaper change: Apply petroleum jelly to the penis to prevent irritation of the site. Cleanse site to prevent infection. Monitor the site for bleeding.
- The baby may be fussy after the circumcision. Advise his mother to calm him by breastfeeding, providing a pacifier to suck on, swaddling, or rocking him gently.
- A film of yellowish material may form over the glans by the second day after circumcision. This is normal granulation tissue and should not be removed.
- Wait to immerse baby in water for tub bath until after the circumcision is completely healed.

Newborn Complications and Problems

Perinatal Acidosis (Asphyxia)

Perinatal acidosis (asphyxia) is the deprivation of oxygen to a neonate during the process of birth resulting in fetal hypoxia that may lead to organ damage.

Risk Factors

- Prematurity, low birth weight
- Sepsis
- SGA
- Meconium aspiration syndrome
- Persistent fetal circulation

Table 6–4 **Procedure Highlight: How to Swaddle a Newborn**

1. Lay a blanket on a flat surface and fold down the top corner (about 6 inches).
2. Place infant on his or her back with his or her head on the fold.

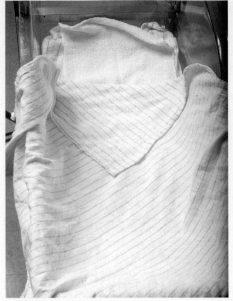

Place the blanket in the crib and fold the top corner.

3. Pull the left corner across the infant's body; then tuck the leading edge under his or her back on the opposite side.

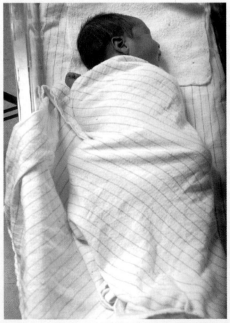

Place the infant on top of the blanket, fold the left corner over, and tuck under the infant's right arm.

Table 6–4 **Procedure Highlight: How to Swaddle a Newborn—cont'd**

4. Pull the bottom corner up under the infant's chin.

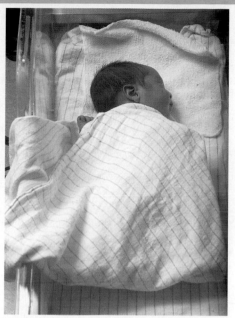

Fold the bottom of the blanket and tuck as shown.

5. Bring the right corner over the infant's body and tuck it under the back on that side. If the infant prefers to have his or her arms free, you can swaddle him or her under the arms. This gives the infant access to his or her hands and fingers.

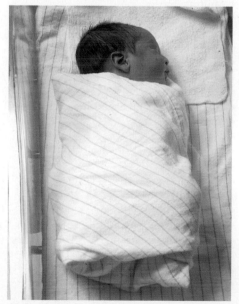

Fold the right corner of the blanket over and tuck as shown.

- Infant born to a substance-abusing mother
- Anemia
- Birth trauma
- Eclampsia
- Advanced maternal age
- Maternal infection, chorioamnionitis
- Cord prolapsed
- Placental abruption
- Multiple births

Clinical Manifestations
- Metabolic acidosis (low pH, excess HCO_3)
- Temperature instability
- Fluctuating or decreased oxygen saturation
- Respiratory distress
- Irritability or lethargy
- Increased or decreased tone
- Seizure
- Poor feeding
- Mottling
- Hypotonia
- Hyperglycemia

Diagnostic Tests
- Cord pH, arterial blood gases (ABG)
- Electroencephalogram
- Computed tomography (CT) scan of the head, magnetic resonance imaging

Nursing Interventions
- During labor
  - Perform prenatal monitoring to detect fetal distress and asphyxia before birth.
  - Monitor fetal heart rate.

- Monitor for changes in fetal movement.
- Monitor appearance of amniotic fluid for meconium, which suggests fetal distress. Perform sterile vaginal examination to detect *prolapsed* cord.
- During delivery
  - Determine Apgar score immediately upon delivery. A score between 7 and 10 is considered normal; scores less than 7 indicate the need for intervention.
  - Assess cord/ABG to determine presence of acidemia related to tissue hypoxia.
  - Monitor vital signs.
  - Monitor color to detect signs of hypoxia or compromised oxygenation (pallor, cyanosis).
  - Monitor muscle tone (limp, depressed, or absent reflexes).
  - Obtain Apgar scores at 1 and 5 minutes after birth to determine the need for resuscitation or to monitor effectiveness of measures to increase and/or maintain oxygenation.
  - Monitor glucose level and observe for signs of hypoglycemia (e.g., tremors, jitteriness, lethargy, loss of muscle tone, weak cry).
  - Suction the newborn's mouth and nose while still on the perineum if meconium is present in the amniotic fluid to prevent aspiration of meconium.
  - Maintain environmental temperatures within the neutral thermal range to minimize oxygen consumption and nutrient use by the newborn because of increased metabolic rate.
  - Administer oxygen to neonate as ordered to ensure adequate delivery of oxygen to prevent tissue hypoxia.
  - Maintain a patent airway to ensure delivery of oxygen to the lungs by positioning infant for maximum respirations and suctioning as needed.

ALERT!

An infant with hypoxia will have decreased temperature, decreased heart rate (bradycardia), decreased blood pressure (hypotension), and altered respirations (apnea, tachypnea, retractions, grunting, and nasal flaring).

WHY IS MECONIUM IMPORTANT?

Meconium is the newborn's first several stools. It is a viscous substance usually described as having a "tarry" appearance. If passed while in utero, it can block the infant's airway and compromise breathing after delivery.

Cold Stress
Risk Factors
- Prematurity, low birth weight
- Sepsis
- Illness
- SGA

Clinical Manifestations
- Temperature instability
- Fluctuating oxygen saturation
- Metabolic acidosis
- Increased white blood cells
- Mottling
- Hypotonia
- Hyperglycemia

Diagnostic Tests
- Temperature
- Assessment
  - Perform a comprehensive, physical assessment on admission to the newborn or mother–baby unit. This provides a baseline and identifies potential problems that can lead to hypothermia or hyperthermia.
  - Assess the axillary temperature according to the agency's protocol. This is commonly done every 30 to 60 minutes until stable and then for the next 2 hours; then every 8 hours, or more frequently depending on the infant's temperature.

WHY IS NEWBORN TEMPERATURE MONITORING IMPORTANT?

The newborn's temperature is normally unstable initially, requiring frequent monitoring to prevent cold stress or hyperthermia. It should stabilize by the 12th hour after birth.

- Check the newborn's temperature after the first bath. The newborn may have lost heat by radiation, evaporation, conduction, and convection and may require rewarming.
- Assess the heart rate and respiratory rate. Temperature fluctuations cause an increase in the respiratory rate, an increased metabolism of brown fat, and an elevated heart rate.
- Assess mother's and family's knowledge and ability to help maintain a normal temperature. The newborn may be staying in the mother's room and can become exposed to cool temperatures if precautions are not taken.

Nursing Activities to Prevent Cold Stress
- Use a radiant warmer immediately after birth until the newborn's temperature is stable.
- Consider using a radiant warmer when performing procedures (e.g., bathing, assessment, circumcision), as needed.
- Place infant away from air drafts to prevent heat loss by convection.
- Monitor ambient room temperature in the mother's room to avoid convective heat loss.

⭐ **BEST PRACTICES**

When the newborn is under a radiant warmer, a skin probe constantly monitors the temperature, but an axillary temperature should still be taken to ensure accuracy of the equipment and proper contact with the skin probe.

- Preheat the radiant warmer and the linens when preparing for the birth of the baby. This helps to prevent heat loss through conduction.
- At birth, dry the newborn, and place the newborn on mother's chest and cover both with a warm blanket to prevent heat loss through evaporation. Skin-to-skin contact with mother provides heat. The warm blanket adds heat and reduces heat loss by convection and evaporation.
- Use a hat immediately after birth. The head is a large surface area for the newborn, with blood vessels close to the surface; covering it helps prevent heat loss.
- Wrap the newborn in two blankets when moving from the radiant warmer to the open crib to trap body heat in the blankets.
- Postpone the newborn's first bath until temperature is stable and at least 36.5°C (97.7°F); bathe under radiant warmer to prevent heat loss by evaporation, radiation, convection, and conduction. Newborns have an immature neurological system, and the environmental factors can increase heat loss.
- Teach the mother and family to change the diaper, clothing, and linens when wet to prevent heat loss by evaporation.
- Teach the mother and family the importance of keeping the newborn warm by skin-to-skin contact and blankets or clothing, stocking hat, and double-wrapped blankets during this initial period.

> **WHY IS MONITORING FOR INFECTION IMPORTANT?**
>
> Newborns are highly susceptible to infection because of their poor response to pathogenic agents, little or no inflammatory reaction at the portal of entry, and inability to synthesize their own antibodies until about 2 months of age.

Sepsis

Infection is a significant contributor to mortality and morbidity in the neonate during the first month of life.

> **ALERT!**
>
> High-risk infants have a four-fold greater incidence of infection and septicemia (presence of bacteria in the bloodstream) than healthy, term newborns.

Risk Factors
- Prematurity
- Rupture of membranes
- Maternal infection, such as chorioamnionitis
- Bacterial colonization with group B streptococcus on the cervix

Clinical Manifestations

There is a variety of specific and nonspecific signs and symptoms, depending on the type of infection. These include, but are not limited to, temperature instability, lethargy, seizures, hypotonia, feeding intolerance, irritability, hypoglycemia, hyperglycemia, respiratory distress, hypotension, hypertension, tachycardia, pallor, rash, and petechiae.

Diagnostic Tests

- Complete blood cell count (CBC) with differential to detect anemia, leukocytosis, or leukopenia
- X-rays to detect chest and abdominal sources of infection
- Cultures (e.g., blood, urine, tracheal aspirates, wound, cerebrospinal fluid) to identify location and type of infection

Medical Management

- Antibiotic therapy
- Respiratory support
- Fluid and electrolyte management
- Nutritional support
- Immunotherapy
- Blood pressure maintenance
- Hematological supportive therapy
- Pain control

Key Nursing Activities

- Maintain medical and surgical asepsis.
- Monitor for sepsis.
- Maintain hydration.
- Monitor and support nutritional status.
- Administer antibiotics and monitor for therapeutic and adverse effects.

Hypoglycemia

Hypoglycemia is a condition resulting from blood glucose levels less than 40 mg/dL in term infants.

Risk Factors

- Asphyxia
- Cold stress
- Increased work of breathing
- Sepsis
- Premature or SGA
- Infants of mothers with diabetes or gestational diabetics
- LGA

Clinical Manifestations

There is a variety of specific and nonspecific signs of hypoglycemia, depending on blood glucose level and whether the infant is term or preterm. These include, but are not limited to, cyanosis, pallor, sweating, tachypnea, retractions, low oxygen saturation, tremors, jitters, twitches, seizures, lethargy, and poor feeding.

Medical Management

- Glucose supplementation, enteral or parenteral
- Glucose bolus as per orders

Key Nursing Activities

- Monitor blood glucose levels to detect hypoglycemia, which is associated with blood glucose levels less than 40 mg/dL in term infants. Infants exposed to high maternal glucose levels experience

development of pancreatic hyperplasia
and resultant hyperinsulinemia. When
the umbilical cord is severed, the infant is
no longer exposed to the high maternal
glucose levels. This, in combination with
the infant's hyperinsulinemia, produces a
rapid decrease in blood glucose levels.

> **WHY IS COLD STRESS IMPORTANT?**
>
> Cold stress increases glucose utilization and intensifies hypoglycemia.

- Monitor the infant's core temperature.
- Feed neonate as early as possible or ad-
  minister glucose/glucagon as needed. Glucagon produces rapid increases in serum glucose levels and prevents complications from
  hypoglycemia.

Jaundice

Physiological jaundice does not appear until the second or third day of
life, when serum bilirubin (a by-product of RBC catabolism) levels reach
5 to 7 mg/dL. No treatment is required unless bilirubin levels increase
higher or faster than normal.

Pathological jaundice occurs when total bilirubin levels increase by
more than 5 mg/dL per day, exceed 12 mg/dL in a full-term infant or
10 to 14 mg/dL in preterm infants, and produce visible jaundice within
the first 24 hours following birth. Unconjugated bilirubin is highly toxic
to neurons; therefore, the infant with severe hyperbilirubinemia is at
increased risk for *kernicterus* (bilirubin encephalopathy), which is associated with total bilirubin levels greater than 20 mg/dL in normal term
infants.

Risk Factors

Hemolytic disease of the newborn may be caused by maternal/fetal Rh
or ABO incompatibility, infection, glucuronyl transferase deficiency,
polycythemia, biliary atresia, liver impairment, hypoglycemia, and
preterm birth.

Clinical Manifestations

There is a variety of specific and nonspecific signs and symptoms, depending on the type of infection. These include, but are not limited to,
increased total and direct serum bilirubin levels, jaundice, yellow
(icteric) sclera, lethargy, and poor feeding.

Diagnostic Tests

- Determine blood type and Rh status of infant in the event that an
  exchange transfusion is necessary
- Direct Coombs test to establish diagnosis of hemolytic disease
  in newborn; positive result indicates infant's RBCs have been
  sensitized (coated with antibodies)
- Indirect Coombs test measures the amount of Rh-positive antibodies
  in the mother's blood
- Total and direct bilirubin to establish diagnosis of hyperbilirubinemia: total serum bilirubin levels greater than 12 to 13 mg/dL,
  increase in total bilirubin levels more than 5 mg/dL per day, and

direct bilirubin more than 1.5 to 2 mg/dL establish the diagnosis of hyperbilirubinemia; serum bilirubin levels alone do not predict the risk for brain injury caused by kernicterus, although it is associated with levels greater than 20 mg/dL in normal term infants

- CBC with differential to detect hemolysis, anemia (Hb < 14 g/dL), or polycythemia (Hct > 65%); Hct less than 40% (cord blood) indicates severe hemolysis
- Total serum protein to detect reduced binding capacity (< 3.0 g/dL)
- Serum glucose to detect hypoglycemia (< 40 mg/dL)
- Carbon dioxide (CO_2) combining power—to detect hemolysis, which is consistent with decreased CO_2 combining power
- Kleihauer–Betke test to detect fetal erythrocytes in maternal blood
- Increased reticulocyte count is consistent with increased hemolysis

Medical Management

- Early feeding or frequent breastfeeding to prevent enterohepatic circulation
- Adequate hydration
- Phototherapy
- Phenobarbital to enhance conjugation and excretion of bilirubin
- Administration of heme-oxygenase inhibitors and albumin
- Exchange transfusion for kernicterus (rarely used)
- Correction of underlying problems (sepsis, acidosis, etc.)

Key Nursing Activities

- Be aware of maternal and fetal blood types. Review maternal record for presence of antibody, indicating an immune response by the newborn. ABO and Rh incompatibility may result in jaundice.
- Review newborn history and assess for pyloric stenosis, urinary tract infection, sepsis, bacterial or viral meningitis, TORCH infection, cephalohematoma, asphyxia, hypothermia, and hypoglycemia. These conditions predispose the infant to hyperbilirubinemia.
- Observe for jaundice, especially in the sclera and mucous membranes. Jaundice occurs first in the head and progresses gradually to the abdomen and extremities. A general rule to estimate bilirubin level in the first week of life may be figured by using the rule of 5's, whereby jaundice of the sclera, buccal membranes, and face is approximately a bilirubin level of 5 mg/dL. Jaundice visible to the chest at the nipple line is grossly equal to 10 mg/dL. Yellow skin to the level of the umbilicus usually means a bilirubin level of 15 mg/dL. Jaundice extending past the groin indicates a dangerously high bilirubin level of ≥18 to 20 mg/dL. This assessment should be reported to a primary care provider for intervention.

- Assess for excessive bruising. The by-product of RBC breakdown occurring with bruising is a form of bilirubin. Infants with extensive scalp or skin bruising related to traumatic birth process are likely to have higher bilirubin levels.
- Assess the infant's skin color in daylight. Artificial lighting can distort the actual skin color.
- Differentiate between physiological and pathological jaundice. In a normal newborn, jaundice first appears after 24 hours and disappears by the end of the seventh day. If jaundice appears during the first 24 hours of life or persists beyond 7 days, it usually is a sign of a pathological process.
- Review birth records for bilirubin levels. A serum level of unconjugated bilirubin of 2 mg/dL is normal in cord blood. In physiological jaundice, the level will peak at greater than 6 mg/dL by 72 hours of age. No toxicity occurs at these levels.
- Assess if the newborn voided or had a stool since birth. Bilirubin is eliminated in feces and urine.
- Natural sunlight through a window can help to reduce bilirubin level through the skin. Care must be given to avoid overheating the infant.
- Feed infant within the first hour of birth. Feeding helps to prevent hyperbilirubinemia by promoting hydration and stimulating intestinal activity and passage of meconium, helping to keep the serum bilirubin level low (bilirubin is eliminated in the urine and feces).
- Provide thermoneutral environment; prevent cold stress. Cold stress can result in acidosis, which weakens the ability of albumin to bind bilirubin and increases the level of free bilirubin.
- Monitor effectiveness of phototherapy.
- Teach parents how to assess and report jaundice.

Infant of a Diabetic Mother

- The infant of a diabetic mother (IDM) is at high risk for a number of conditions, but especially hypoglycemia. Most infants of diabetic mothers are LGA, but women with poorly controlled diabetes with vascular compromise may give birth to infants who are SGA. The chronic exposure of the fetus to high maternal glucose levels causes a production of higher than normal fetal insulin. Infants of diabetic mothers often have immature lungs.
- After birth, infants of diabetic mothers become hypoglycemic because fetal insulin levels do not adjust rapidly to the loss of maternal glucose supply.
- High maternal glucose and fetal insulin levels may result in congenital malformations that are otherwise rarely seen: sacral agenesis and anencephaly. Infants of diabetic mothers are at increased risk for congenital heart defects.
- Macrosomia places the infant at risk for preterm birth and traumatic delivery.

Risk Factors
- Previous history of infant weighing more than 9 lbs., unexplained stillbirth or spontaneous abortion, polyhydramnios, recurrent maternal candida vaginitis, maternal pregnancy-induced hypertension
- Enlarged placenta and umbilical cord, LGA infant with doughy skin and organomegaly, SGA infant, hypoglycemia, hypocalcemia, hypomagnesemia, polycythemia, hyperbilirubinemia, respiratory distress (tachypnea, cyanosis, retractions, grunting, nasal flaring)

Diagnostic Tests
- Serum glucose
- CBC
- Total bilirubin
- Serum electrolytes
- Ultrasound
- Prenatal lecithin-to-sphingomyelin ratio to assess fetal lung maturity; insulin interferes with lecithin synthesis that is needed for fetal lung maturation

Clinical Manifestations
- Macrosomia
- Hypoglycemia (jittery, sweating if term or older)
- Jaundice
- Congenital heart defect, murmur

Medical Management
- Correct hypoglycemia.
- Correct hypocalcemia and hypomagnesemia.
- Administer phototherapy.
- Administer fluid therapy.
- Maintain oxygenation and ventilation.

Key Nursing Activities
- Identify the woman at risk for diabetes.
- Detect and manage hypoglycemia and other complications in newborn.
- Provide emotional support for parents. Listen with empathy and acceptance.

Infant Born to a Mother Who Abuses Substances During Pregnancy

Infants born to women who use tobacco, alcohol, or illicit substances during pregnancy are at risk for numerous complications before and after birth. Narcotics readily pass the placental barrier, affecting the fetus before delivery. After delivery, the infant who has been exposed to intrauterine chemical substances can experience withdrawal symptoms (neonatal abstinence syndrome). Smoking is associated with significant low-birth-weight abnormalities, and maternal alcohol abuse is associated with fetal alcohol syndrome and fetal alcohol effects.

Clinical Manifestations
- Congenital defects include intrauterine growth retardation, small eyes, low nasal bridge, hypoplastic philtrum, thin upper lip, short nose, micrognathia, microcephaly, and others.
- Behavioral signs include poor postnatal growth, poor coordination, decreased tone, cognitive impairment, vomiting, mottling, irritability as a newborn, seizures, hyperactivity, poor feeding and sleeping, increased response to stimuli, gaze aversion, rhinorrhea and nasal congestion, decreased orientation to faces and voice, and poor state control as a newborn.
- Long-term effects later involve learning difficulties, impulsivity, memory deficits, poor judgment, and altered social patterns.

Diagnostic Tests
- Abstinence scoring
- Toxicology screen (infant blood, urine, and meconium; maternal blood and urine)
- Ultrasound
- HIV testing
- CBC
- Serum calcium
- Serum glucose
- Bilirubin

Medical Management
- Supportive care
- Pharmacological treatment with paregoric, lorazepam (Ativan), or phenobarbital
- Diazepam (Valium) to suppress narcotic withdrawal

Key Nursing Activities
- Decrease external stimuli. White noise or noise reduction techniques can be used to decrease environmental stimuli to calm infant and prevent overstimulation in infants with central nervous system (CNS) irritability that can precipitate seizures.
- Swaddle infant tightly in flexed position with arms midline. This provides a sense of security for the infant and prevents skin abrasions.
- Rock gently in vertical position.
- Provide opportunities for non-nutritive sucking. Use of a pacifier helps satisfy the increased need for sucking, calms the infant, and facilitates behavior organization.
- Feed small quantities in upright position and burp frequently to minimize vomiting and regurgitation and the potential for aspiration.
- Keep infant's chin tucked downward and support chin or chin and cheeks to facilitate the suck-swallow reflex and reduce the risk for aspiration should vomiting occur.
- Encourage kangaroo care, which provides sense of security and has a calming effect.
- Cluster care of infant to minimize handling and stimulation of infant and to decrease the potential for seizures related to overstimulation.

- Provide skin care and apply barrier dressings to elbows and knees to prevent excoriation related to increased activity.
- Change infant's position and use sheepskin to avoid development of pressure areas.
- Administer medications as prescribed for seizures, CNS stimulation, or insomnia.

For a more detailed discussion of infants born to compromised mothers, see Chapter 11 "Substance Abuse."

Prematurity

Infants born before the 37th week of gestation are considered preterm (premature).

Risk Factors

There is a variety of specific and nonspecific risks for prematurity, depending on gestational age. These include but are not limited to a lack of prenatal care, poor prenatal care, uterine enlargement (e.g., multiple gestation, uterine anomalies), cervical incompetence, chronic maternal diseases, tobacco smoking, anemia, substance abuse, sexually transmitted diseases, group B streptococcus infection, placenta previa, and abdominal trauma. Infants with congenital anomalies also are more at risk for a preterm birth.

Clinical Manifestations

- Abundant vernix and lanugo; head disproportionately large (>3 cm greater than chest size); poorly formed ear pinna with minimal cartilage; flat areola; absent sole creases; thin, ruddy skin with visible veins; poor tone; fused eyelids, undescended testes in males; prominent clitoris and labia minora in females
- Possible long-term effects of preterm birth include retinopathy of prematurity, bronchopulmonary dysplasia, attention-deficit disorder, developmental and learning delays, and hearing loss

Diagnostic Tests

- Lecithin-to-sphingomyelin ratio: performed on amniotic fluid to estimate fetal lung maturity
- Phosphatidylglycerol/phosphatidylinositol to evaluate fetal maturity
- Ultrasound
- Serum glucose
- Serum calcium
- Cord blood bilirubin levels
- CBC
- Serum electrolyte levels: to determine potassium, sodium, magnesium, and other electrolyte levels
- Erythrocyte sedimentation rate
- ABG
- Fibrinogen levels
- Blood and/or body fluids cultures

- Urinalysis, culture, and specific gravity
- Stool analysis
- Cranial ultrasound

Medical Management
- Maternal steroid administration, if meets criteria
- Artificial surfactant administration, if meets criteria
- Diagnosis and treatment of infection
- Assisted ventilation and oxygen therapy
- Fluid/electrolyte therapy
- Correction of acid–base imbalances
- Enteral and parenteral nutrition
- Phototherapy
- Medication or surgical closure of patent ductus arteriosus (PDA)
- Temperature regulation
- Respiratory support

Key Nursing Activities
- Conduct a gestational age assessment. Differentiate between preterm and SGA infant.
- Monitor for and prevent complications (e.g., hypothermia, hypoglycemia, respiratory distress syndrome [RDS], hyperbilirubinemia).
- Provide neutral thermal environment.
- Monitor and support hydration and nutritional status.
- Monitor and support cardiorespiratory status, including blood gas analysis, pulse oximetry, chest radiographs as needed, cardiorespiratory monitoring, oxygen therapy, surfactant, and mechanical ventilation as needed.
- Monitor for apnea and bradycardia.
- Position therapeutically to maintain a neutral airway, prevent reflux, and optimize lung expansion.
- Group activities to provide rest periods; minimize stimulation as needed.

Post-maturity

An infant born after 42 weeks' gestation is considered *postterm*. The term *postmature* refers to the infant born after 42 weeks of gestation who shows the effects of progressive placental insufficiency. Most postterm infants are healthy and born at weights that exceed 4 kg. Their large size, however, increases the risk for traumatic or cesarean births. Meconium staining and aspiration are common. Long-standing hypoxia results in polycythemia and hyperbilirubinemia; utilization of glycogen stores in utero results in hypoglycemia; and wasting of subcutaneous stores of fat leads to hypothermia.

Risk Factors
- Women with a history of prolonged pregnancies, as well as primiparas and grand multiparas, seem to be at greatest risk.
- Postterm delivery may also be a function of incorrect dating of the pregnancy (and, therefore, not truly postterm).

Clinical Manifestations

There is a variety of specific and nonspecific signs of postmaturity, depending on gestational age. Infants with postmaturity syndrome are SGA, with dry, cracked, parchment-like wrinkled skin; wide-eyed alert expression; long, thin extremities; long nails; profuse scalp hair; absence of vernix and lanugo; and meconium-stained skin. There usually is a history of oligohydramnios and cord compression.

Diagnostic Tests

- Biophysical profile to evaluate fetal well-being
- Nonstress test reflects the function of the fetal brainstem, autonomic nervous system, and heart
- Contraction stress test assesses fetal heart rate in response to uterine contractions
- Doppler flow studies identify fetal heart and great vessel abnormalities and variations in blood flow
- Electronic fetal monitoring identifies fetal heart tone variations such as decelerations, decreasing baseline variability, or increasing baseline rate
- Gestational age assessment
- CBC
- Serum glucose
- Bilirubin to detect hemolytic anemia (erythroblastosis fetalis) or congenital icterus

Medical Management

- Induction of labor
- Cesarean birth if cephalopelvic disproportion is present
- Supportive care for infant

Key Nursing Activities

- Monitor for and detect complications related to placental insufficiency.
- Assess for birth trauma.
- Prevent complications of birth trauma.
- Maintain neonate's body temperature.
- Offer emotional support to mother/partner.
- Estimate gestational age. Infants born postmature are at increased risk for macrosomia. A large fetus is more likely to suffer birth trauma than the smaller, less mature fetus.

Meconium Aspiration Syndrome

Meconium is passed in utero when the anal sphincter relaxes as a result of the hypoxic insult. Either in utero or after delivery the infant gasps and aspirates meconium into the tracheobronchial tree, resulting in airway occlusion, atelectasis, and pneumonitis. Aspiration of meconium can trigger persistent pulmonary hypertension, which can result in respiratory failure and circulatory collapse.

Risk Factors

- Intrauterine asphyxia
- Intrauterine stress

Clinical Manifestations
- Yellow or green amniotic fluid
- Meconium-stained cord, meconium-stained skin and nails of newborn, meconium visualized beyond the glottis
- Intrauterine growth retardation
- Patchy infiltrates, pulmonary interstitial emphysema, or pneumothorax on chest radiograph
- Hypoxemia, hypercarbia, and acidosis
- Tachypnea, cyanosis, and decreased peripheral perfusion
- Systolic murmur and other abnormal heart sounds

Diagnostic Tests
- Postnatal intubation and visualization of trachea to identify meconium in the tracheobronchial tree
- Chest radiograph to identify the presence of pneumonitis, pneumothorax, infiltrates, hyperexpansion, and atelectasis
- Blood gases to detect metabolic and respiratory acidosis and hypoxia
- Electrocardiography to aid in diagnosis cor pulmonale

Medical Management
- Early identification of the compromised fetus
- Suctioning of the oropharynx while the head is still on the perineum
- Intubation and suction of the trachea after complete delivery and before the first breath
- Oxygen therapy
- Assisted ventilation (conventional or high frequency)
- Nitric oxide therapy
- Antibiotics
- Extracorporeal membrane oxygenation
- Vasopressors
- Volume expanders
- Correction of acidosis
- Paralyzing agents

Key Nursing Activities
- Review prenatal and labor/birth history for risk factors for intrauterine and birth hypoxia.
- Assess for meconium-stained amniotic fluid during labor and birth.
- Assess newborn for meconium-stained umbilical cord and nails.
- Assess for (visualize) meconium below the vocal cords to establish that meconium has been aspirated into the trachea and bronchi.
- Assess respiratory status to detect respiratory distress. Tachypnea, apnea, grunting, retractions, nasal flaring, crackles, rhonchi, and decreased or absent breathing sounds indicate respiratory distress. Aspiration of meconium into the lungs causes pneumonitis (localized lung inflammation), which disrupts surfactant production and decreases lung compliance (elasticity). Pneumonitis prevents

the lungs from fully expanding, causing the condition known as atelectasis. Both conditions inhibit the exchange of oxygen and carbon dioxide and ultimately intensify the work of breathing.

- Assess vital signs. Heart rate increases as it attempts to compensate for the hypoxia. Bradycardia occurs with decompensation. Hypotension may be associated with asphyxia and shock.
- Assess color and perfusion. Pallor, poor perfusion, and dusky color are associated with poor oxygenation and peripheral vasoconstriction, secondary to hypoxemia.
- Monitor ABG to detect hypoxemia, hypercapnia, respiratory or metabolic acidosis. Atelectasis and air trapping decrease gas exchange, leading to decreased oxygenation, increased CO_2 retention, and acid–base imbalance.
- Monitor radiology studies to detect atelectasis, patchy lung infiltrates, or air leak.
- Administer oxygen as prescribed.
- Maintain hydration and humidify oxygen, which helps to mobilize secretions by keeping them thin, so they can be coughed out or suctioned. Thick secretions can block the area and contribute to the development of hypoxia.
- Perform chest physiotherapy to help mobilize secretions, so they do not block the airway and contribute to hypoxia.
- Suction as needed to remove secretions to maintain a patent airway and enhance oxygenation.
- Provide a neutral thermal environment as increased environmental temperature contributes to increased body temperature, which increases metabolic demands and oxygen consumption. The same is true for an environmental temperature that is too cool.
- Correct acid–base imbalances and metabolic disorders to facilitate perfusion and oxygenation of tissues.
- Administer paralytic agents or sedatives to facilitate breathing if assisted ventilation becomes necessary.
- Administer vasopressors, pulmonary vasodilators, and volume expanders to promote circulation in the presence of fetal circulation.
- Administer antibiotics as prescribed to prevent infection from retained meconium in the lung. Meconium is a waste product that irritates the lung parenchyma and leads to lung inflammation (pneumonitis) and infection from retained secretions and inadequate alveolar expansion. Prevention or elimination of infection reduces inflammation and prevents hypoxia.
- Suction the neonate while the head is still on the perineum to remove meconium from the mouth, which reduces the risk for aspiration.
- Avoid stimulating respirations in a meconium-stained infant to decrease the risk for aspiration. Once meconium has been visualized

and aspirated from the lungs, the infant can be suctioned and then stimulated to breathe.

- Prevent cold stress, which increases metabolic demands and oxygen needs.
- Cluster neonatal care to prevent oxygen consumption because of increased activity and stress.
- Avoid high inflating pressures to ventilate infant. High pressures increase the risk for airway trauma and air leaks.
- Administer paralytic agents or sedatives as prescribed, if needed, to prevent infant from fighting assisted ventilation and increased intrapulmonary pressures to maximize ventilation and oxygenation.
- Perform chest physiotherapy and suctioning as needed to maintain a patent airway and prevent further respiratory compromise.
- Provide emotional support for parents.

Respiratory Distress Syndrome

RDS occurs primarily in preterm infants as a result of surfactant deficiency. It is characterized by compromised lung expansion, poor gas exchange, and ventilatory failure.

Risk Factors
- Prematurity
- Perinatal acidosis
- Sepsis
- Maternal infection
- Maternal diabetes
- Preterm, premature, prolonged rupture of membranes
- Maternal substance abuse during pregnancy
- Meconium aspiration

Clinical Manifestations
- Grunting, flaring, retractions, increased work of breathing
- Adventitious breath sounds (rales and rhonchi)
- Hypercarbia, hypoxemia, acidosis
- Reduced oxygen saturation
- Poor perfusion and hypotension
- Low tone
- Apneic episodes

Diagnostic Tests
- ABG
- Oxygen saturation
- Chest radiograph
- CBC
- Blood culture
- Blood glucose and serum calcium

Medical Management
- Surfactant therapy
- Antibiotic therapy

- Oxygen therapy and ventilation
- Correction of acidosis

Key Nursing Activities
- Monitor the infant's respiratory status, clinically as well as by oxygen saturation, ABG, and chest x-ray.
- Monitor the infant's vital signs. Maintain adequate oxygenation.
- Suction as needed to remove secretions to maintain a patent airway and enhance oxygenation.
- Administer medications as prescribed.
- Decrease stimulation; cluster care.
- Offer emotional support to families of infants with RDS.
- Maintain a neutral thermal environment.
- Maintain intravenous (IV) access and administer fluid therapy as prescribed.

Necrotizing Enterocolitis

Necrotizing enterocolitis (NEC) is a feeding complication, occurring primarily in preterm infants wherein the tissue in a portion(s) of the bowel dies.

Risk Factors
- Prematurity
- Perinatal acidosis
- Sepsis
- Maternal infection
- Maternal diabetes
- Preterm, premature, prolonged rupture of membranes
- Maternal substance abuse during pregnancy
- Meconium aspiration

Clinical Manifestations
- Feeding intolerance, emesis, gastric residuals
- Abdominal distention
- Bloody stools
- Abdominal tenderness
- Visible loops of bowel
- Abdominal discoloration
- Hypotension
- Low tone
- Temperature instability
- Grunting, flaring, retractions, increased work of breathing

Diagnostic Tests
- Abdominal radiograph shows dilated loops of bowel, interstitial pneumatosis in bowel wall, portal venous gas, pneumoperitoneum (free air outside the bowel within the peritoneal cavity)
- Paracentesis may help to confirm the presence of intestinal gangrene in infants with NEC when there is no evidence of pneumoperitoneum
- ABGs

- Oxygen saturation
- Stool culture, rotavirus assay
- CBC, blood culture
- Blood glucose

Medical Management
- NPO, parenteral nutrition to allow the bowel to rest
- Gastric decompression and intermittent suction
- Surgical intervention may be necessary (bowel resection, colostomy/ileostomy)
- Antibiotic therapy
- Oxygen therapy and ventilation
- Vasopressors might be able to support blood pressure, if necessary.
- Correction of acidosis

Key Nursing Activities
- Monitor blood pressure for hypotension.
- Provide comfort measures to the baby.
- Provide oxygen therapy as needed. Monitor closely.
- Monitor blood gases and oxygen saturation.
- Administer IV therapy and parenteral nutrition, as prescribed. There is insufficient evidence to recommend a specific placement location for the tip of the umbilical artery catheter. Umbilical artery catheter position (high versus low) has not been found to affect the incidence of NEC.
- Encourage breast feeding when feedings are resumed. Breast milk has a protective function.
- There is insufficient evidence to recommend either the use or avoidance of probiotics. Clinical trials of the effects of probiotics on the risk for NEC have shown inconsistent benefit.
- Slowly reintroduce feedings in strength and volume, as tolerated. There is insufficient evidence to recommend a specific rate of feeding volume advancement.
- There is insufficient evidence to support bolus versus continuous tube feeding as a method to reduce the risk or recovery from NEC.
- Offer emotional support to parents. You might need to prepare them for surgery.

Patent Ductus Arteriosus
PDA is the connection between the pulmonary artery with the aorta, which allows mixing of well-oxygenated with poorly oxygenated blood.

Risk Factors
- Prematurity
- Genetic disorders, such as Down syndrome
- Rubella exposure of mother during pregnancy

Clinical Manifestations
- Tachycardia
- Continuous machinery murmur best heard at the second or third intercostal space at the upper left sternal border

- Hyperdynamic precordium
- Bounding pulses
- Tachypnea, grunting, retractions, nasal flaring, crackles, rhonchi, RDS
- Acidosis, hypoxemia
- Poor perfusion, hypotension
- Cardiac enlargement, increased pulmonary vascularity, pulmonary edema

Diagnostic Tests
- ABGs
- Oxygen saturation
- X-ray

Medical Management
- Oxygen therapy or ventilation
- Prostaglandin inhibitor medication (indomethacin)
- Management of congestive heart failure, if occurs
- Fluid restriction

Key Nursing Activities
- Daily weights at the same time.
- Monitor blood pressure for hypotension.
- Administer prostaglandin inhibitor, as prescribed.
- Provide oxygen therapy as needed. Monitor closely.
- Suction the oropharynx and trachea as needed.
- Monitor blood gases and oxygen saturation.
- Provide IV therapy, if prescribed.
- Provide emotional support to the family.

Small for Gestational Age

SGA describes infants with birth weights below the 10th percentile for length, weight, or head circumference for gestational age. Intrauterine growth retardation may be symmetrical, affecting all parameters of growth, or asymmetrical. Asymmetrical growth usually results in sparing of brain growth and head circumference and indicates longer standing insult to the fetus.

Risk Factors
- Intrauterine exposure to maternal substances (tobacco, drugs, alcohol)
- Maternal diabetes
- Maternal pre-eclampsia
- Maternal chronic systems failure (renal, cardiac, etc.)
- Maternal anemia, thrombocytopenia
- Uteroplacental insufficiency (poor circulation to the growing fetus)
- Multifetal gestation (twins, triplets, etc.)
- Intrauterine viral infection (TORCH)
- Fetal chromosomal abnormalities
- Cord prolapse, cord thrombosis

Clinical Manifestations
- Weight, length, and/or head circumference below the 10th percentile
- Hypoglycemia, jittery
- Polycythemia (elevated Hct, ruddy color)
- Temperature instability
- Meconium staining
- Perinatal asphyxia, hypoxemia

Diagnostic Tests
- Ultrasound to estimate fetal measurements
- Doppler studies to determine flow through the umbilical cord to the fetus
- Pattern of maternal weight gain
- Gestational assessment with anthropometrics plotted on growth chart (see Fig. 6–17, growth chart for newborns 20 to 44 weeks' gestation)

Medical Management
- Follow developmental screening
- Nutrition
- Glucose management
- Oxygen support as needed

Key Nursing Activities
- Monitor parameters of growth. Metabolic needs are increased for catch-up growth.
- Support neutral thermal environment. Temperature-controlled isolette or radiant warmer might be necessary initially, depending on the extent of growth impairment.

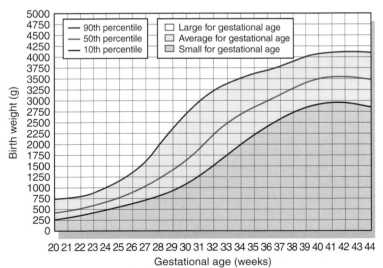

FIGURE 6-17: Gestational age measurement chart.

- Monitor blood sugar closely. Frequent feedings of small amounts are more readily tolerated and help prevent hypoglycemia, which can occur rapidly in the SGA infant with decreased glycogen stores.
- Encourage frequent breastfeeding, or bottle- or gavage-feed every 3 to 4 hours or more, depending on gestational maturity, pattern of weight gain, and any other complications.
- Monitor feeding tolerance, suck, and swallow. May require occupational therapy consultation.
- Assess for signs of sensory overload. SGA infants may have impaired tolerance for stimulation. Sensory overload may manifest as crying, irritability, restlessness, or facial grimacing.
- Encourage parents to provide developmental care at home and follow up with developmental evaluation.

Large for Gestational Age

LGA is birth weight greater than the 90th percentile for gestational age. At term, that would be 4 kg.

Risk Factors
- Infant of a diabetic mother
- Familial tendency
- Genetic abnormality (e.g., Marfan syndrome)

Clinical Manifestations
- Macrosomia
- Tremors from hypoglycemia or hypocalcemia
- May show signs of birth trauma (e.g., fractured clavicle, cephalohematoma, palsy, bruising)
- Signs of respiratory distress
- Hypotonia
- Ruddy (polycythemia)
- May have meconium-stained nail beds or skin

Diagnostic Tests
- Anthropometric measurements (weight, length)
- Blood glucose
- Serum calcium
- CBC

Medical Management
- Cesarean birth may be necessary
- Glucose management
- Management of respiratory distress, meconium aspiration, or other complications, if occurs

Key Nursing Activities
- Monitor glucose closely.
- Provide early feedings or IV therapy, as prescribed.
- Monitor for signs of respiratory distress.
- Support respiratory status with oxygen therapy, as prescribed.
- Anticipate elevated bilirubin if bruising is extensive.
- Provide emotional support to parents as needed.

Congenital Anomalies in Newborns

Congenital anomalies, also referred to as *birth defects*, may have several different causes such as genetics, viral infection in utero, or pregnancy complications. However, for some congenital anomalies, there is no known cause.

Cleft Lip/Palate

Cleft lip/palate is the incomplete closure of the maxillary and mandibular tissue during embryonic development.

Causes
- Unknown in most cases
- Exposure to teratogens, such as medication to treat acne (isotretinoin [Accutane]), cancer (methotrexate), or seizures
- Familial tendency

Clinical Manifestation

Cleft lip is unilateral or bilateral notching of the vermillion of the lip or a complete cleft extending through the lip to a nare. Also observed are:
- Asymmetry of the nares
- Flattening of the midfacial contour

Cleft palate is midline fissure or opening in the hard or even into the soft palate (roof of the mouth). Typically involves:
- Coughing and choking with feeding
- Difficulty forming a seal for sucking
- Congestion
- Reflux
- Failure to thrive when a cleft palate is unrepaired and feeding difficulties persist

Diagnosis
- History
- Physical examination
- Prenatal ultrasound

Treatment
- Multiple-stage, surgical closure to correct the defect
- Special feeding appliances
- Oral care
- Monitoring growth

⭐ **BEST PRACTICES**

Because of the opening in the palate and poor seal with feeding, the infant is at high risk for airway obstruction and aspiration. Careful positioning, burping, and feeding techniques are important for preventative care. Suction should be readily available to clear the airway as needed. During the newborn period, hold the baby upright with the head and chest tilted slightly backward to aid in swallowing and to reduce the risk for choking and aspiration.

Myelomeningocele

Myelomeningocele is failure of the vertebrae and spinal canal to close before birth. This condition is also known as a type of spina bifida.

Causes
- Unknown
- Low levels of folic acid in the mother's body early in pregnancy
- Familial risk
- Viral trigger (theorized)

Clinical Manifestation
- Saclike
- Hydrocephalus
- Loss of bladder or bowel control
- Partial or complete paralysis of the legs
- Weakness of the feet, legs, or hips
- Hair tuft or dimpling at the sacral area

Diagnosis
- Prenatal
  - Maternal blood test (drawn usually between the 16th and 18th week; Alpha Feto Protein (AFP), human chorionic gonadotropin, unconjugated estriol, Inhibin A)
  - Fetal ultrasound
  - Amniocentesis
- Postnatal
  - Neurological examination
  - X-ray
  - Ultrasound, CT, or magnetic resonance imaging of the spinal area and head

Treatment
- Surgical closure of the spinal defect
- Surgical drain or ventriculoperitoneal shunt if hydrocephalus involved increased intracranial pressure (ICP)
- Bladder training, Credé maneuver, or intermittent catheterization to drain the bladder of urine if there is loss of bladder control
- Bowel training and high-fiber diet may improve bowel function
- Orthopedic or physical therapy is needed to treat neuromuscular weakness or paralysis; the extent of support, including bracing, depends on the type of defect and level of spinal cord involvement.
- Home care and follow-up support are needed to provide emotional support for the caregivers, to prevent complications, and to monitor growth and development
- Genetic counseling is recommended for future pregnancies because of the familial link.

ALERT!

Hydrocephalus is commonly associated with spinal cord defects, such as myelomeningocele. Untreated ICP can lead to significant cognitive or developmental impairment. Be sure to follow head growth and assess closely for signs of ICP.

Omphalocele

Omphalocele is a midline abdominal defect at the umbilicus in which the infant's intestine and other abdominal organs are born within a thin sac outside the body.

Causes
- Unknown
- Chromosomal abnormality associated

Clinical Manifestation
- Membranous sac containing intestine and possibly liver and spleen born outside the abdominal cavity at the base of the umbilicus
- Similar to gastroschisis, except the abdominal organs with omphalocele are within a sac; in gastroschisis, the intestines are not

Diagnosis
- Prenatal ultrasound
- Amniocentesis
- Physical examination after birth
- Decreased bowel sounds
- Feeding problems
- Bilious vomiting

Treatment
- Surgical closure of the abdominal wall
- Synthetic sac covering the omphalocele might be necessary to slowly introduce the abdominal contents back into the abdominal cavity
- Genetic testing

Diaphragmatic Hernia

A diaphragmatic hernia is an abnormal opening in the diaphragm that allows the abdominal organs, such as intestine, liver, and spleen, to protrude into the chest cavity; this does not allow the lung to develop fully on the affected side.

Causes
- Unknown in most cases
- Familial tendency

Clinical Manifestation
- Severe respiratory distress
- Respiratory acidosis
- Hypotension
- Cyanosis
- Tachycardia
- Tachypnea

WHY IS KNOWING ABOUT SPINA BIFIDA IMPORTANT?

- Frequent urinary tract infections can occur when bladder control is impaired.
- Pressure sores are common for children with paralysis and reduced or lost sensation to the lower legs and sacrum.
- Meningitis is a risk, particularly when a drain is in place.

ALERT!

Approximately 25% to 40% of omphaloceles have other associated congenital defects; they are often associated with chromosomal abnormalities and other midline defects, such as congenital heart disease or diaphragmatic hernia.

WHY IS KNOWING ABOUT OMPHALOCELE SURGERY IMPORTANT?

Replacing too much intestine and other organs into the abdominal space too quickly can lead to compression of the superior vena cava, which affects blood pressure and circulation to and from the heart.

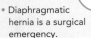
- Bowel sounds in the chest
- Absent breath sounds on the affected side

Diagnosis

- Prenatal ultrasound: shows abdominal contents in the chest cavity; polyhydramnios (excessive amniotic fluid)
- Postnatal radiograph

Treatment

- Surgical repair of the diaphragm and placement of the organs back into the abdominal cavity
- Mechanical ventilation
- Extracorporeal membrane oxygenation necessary for severe cases
- Vasopressors for hypotension
- IV fluids

Tracheoesophageal Fistula

TEF is a defect between the upper part of the esophagus and the trachea.

Causes

- Congenital
- Acquired, including malignancy, infection, trauma after endotracheal intubation, trauma secondary to malpositioned tracheostomy tube, ruptured diverticula

Clinical Manifestations

- Excessive mucous secretions
- Periodic breathing and cyanosis
- Choking
- Abdominal distention after birth
- Vomiting
- Endotracheal tube suctioning of stomach contents
- Failure to pass a nasogastric tube
- Clinical symptoms of aspiration pneumonia (rales, rhonchi, respiratory distress, retractions, tachypnea)
- Symptoms worsen during feeding

Diagnosis

- Prenatal ultrasound reveals polyhydramnios
- Postnatal chest radiograph shows tracheal deviation or aspiration pneumonia
- CT scan
- Flexible esophagoscopy or bronchoscopy

Treatment

- Surgical repair in the first few days of life, depending on birth weight, pneumonia, or other abnormalities
- Parenteral nutrition

- Gastrostomy tube for feedings
- Mechanical ventilation

Congenital Cardiac Defects

Congenital cardiac defects are due to abnormalities of the structure of the heart and great vessels of a newborn.

Common Causes

- *Hypoplasia*, including hypoplastic left-heart syndrome. This is a significant cyanotic heart defect because the left ventricle is the chamber for pumping blood to the body. If the pumping chamber is underdeveloped, the body does not receive the blood it needs; hypoxemia and acidosis develop.

ALERT!

The abnormal connection between the trachea and esophagus may lead to respiratory distress and aspiration pneumonia. Notify provider if infant shows signs of respiratory distress with feeding or if you suction material that appears to be formula from an endotracheal tube.

- *Obstruction defects*
  - Aortic valve stenosis is a narrowing of the valve that allows blood to flow from the left ventricle into the aorta and then out to the rest of the body.
  - Pulmonary valve stenosis is a narrowing of the pulmonary valve that allows blood to flow from the right ventricle to the lungs.
  - Coarctation of the aorta is the narrowing of the aorta, causing decreased blood flow to the lower body.
- *Septal wall defects*
  - Failure of the walls (septum) of the heart to close before birth. Many of these defects are small and will close over time without treatment. Some large defects must be closed surgically.
  - Patent foramen ovale is an opening in the septal wall between the right and left atria.
  - Ventricular septal defect is an opening in the septal wall between the right and left ventricles.
- Defects of the great vessels
  - Coarctation of the aorta
  - Total or partial anomalous pulmonary venous return
  - Interrupted aortic arch
- *Conduction defects*
  - Wolff–Parkinson–White syndrome is a rapid heart rate because of extra pathways that conduct electrical patterns in the heart.
  - Supraventricular tachycardia is a rapid heart rate, usually more than 220 bpm in infants.
- *Cyanotic heart lesions*
  - Shunting of blood *away from* the lungs, causing oxygen-poor blood to be pumped through the pulmonary artery to the lungs (right-to-left shunt); poorly oxygenated blood is circulated to the body, leading to hypoxia and acidosis.

- Persistent truncus arteriosus is a heart defect where one large vessels leads out of the heart, instead of two separate vessels; this creates mixing of well-oxygenated with poorly oxygenated blood
- Total or partial anomalous pulmonary venous return
- Tetralogy of Fallot is a congenital heart condition that involves four defects; some infants have cyanotic episodes, called "tet spells."
- Tricuspid atresia is a defect where the tricuspid valve is under-developed, resulting in poor blood flow through the heart and into the lungs.
- Hypoplastic left-heart syndrome
- Transposition of the great vessels is a reversal of the pulmonary artery and aorta with the heart; this causes oxygen-rich blood to circulate to the lungs and heart but not to the rest of the body.
- Pulmonary atresia
- *Acyanotic heart lesions*
  - Shunting of blood *to* the lungs, causing overflow of congestion in the pulmonary system and heart failure (left-to-right shunt); the shunting increases the pressure in the pulmonary (pulmonary hypertension) and leads to insufficient blood supply to the body (congestive heart failure) and acidosis
  - Patent foramen ovale
  - PDA
  - Ventricular septal defect

Clinical Manifestations
- Poor feeding
- May be cyanotic, depending on the lesion
- Murmur or abnormal heart sounds (gallop, single S2, split, or thrill, depending on the lesion)
- Metabolic acidosis
- Poor growth
- Respiratory distress
- Hyperactive precordium
- Poor peripheral perfusion
- Difference in pulses (upper versus lower extremities)
- Bounding or weak pulses
- Hypoxemia
- Shock

Diagnosis
- Chest radiograph
- Blood gas analysis
- Electrocardiogram
- Echocardiogram
- Cardiac catheterization

- Monitoring oxygen saturation both preductal (right hand) and postductal (foot)
- Oxygen challenge test with 100% F_{IO_2}

Treatment

- Surgical repair, depending on the cardiac defect
- Balloon septostomy to create a temporary shunt for keeping adequate blood flowing when there is obstruction or hypertension in the cardiopulmonary system
- Prostaglandin E_1 (if PDA) to keep ductus arteriosus open for ductal-dependent lesions
- Vasopressors if shock is present
- Mechanical ventilation or oxygen support if CHD is cyanotic type or hypoxia, hypoventilation, or acidosis is present

7 Contraceptive Counseling

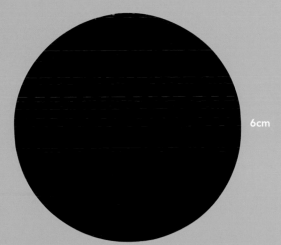

6cm

CHAPTER 7

Contraceptive Counseling

To provide thorough contraceptive counseling for our patients, we must educate ourselves on the wide range of available birth-control options. Empowering our patients with knowledge about which options are most effective, safe, affordable, and best suited to their lifestyle can help increase proper and consistent use.

WHY IS CONTRACEPTIVE COUNSELING IMPORTANT?

- Approximately 3.1 million pregnancies each year are unintended—that is, half of all pregnancies annually.
- Half of these unintended pregnancies are the result of failed contraception.
- Of these pregnancies, four in 10 are terminated. Therefore, it is our responsibility as health-care practitioners (HCPs) to educate patients about the various types of birth control, so they can choose the method that is most effective, safe, affordable, and suited to their lifestyle.

Methods of Contraception

This section discusses the various methods of contraception and family planning, including hormonal, nonhormonal, fertility awareness-based methods, and sterilization. The effectiveness, advantages, and disadvantages of each method are reviewed. Information on how the particular method works to prevent pregnancy and instructions for use of the method are also included. In addition, verbatim nurse–patient interactions (shown in italics in "Patient Education" sections) are provided as models for readers.

Abstinence

Abstinence is defined by some as the avoidance of any sexual activity involving contact between the male and female genitals. Couples can still engage in oral–genital contact, masturbation, or penile–anal intercourse. Others define abstinence as refraining from *any* type of sexual activity, including masturbation.

Effectiveness

Abstinence is the only form of contraception that is 100% effective at preventing pregnancy.

SPEAKING OUT

Discussing with your patients their risks for using a particular form of birth control is absolutely necessary. The most serious risk—death—from the use of birth control in a nonsmoker between the ages of 15 and 34 years is 1 in 1,667,000 per year; in nonsmoking women aged 35 to 44, it is 1 in 33,300 per year. However, the risk for death from pregnancy is 1 in 8700. To put this in perspective, the risk for death from an automobile accident is 1 in 5000 per year and in an airplane crash is 1 in 250,000.

TIPS

OUTERCOURSE, OF COURSE!

Outercourse is the exact opposite of intercourse. Using this method, a couple may engage in a wide range of activities to express themselves sexually without actual penile–vaginal intercourse. If your patient desires to avoid pregnancy and does not want to use any form of birth control, you may want to present this option.

Continued

Advantages of Use

- Not only is abstinence the most effective form of contraception in preventing pregnancy, it is free.
- Abstinence may be the best option for women in a variety of special circumstances, including those who have medical issues and are not able to take hormonal birth control, those who are receiving treatment for an STI and/or are awaiting partner treatment, and postpartum women who are advised pelvic rest for 4 to 6 weeks after giving birth, especially if vaginal laceration, episiotomy, or both are present.

Disadvantage of Use

For some individuals, abstinence may not provide sexual gratification.

Patient Education

- Discuss the benefits of abstinence with the patient, and note that it is the only type of birth control that is 100% effective at preventing pregnancy.

- Discuss ways in which the patient and her partner can express themselves sexually without having intercourse. These activities may include hugging, holding hands, massaging, kissing, dancing, sharing sexual fantasies, using erotic books or videos, and solo or mutual masturbation.

TIPS—cont'd

However, because there may still be contact with bodily fluids, the patient needs to know that outercourse may not be effective in preventing sexually transmitted infections (STIs).

- In case the desire or opportunity arises to engage in sexual intercourse, discuss with your patient the need for a backup plan for contraception. She may want to obtain a prescription from her HCP for hormonal birth control or buy over-the-counter products such as female or male condoms. In addition, depending on the type of emergency contraceptive pill (ECP) and the age of the patient, ECPs are also available by prescription or possibly over-the-counter. Options include, but are not limited to, Plan B One-Step, Next Choice, Next Choice One Dose, Levonorgestrel, and Ella.

Coitus Interruptus (Withdrawal Method)

Coitus interruptus (also known as *withdrawal*) is a simple method in which the penis is withdrawn from the vagina before ejaculation.

Mechanism of Action

Fertilization is avoided by withdrawing the penis from the vagina before ejaculation of seminal fluid.

QSEN APPLICATION

Patient-centered care includes attitudes such as:
- Respecting patient's preferences for degree of active engagement in care process
- Respecting patient's right to access to personal health records
- Valuing seeing health-care situations "through patients' eyes"
- Respecting and encouraging individual expression of patient values, preferences, and expressed needs
- Valuing the patient's expertise with her health and symptoms
- Seeking learning opportunities with patients who represent all aspects of human diversity
- Recognizing personally held attitudes about working with patients from different ethnic, cultural, and social backgrounds
- Willingly supporting patient-centered care for individuals and groups whose values differ from own

In this chapter, together with information about care of pregnant women and newborns, QSEN competencies assure delivery of the best nursing care.

http://qsen.org/competencies/pre-licensure-ksas/#patient-centered_care

Effectiveness

Withdrawal has low effectiveness (possibly only 27% effective).

Advantages of Use

- Convenient and free
- No need to consult an HCP for a prescription

Disadvantages of Use

- Withdrawal is not highly effective in preventing pregnancy.
- Pre-ejaculate fluid containing infectious pathogens and semen may be released before full ejaculation without the male partner's knowledge, potentially exposing the female partner to STIs or pregnancy.
- Patient must rely on her male partner to withdraw his penis before ejaculation.
- Because there is still penile–vaginal penetration, exposure to STIs via an infected sore, vaginal fluid, or pre-ejaculate fluid—even without ejaculation—may occur.

Patient Education

- *The efficacy of coitus interruptus is low and is not a reliable form of contraception or STI prevention. Other forms of contraception are more reliable in preventing pregnancy. Barrier methods, such as condoms, should also be used to decrease the risk for acquiring an STI.*
- *Should you engage in intercourse again within a short period of time after the last encounter, your male partner needs to urinate and wipe the tip of his penis of any semen that is left over from the first encounter.*

Hormonal Options

Combination: Estrogen and Progesterone

Birth control that contains both estrogen and progesterone hormones is very effective at preventing pregnancy. Hormonal birth control is currently available through several different delivery methods: oral, transdermal, and intravaginal.

Effectiveness

Combination estrogen and progesterone birth control is 91% to 99% effective.

Mechanism of Action

The combination of the hormones estrogen and progesterone suppresses ovulation, thickens cervical mucus (which impedes sperm penetration into the uterus), and changes the endometrium (making it an inhospitable host for implantation).

Advantages of Use

- Decreased pain and bleeding associated with menses, and fewer symptoms of premenstrual syndrome (PMS)
- Improvement of endometriosis symptoms, menstrual migraines, acne, and hirsutism
- Reduced risk for ovarian and endometrial cancer
- No interruption in lovemaking

Disadvantages of Use

- May have unpredictable bleeding patterns in the first few months of using combined oral contraceptives (COCs), as well as headaches, breast pain, mood swings, depression, and nausea
- Inconvenient and easy to forget to take the pill consistently at the same time each day
- May not be the most private choice because the pill must be kept somewhere accessible to the patient every 24 hours
- Cost may be high; in many states, insurance providers do not absorb the cost of contraceptive coverage, and the patient may have to pay out of pocket.
- Does not protect from STIs
- Prescription from an HCP is required.
- Increased risk for myocardial infarction (MI) and stroke for smokers
- Increased risk for venous thromboembolism, especially in obese, sedentary women
- Increased risk for high blood pressure
- Decreased libido
- Possible drug interactions with certain medications

Patient Education

- *Keep the instructions that come with your pill/patch/ring pack. If you miss taking a pill/applying a patch/placing a ring, follow the instructions that came with your pack. Remember that not all pills are the same, and the instructions are specific to the type of pill you are taking. If you have questions about what to do, call your HCP and abstain from sex or use a backup method of contraception. If you think you had sexual intercourse without proper protection, you may want to consider taking emergency contraception. Call 1-888-NOT-2-LATE.*
- *Remember, the pill/patch/ring does not protect you from any type of STIs, such as syphilis, hepatitis, and HIV. You will need to use condoms correctly and consistently with each sexual encounter.*
- *If you want to avoid pregnancy, do not take a break from taking the pill/patch/ring.*
- *Smoking increases rare, but serious, complications associated with taking contraception with both estrogen and progesterone. You should not smoke while on the pill/patch/ring. Your HCP may need to prescribe an alternative form of contraception if you continue smoking.*

- *If you are prescribed new medications or are diagnosed with a new medical condition, you need to let your HCP know that you are using a contraceptive pill/patch/ring.*
- Go over the ACHES warning signs with the patient and instruct her to contact her HCP if she experiences any of the symptoms.
- Discuss with the patient that possible menstrual irregularities associated with pill/patch/ring use are common in the first 3 months of use.

Combined Oral Contraceptive

Combined oral contraceptives (COCs), or "The Pill," were introduced in the United States in the 1960s. COCs are the most widely used form of birth control in the United States, and 75 million women worldwide use COCs.

Brands Available in the United States

Dozens of different types of COCs are available in the United States. The following are some examples of COCs:

- **20 mcg (lowest amount of estrogen):** Loestrin 1/20, Mircette, and Alesse
- **30 mcg:** Seasonale, Nordette, Desogen
- **35 mcg:** Ortho-Cyclen 28, Norethin 1/35E-28, Ovcon 35
- **50 mcg:** Ovcon 50, Zovia 1/50, Demulen 1/50

Dosing

The patient needs to take one pill a day, at the same time each day.

Contraceptive Transdermal Patch

Approved by the U.S. Food and Drug Administration (FDA) in 2002, the Ortho Evra patch is the only contraceptive on the market that delivers both estrogen and progestin hormones transdermally.

Dosing

One patch should be applied each week for 3 weeks; no patch is applied the fourth week. Patch may be applied to the upper torso (avoiding the breast), lower abdomen, buttocks, or upper outer arm.

Advantages of Use

- The weekly regimen of the patch may be an easier regimen to remember than a daily pill.
- Reversibility of the patch is prompt. Return to fertility may occur the month after discontinuance.

- Because the patch is administered transdermally, it is ideal for women who are not able to take medications orally.
- Because the Ortho Evra patch is made from polyester, it is safe for women with latex allergies.

- Negative side effects include headache, nausea, breast tenderness, breakthrough bleeding, and skin irritation at application site.

- *Apply the patch to clean, dry skin.*
- *Remember the day you start the patch regimen. That day becomes your "change day." If you start using the patch on a Wednesday, then Wednesday is the day you should change the patch each week.*
- *At the end of the third week, remove the patch for a patch-free week. If your change day is on a Wednesday, you will be patch-free until the next Wednesday. At the end of the patch-free week, apply a new patch on your designated "change day," even if you are still having withdrawal bleeding. Waiting more than 7 days to start the new cycle of patches may put you at risk for ovulation and thus, possible pregnancy.*
- *If the skin under or around the patch becomes irritated, rotate the placement of the patch to different sites.*

Vaginal Contraceptive Ring

Approved in 2001 by the FDA, the NuvaRing is the only contraceptive vaginal ring that has been approved in the United States. It is a flexible ring that contains both estrogen and progesterone hormones.

Patients insert one ring intravaginally for 21 days and then are ring free for 7 days.

- The ring is easy to insert and remove, and most women find it comfortable to use.
- Verifying that the device is in the vagina is easy to do and can be reassuring.
- Reversibility of the NuvaRing is prompt. Return to fertility may occur 17 to 19 days after it is discontinued.
- The ring may be used with tampons.
- Because the hormones in the ring are administered intravaginally, it is ideal for women who are not able to take medications

---

⭐ BEST PRACTICES

NuvaRing is for one-time use only and needs to be discarded after use. The ring does not have to be placed around the cervix. As long as the ring is in the vaginal canal, the hormones in the ring will be absorbed through the vaginal walls.

orally. Also, the intravaginal route increases the bioavailability of hormones; therefore, a lower hormonal dose is used compared with the dose in COCs and the contraceptive patch. With a lower total dosing, adverse effects are reduced as well.

- The ring is safe for women with latex allergies.

Disadvantages of Use

- Bleeding between periods
- Nausea and vomiting
- Vaginal irritation
- Breast tenderness

Patient Education

The nurse should provide careful instructions on using the ring.

- *Store your NuvaRing at room temperature (between 59°F and 86°F, or 15°F and 30°C).*

ALERT

Although rare, there is a risk for toxic shock syndrome (TSS) with NuvaRing use. Patients need to be counseled on the signs and symptoms of TSS. These include:

- Fever
- Malaise
- Diarrhea

ALERT

Smoking while using the Nuva Ring may increase your risk for cardiovascular side effects. Patients more than 35 years old who smoke more than 15 cigarettes a day are at an increased risk.

- *Insertion: Before opening the packet and handling the NuvaRing, make sure you wash your hands thoroughly. Put the NuvaRing in between your thumb and index finger, and squeeze. Find a comfortable position — standing with one leg up, lying down, or squatting. Insert the folded NuvaRing into the vagina. As long as it is in the vaginal canal and you are comfortable, the ring does not have to end up around the cervix or in a specific location in the vagina. Leave the ring in place for 21 days.*
- *Before removing the ring, wash your hands thoroughly. Gently hook your finger on the NuvaRing and pull it out. Discard the ring in a trash receptacle that is out of reach of children and pets. The ring is not flushable.*
- *At the end of the ring-free week, on the same day of the week the previous ring was inserted, insert a new ring in the vagina to start the new cycle even if you still have your period.*

Progestin Only

Progestin-only forms of birth control provide effective contraception without the risks associated with estrogen-containing birth control such as thrombophlebitis, MI, and pulmonary embolism.

Mechanism of Action

- The main mechanism of progestin-only pills (POPs) in preventing pregnancy is suppressing ovulation; therefore, no egg is released for the sperm to fertilize.
- Cervical mucus also thickens, which prevents penetration of sperm.

- Ciliary activity in the fallopian tubes is decreased, which may impede sperm from fertilizing the egg.

- The woman does not need to rely on her partner for birth control and can independently take charge of her undesired fertility.
- There is decreased pain related to the menstrual cycle and endometriosis.
- Lovemaking does not have to be interrupted.

- Unpredictable bleeding patterns
- Does not protect from STIs
- Possible weight gain

Injectable Contraceptives

Depot-medroxyprogesterone acetate (DMPA) or Depo-Provera, an intramuscular injection, and a lower-dose depo-subQ Provera 104, a subcutaneous injection, are injectable forms of contraception that contain only the hormone progestin. Both need to be administered by a nurse or an HCP every 12 weeks.

- **Depo-Provera:** 150 mg/1 mL intramuscular injection once every 12 weeks
- **Depo-subQ Provera dose:** 104 mg/0.65 mL subcutaneous once every 12 weeks

Injectable contraceptives are 91% to 99% effective.

- Convenient dosing; patient does not have to remember to buy, take, or refill any medication for 3 months
- Method may provide more privacy for the patient. There is little visual evidence at the injection site.
- Reversibility; return to ovulation within 9 to 10 months after last dose

- Decrease in bone density with long-term use
- Increased likelihood of depression
- Clearance of medication from body may take 6 to 8 months; if a woman experiences an allergic reaction, adverse effects, or unwanted symptoms, she cannot reverse the effects of DMPA

- It is imperative that a woman is given proper counseling about the menstrual irregularities that could be expected from DMPA use. *You may experience spot bleeding between your periods, longer periods, or no periods at all while on Depo-Provera.*
- Scheduling the next appointment for the patient before she leaves the health facility may increase her likelihood of returning for a follow-up shot. *May we schedule your appointment in 12 weeks for your next Depo-Provera shot before you go?*

- *Depo-Provera will not protect you from STIs. To protect yourself from infections such as gonorrhea, chlamydia, HIV, and hepatitis, you will need to use a condom correctly and consistently every time you have sexual intercourse.*

Implantable Contraceptive

The only implantable contraceptive available in the United States is the single-rod Nexplanon. Nexplanon is 4 cm long and 2 mm in diameter, and contains 68 mg of the hormone progestin. It is inserted in the inner aspect of the patient's upper nondominant arm. Nexplanon is effective for 3 years after insertion.

Effectiveness

Nexplanon is 99% or more effective.

Advantages of Use

- Convenience is a primary advantage of Nexplanon. The patient does not have to remember to buy, take, or refill any medication for 3 years.
- Method may provide more privacy for the patient. Placed in the inner aspect of the upper arm, Nexplanon is barely noticeable.

Disadvantages of Use

- Adverse effects include mood swings, depression, headaches, yeast infection, abdominal pain, vaginal discharge, and breast pain.
- Upfront cost is high.
- HCP needs to place and remove the Nexplanon rod.
- Because the insertion and removal of the Nexplanon rod is a surgical procedure requiring a tiny incision, scarring may form at the site of implantation.

Patient Education

- Once the HCP places the Nexplanon, the patient should be instructed to palpate the rod under the skin for reassurance of placement.
- A reminder card will be filled out by the HCP and given to the patient after insertion. *Keep this reminder card in a safe place. The date of insertion, the date scheduled for removal, which arm the rod was inserted in, the name of the HCP, and the lot number of the device is written on this card.*
- *Once the rod is removed and you are planning to have a baby, the likelihood of you being able to get pregnant is as early as 6 weeks. If you want to continue to avoid pregnancy, you can opt to get a new Nexplanon placed right away or switch to another birth-control method.*
- *When you see other HCPs and are asked what medications you are taking, do not forget to let them know that you have a contraceptive called Nexplanon implanted in your arm.*
- *Contact your HCP if you experience any signs and symptoms of an infection at the site of insertion: redness, swelling, tenderness, warmth, or a foul-smelling discharge.*

Mirena Intrauterine Device

Two types of intrauterine contraceptives, T-shaped devices inserted into the uterus by an HCP, are available in the United States: the Copper T 380 (ParaGuard IUD) introduced in 1988, and the levonorgestrel IUD (Mirena), first sold in the United States in 2001. The Mirena IUD contains the hormone progestin and is effective for 5 years.

Effectiveness
IUDs/IUSs are 99% or more effective.

Mechanism of Action
- The levonorgestrel (a progestin) in the Mirena IUD thickens the cervical mucus and changes the endometrial lining.

Advantages of Use
- Highly effective and safe
- Long-lasting but reversible
- Convenient: no need to remember to take anything on a periodic basis
- May have upfront expense, but then there is nothing to buy for 5 years
- Privacy of choice

Disadvantages of Use
- Discomfort and cramping following insertion
- Irregular and breakthrough bleeding
- Rare possibility of uterine perforation
- Increased risk for ectopic pregnancy
- 2% to 10% rate of IUD expulsion in the first year of insertion
- No protection against STIs
- Provider dependent

Patient Education
- Because the IUD increases the risk for ectopic pregnancy, the patient should be instructed to come in for evaluation if she suspects a pregnancy.
- There is a small risk for infection during the insertion process, but the patient is not at a greater risk for pelvic inflammatory disease (PID) due to the IUD alone.
- Teach the patient to check for the strings coming out of her cervix, and if she does not feel the strings, she will need to alert the HCP to confirm that the IUD was not expelled.

Progestin-Only Pills

Introduced in 1973, there are only a few brands of oral contraceptive pills that do not contain estrogen; these are called *POPs*, or "mini-pills."

Brands Available in United States
POPs currently available in the United States are Micronor, Nor-QD, and Ovrette.

Effectiveness
POPs are 91% to 99% effective.

Advantages of Use
- Highly effective but may be contingent on POPs being taken at the same time each day

- Can be used safely by most women 35 years and older
- Can be used by most women who smoke

- Inconvenient and easy to forget to consistently take the pill at the same time each day
- Prescription from an HCP is required

The nurse should give the client detailed instructions on how to take the pills.
- *For the first 48 hours after taking your first pill, you will need to abstain from sexual intercourse or use a backup method of birth control such as condoms.*
- *Because there are no hormone-free days with this type of pill, you will need to make sure your next pack is available by the time you are done with your current pill pack. There should not be any breaks between packs.*

Nonhormonal Options
Nonhormonal options include the following:
- Barrier methods
- Copper intrauterine device

Barrier Methods
- No hormones; therefore, no adverse effects, such as irregular menstrual bleeding or increased risk for thromboembolic events associated with some hormonal contraception
- Quick reversibility

- Lovemaking may be disturbed
- Effectiveness not as high as with COCs, injectables, or the contraceptive patch or ring
- Need to remember to use for each sexual encounter

Condom, Female
The Reality female condom made of polyurethane was approved by the FDA in 2003, and the FC2 female condom made of synthetic rubber was approved in early 2009.

Female condoms are 81% to 90% effective.

- The Reality condom may be used by women with latex allergies.
- A female-controlled birth-control method that also provides STI protection
- No need for prescription
- The Reality condom may be inserted ahead of time, so it does not interrupt lovemaking.

- Allergy/sensitivity to polyurethane
- May be cumbersome and nondiscreet

- The Reality condom comes coated with nonspermicidal lubricant on both the inside and outside parts of the sheath, and may be inserted up to 8 hours before sexual intercourse.
- *Insert the flexible ring with the closed part of the sheath into the vagina; the other ring lies outside of the vaginal opening.*

Vaginal Barriers

Approved by the FDA in 2003, the FemCap is a soft cap made of rubber that comes in three different sizes to fit the cervix. Lea's Shield is a rubber disk that is dome shaped to cover the cervix; it was approved by the FDA in 2002.

Effectiveness

Vaginal barriers are 80% effective.

Advantage of Use

A vaginal barrier may have a high cost upfront, but it is reusable.

Disadvantages of Use

- Latex allergy/sensitivity
- Risk for toxic shock syndrome (TSS)
- Increased risk for urinary tract infection (UTI)

Patient Education

- *Apply spermicide on the inside of the FemCap or Lea's Shield before inserting. Press against the cervix for a complete seal to act as a barrier against sperm.*
- *If additional acts of intercourse are to occur, apply additional spermicide with Lea's Shield without removing the device. No additional spermicide is needed for FemCap.*
- *Leave the FemCap in place for 6 hours and the Lea's Shield for 8 hours. The FemCap and Lea's Shield may be left in for up to 48 hours.*
- *After pregnancy or childbirth, you will need to be refitted for a new FemCap. You do not need to be refitted if you are using Lea's Shield.*

Diaphragm

The diaphragm is a rubber dome that was first described by a German gynecologist in the 1880s and was introduced in the United States by Margaret Sanger in 1916.

Effectiveness

A diaphragm is 81% to 90% effective.

Mechanism of Action

A diaphragm serves as a barrier that protects the cervix from sperm.

Advantage of Use

A diaphragm may have a high cost upfront, but it is reusable.

Disadvantages of Use

- Does not offer complete protection against STIs because the vaginal mucosa is still exposed to semen and penis
- Latex allergies/sensitivity; however, a silicone option is available
- Need for refitting if there is weight gain and after delivery of a baby
- Increased risk for UTI

- The nurse should teach the client how to use the diaphragm: *Apply spermicide on the inside dome of the diaphragm and insert the diaphragm before having sexual intercourse (up to 6 hours prior). The diaphragm needs to be left in place for 6 hours after intercourse. If another sexual encounter is expected, the diaphragm may be left in for 24 hours, but additional spermicide should be inserted with an applicator for better protection.*
- There are different types of diaphragms, and the HCP should fit the client for the right kind and size. The nurse or other HCP should teach the patient how to insert, remove, and check for proper positioning of the diaphragm at the office.
- The HCP should also ask the client if she is allergic to latex, and if she is, prescribe a type of diaphragm made of silicone instead of latex.

Sponge

The sponge was introduced in the United States in 1983, but production was discontinued in 1995. The Today sponge was re-introduced to the U.S. market in 2005.

Effectiveness

The sponge is 81% to 90% effective.

Advantage of Use

The sponge is available over the counter.

Disadvantages of Use
- Cost; the sponge is not reusable; a new one needs to be used each time
- Less effective in parous women

Patient Education
- *Moisten the sponge with tap water, squeeze, and insert it in the vagina before intercourse. It needs to stay in place for 6 hours after sex and may be left in the vagina for 24 to 30 hours.*
- *The vaginal sponge already contains the spermicide nonoxynol-9, and there is no need to re-apply spermicide with additional acts of intercourse.*

Condom, Male

Male condoms are the third most widely used method of birth control. More than 13 million reproductive-age women have their partner use this method to prevent pregnancy and provide protection against STIs.

Effectiveness

The male condom is 81% to 90% effective.

Types
- Latex
- Natural membrane (lambskin)
- Synthetic (polyurethane)

Advantages of Use
- Low cost and easy access
- No need for a prescription
- Provides some protection against STIs

Disadvantages of Use
- Latex allergy or sensitivity
- Some men complain of having problems with erection and decreased sensation with condom usage.
- Male partners may not be cooperative with condom use.

ALERT

Natural membrane (lambskin) condoms are more porous than latex condoms and may not provide the same efficacy in preventing STIs, such as HIV, herpes simplex virus, and hepatitis.

Patient Education
- *Condoms provide some protection against STIs. I encourage you to use condoms each time you have oral, vaginal, or anal sex to decrease your risk for STIs, even if you are already using another form of birth control, such as COCs, Depo-Provera, Nexplanon, or intrauterine device (IUD).*
- *If you are sexually active, have condoms on hand and ready for use with every sexual encounter. Have backup condoms available in case slippage or breakage occurs.*
- Pregnant women and their partners should continue to wear condoms for STI prevention and to protect themselves and the fetus from infection.
- *Preventing STIs now may contribute to the preservation of your future fertility. If left untreated, some STIs may lead to pelvic inflammatory disease (PID) and increase the risk for infertility and ectopic pregnancy.*
- *Before genital contact, a new condom should be placed at the tip of an erect penis. While holding the tip of the condom (also called the reservoir pouch to collect semen upon ejaculation), the condom is rolled down to the base of the penis. After ejaculation, the condom should be held at the base of the erect penis while the penis is withdrawn from the vagina to prevent leakage or slippage of the condom. The condom should then be discarded in a receptacle out of the reach of children and animals (see Fig. 7–1).*

TIP

Do not use a female condom or another male condom for a second layer of protection because the two condoms may create friction and lead to breakage or slippage.

Spermicide
Spermicide comes in different forms: foam, cream, gel, suppository, and film.

Mechanism of Action
Spermicides help prevent sperm from fertilizing the egg by blocking the cervix and making the sperm immotile.

Effectiveness
Spermicides are moderately effective (80%)

Advantages of Use
- Available over the counter
- Easy to use

TIP

Oil-based lubricants, such as petroleum jelly (Vaseline), vaginal infection medications, massage oil, cooking oil (vegetable, peanut, canola, olive), body lotion, and suntan lotion may decrease the integrity

Continued

TIP—cont'd

of latex condoms, which
may lead to breakage.
Polyurethane condoms
are not affected by these
oil-based lubricants.

Water-based lubricants,
such as Slippery Stuff, K-Y
Jelly, and Astroglide, do
not have an effect on latex
or polyurethane condoms
and are considered safe for
use with either type of condom. Although saliva does
not break down condoms
and may be an alternative
lubricant, it may carry
pathogens such as herpes,
which can be transmitted
from one partner to the
other if used as lubrication.

Disadvantages of Use
- Irritation/sensitivity/allergy
- Increased risk for UTI

Patient Education

You need to insert the spermicide 5 to 90 minutes before intercourse, depending on the type of spermicide used.

ParaGard Intrauterine Device

Copper T 380

The Copper T 380 does not contain hormones and is effective for 10 years, though more recent studies have shown effectiveness for as many as 12 years.

Effectiveness

IUDs are 99% or more effective.

Mechanism of Action
- ParaGard prevents sperm from fertilizing the egg by increasing macrophages, prostaglandins, copper ions, and enzymes in the uterus and fallopian tubes.

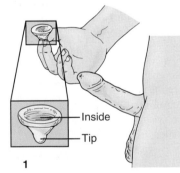

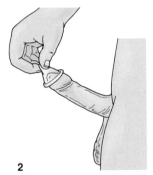

— Inside

— Tip

1

2

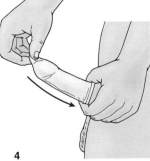

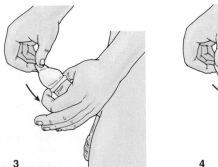

3

4

FIGURE 7-1: How to use a male condom.

- Highly effective and safe
- Long-lasting but reversible
- Convenient: no need to remember to take anything on a periodic basis
- May have upfront expense, but then there is nothing to buy for 10 years
- Privacy of choice

- Discomfort and cramping following insertion
- Irregular bleeding
- Rare possibility of uterine perforation
- Increased risk for ectopic pregnancy
- 2% to 10% rate of IUD expulsion in the first year of insertion
- No protection against STIs
- Provider dependent

- Because the IUD increases the risk for ectopic pregnancy, the patient should be instructed to come in for evaluation if she suspects a pregnancy.
- There is a small risk for infection during the insertion process, but the patient is not at a greater risk for PID due to the IUD alone.
- Teach the patient to check for the strings coming out of her cervix, and if she does not feel the strings, she will need to alert the HCP to confirm that the IUD was not expelled.

Fertility Awareness-Based Methods

Fertility awareness-based methods include the calendar days method, standard days method, billings ovulation method, symptothermal method, and two-day method.

Effectiveness

Fertility awareness-based methods are 80% effective.

Mechanism of Action

The mechanism of action of fertility awareness-based methods identifies the fertile days in a woman's cycle, so sexual intercourse can be avoided during those days (see Fig. 7–2).

Types of Fertility Awareness-Based Methods

The nurse should explain the different types of fertility awareness methods and provide patients with instructions on how to use each method.

- **Billings ovulation method:** based on amount and consistency of cervical mucus
- **Calendar days method:** based on record of menstrual cycle for 6 months to 1 year
- **Standard days method:** based on expected days of ovulation in each cycle

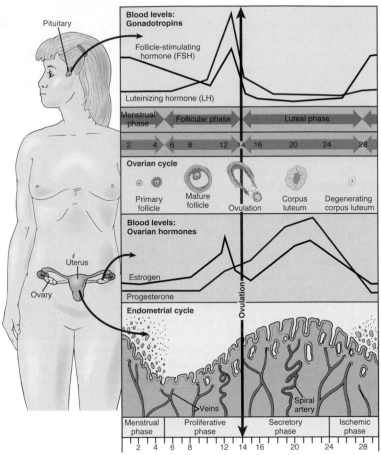

FIGURE 7-2: The menstrual cycle.

- **Symptothermal method:** based on cervical mucus and basal body temperature (BBT)
- **Two-day method:** based on cervical mucus presence or absence

Advantages of Use

- No exogenous hormones involved
- Inexpensive method; may only need to buy a calendar and thermometer
- Reversible; can use same method to identify fertile days to increase chance of pregnancy

Disadvantages of Use

- No protection against STIs
- During potential fertile days (which may be one-third of the woman's cycle), woman may not engage in sexual intercourse

- **Billings ovulation method:** *Starting the first day after your period ends, track the amount and texture of your cervical mucus. The secretions start off as sticky with a cloudy color. During your fertile days, the secretions will change to clear, slippery, copious in amount, and stretchy. Avoid sex 3 days before and 2 to 3 days after this type of cervical secretion.*
- **Calendar days method:** *Keep track of your cycle for 6 months to 1 year, making note of your shortest and longest menstrual cycles. Subtract 18 days from the shortest cycle and 11 days from the longest cycle. The numbers that you get are the start and end of the days you are fertile. For example, if your shortest cycle is 26 days and your longest cycle is 32 days, your fertile days are day 8 through day 21, and you should avoid sexual intercourse on those days.*
- **Standard days method:** *Count the first day of your period as day 1 and avoid sexual intercourse between days 8 and 19.*
- **Symptothermal method:** *Combined with the ovulation method, take your BBT every morning at the same time before getting out of bed and record your BBT readings on a chart. Around the time of ovulation, there will likely be a 0.4°F increase in your BBT, which will remain elevated until the start of the next menstrual cycle.*
- **Two-day method:** *If you noticed any type of cervical secretions today or yesterday, you should consider yourself fertile today and avoid sexual intercourse. If you did not notice the presence of cervical mucus, you are likely not fertile at this time.*

Permanent Forms of Contraception

Tubal Ligation

Tubal ligation is a form of permanent female sterilization performed surgically by a medical doctor (see Fig. 7–3).

Mechanism of Action

In tubal ligation, there is mechanical blockage or cutting of the fallopian tubes to inhibit sperm from fertilizing an egg.

QSEN APPLICATION

Integration of evidence-based practice includes knowledge such as:
- Examining how the safety, quality, and cost-effectiveness of health care can be improved through the active involvement of patients and families
- Examining common barriers to active involvement of patients in their own health-care processes
- Describing strategies to empower patients or families in all aspects of the health-care process

In this chapter, together with information about care of pregnant women and newborns, QSEN competencies assure delivery of the best nursing care.

http://qsen.org/competencies/pre-licensure-ksas/#patient-centered_care

---

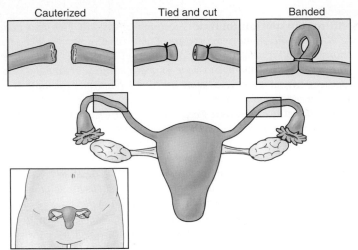

FIGURE 7-3: Bilateral tubal ligation.

Essure

Essure is a form of female sterilization approved by the FDA in 2002.

Mechanism of Action

Small metallic coils are inserted transcervically into the fallopian tubes. Scarring occurs, blocking the fallopian tubes and preventing sperm from fertilizing the egg.

Vasectomy

Vasectomy is a form of male sterilization that is safe and effective. It is performed in an outpatient facility using local anesthetics.

Mechanism of Action

The man's vas deferens is cut, tied, or sealed to prevent sperm from traveling to the penis from the testicles (see Fig. 7-4).

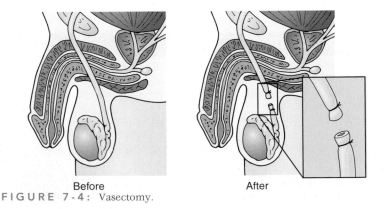

Before   After

FIGURE 7-4: Vasectomy.

Permanent forms of contraception are >99% effective.

- Permanence of procedure
- Highly effective and safe
- Choice can be made privately
- Overall cost-effectiveness
- Nonhormonal option
- Lovemaking does not have to be interrupted.

- The procedure is permanent.
- If failure of method occurs, there is increased risk for ectopic pregnancy.
- Procedure offers no protection against STIs.
- There is a high occurrence of regret associated with tubal ligation.
- Essure is not immediately effective. The woman must use another form of birth control for 3 months after the surgery and confirm with her HCP that coil placement and blockage have occurred before using it as a sole method of birth control.
- Permanent forms of birth control may not be available to women under 21.
- A vasectomy is not immediately effective in preventing pregnancy. Need to use backup birth control for 12 weeks and/or 15 to 20 ejaculations. May need confirmation that semen does not contain sperm for reassurance that the surgery was successful.
- There may be mild-to-moderate pain after these procedures.

Postpartum Use of Birth Control

Hormonal Birth Control
Hormonal birth control includes both combined birth control and progestin-only birth control.

Combined Birth Control
Combined birth control includes COC, contraceptive patch (Ortho Evra), and contraceptive ring (NuvaRing). If the woman is exclusively breastfeeding, she may wish to delay using combined birth control until 6 months postpartum because of the theoretical risk of decreasing the supply of breast milk. If the woman is supplementing breastfeeding with formula, the American Academy of Pediatrics supports starting COCs sooner, but no earlier than 3 to 4 weeks postpartum. If the woman is not breastfeeding, she may start combined birth control at 3 to 4 weeks postpartum, but no sooner as she is still in a hypercoagulable state.

Progestin-Only Birth Control
Progestin-only birth control includes POPs (Micronor), contraceptive implant (Nexplanon), injectables (Depo-Provera, depo-subQ), and Mirena IUS. If the woman is breastfeeding, it is recommended to delay use of progestin-only birth control until 6 weeks postpartum because

of the theoretical risk for a decrease in breast milk production. The nurse needs to collaborate with the HCP and patient regarding risks and benefits. If the woman is not breastfeeding, Nexplanon and Depo-Provera may be inserted/administered immediately postpartum. POPs may be started sooner than 6 weeks postpartum. Mirena IUS should not be inserted earlier than 3 weeks postpartum.

Nonhormonal Birth Control

Nonhormonal birth control methods include abstinence, barrier methods and spermicide, copper IUDs, sterilization, and several other methods.

Abstinence, Coitus Interruptus, Fertility Awareness-Based Methods, and Lactational Amenorrhea Method

Regardless of whether the patient is breastfeeding, the woman may use abstinence, coitus interruptus, fertility awareness-based methods, and lactational amenorrhea method (LAM) immediately postpartum.

Barrier Method and Spermicide

FemCap, Lea's Shield, female and male condoms, and spermicide may be used immediately postpartum regardless of whether the woman is breast-feeding. Use of a diaphragm or sponge should be delayed up to 6 weeks postpartum regardless of whether the woman is breastfeeding because of the increased risk for TSS and the need for refitting the diaphragm.

Copper Intrauterine Device

A copper IUD may be inserted immediately after expulsion of the placenta regardless of whether the woman is breastfeeding. In women who had a spontaneous vertex delivery, the rate of IUD expulsion was 50%. In a study of women who had a cesarean section, there was no expulsion of an IUD when it was placed through the hysterotomy site transoperatively. In delayed postpartum insertion, the IUD is inserted within 48 hours after delivery. An IUD can also be inserted after discharge in the outpatient OB/GYN setting.

Sterilization: Tubal Ligation, Essure, and Vasectomy

A tubal ligation may be done during a caesarean section or after a vaginal delivery before discharge, or it may be done at 6 weeks (or later) postpartum regardless of whether the woman is breastfeeding. Essure is typically done after 6 weeks postpartum regardless of whether the woman is breastfeeding. A vasectomy is done on the male individual and thus has no effect on lactation.

Emergency Contraception

Emergency contraception helps prevent pregnancy after unprotected sexual intercourse. Emergency contraception does not result in abortion and will not harm an established pregnancy; instead, it either prevents or delays ovulation. There are two options for emergency contraception, in the form of a pill or intrauterine device.

Emergency Contraceptive Pills
Currently, in the United States, about two dozen brands of combined hormonal birth control pills can be taken in specific doses to be used as emergency contraception. Only four products in the United States have been approved specifically by the FDA as emergency contraceptive pills (ECPs): Plan B One-Step, Plan B, Next Choice, and Ella. These ECPs contain progestin only, except for Ella, which contains ulipristal acetate.

Intrauterine Device
The Copper T IUD is used by women as a form of contraception; however, it can also be effectively used as a form of emergency contraception that is inserted by a trained clinician up to 5 days after unprotected sexual intercourse. The device can then be left in place as a form of long-term contraception for 10 years.

Patient Education
- ECPs are not as effective as birth control methods such as the Ortho Evra patch, NuvaRing, Nexplanon, and sterilization. ECPs should not be used as a form of contraception.
- Although ECPs are commonly referred to as the "morning-after pill," women should not delay taking ECPs until the morning after; instead, they should take ECPs as soon as possible after unprotected sex. ECPs can be taken up to 5 days after unprotected sex, but are more effective the sooner they are taken.
- The Copper T IUD is a much more effective form of emergency contraception than ECPs.
- Neither ECPs nor the Copper T IUD protect from STIs.

8 Sexually Transmitted Infections

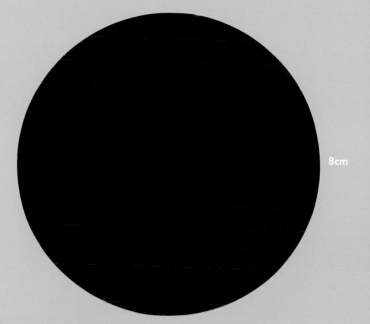

8cm

CHAPTER 8

Sexually Transmitted Infections

As the nurse, you have an important role in educating patients on ways to prevent the spread of sexually transmitted infections (STIs). Obtaining a thorough sexual history from your patient is integral for the following tasks:

- Identifying persons at risk for STIs who need further education and counseling on prevention
- Recognizing asymptomatic and symptomatic individuals who are infected with an STI and referring them to a practitioner for proper diagnosis, treatment, and management
- Counseling and referral for treatment of infected partners
- Providing vaccination for individuals at risk for vaccine-preventable STIs

Counseling and education regarding STIs require skills that foster mutual respect between you and the patient. A matter-of-fact and nonjudgmental approach should be taken to facilitate effective nonbiased communication. Remember to take into consideration the patient's age, educational and developmental levels, sexual orientation, language, culture, and religious background in providing client-centered counseling. A complete sexual health history is essential (see Box 8–1).

This chapter discusses the most common reproductive tract infections, focusing on women but providing some pertinent information about STIs in male individuals. This chapter identifies the causes and most common signs and symptoms for each disease; the diagnostic criteria for the disease; treatment measures; effects of the disease in pregnant, nonpregnant, and lactating women; and its effect, if any, on the fetus or neonate. The effects of treatment for the disease, including the category of safety in which the U.S. Food and Drug Administration (FDA) classifies a drug used during pregnancy, are also included in this chapter.

For more comprehensive treatment regimens, please refer to the Centers for Disease Control and Prevention's (CDC's) Sexually Transmitted Disease Treatment Guidelines 2010 in *Morbidity and Mortality*

Weekly Report and to the CDC Web site for updated information (www. cdc.gov/mmwr/pdf/rr/rr5912.pdf).

Most of the infections discussed in this chapter are transmitted through sexual activity (e.g., vaginal, rectal, oral). In fact, diseases such as gonorrhea, chlamydia, and syphilis are almost exclusively transmitted sexually. However, some diseases such as bacterial vaginosis (BV) and candidiasis may be caused by altered vaginal flora.

Bacterial Vaginosis

BV is the most common cause of malodorous vaginal discharge. However, more than half of women with BV do not have any symptoms. When normal vaginal flora is altered, anaerobic bacteria replace the normally occurring *Lactobacillus* species and cause vaginosis. It is not clear whether BV is transmitted sexually; however, it is linked with having multiple sex partners or a new sex partner, and it rarely affects women who are not sexually active.

SPEAKING OUT

To decrease the risk for STI exposure, patients should be educated on using condoms consistently with every sexual encounter, educated on abstaining from sexual intercourse, counseled to delay sexual debut, and encouraged to be involved in a mutually monogamous relationship and to refrain from having multiple partners.

Cause

Several species of bacteria can cause BV: *Gardnerella vaginalis*, *Mycoplasma hominis*, *Prevotella* species, and *Mobiluncus* species.

Risk Factors

Risk factors for BV include:
- New or multiple sex partners, female or male
- Douching
- Lack of condom use

Signs and Symptoms
- Thin gray–white vaginal discharge
- Fishy odor

Diagnosis

BV is diagnosed in two ways:
1. **Gold standard:** Gram stain
2. **Amsel's criteria:** Three of the four following signs and symptoms are needed to diagnose BV:
   - Homogeneous, thin, white discharge
   - Presence of characteristic clue cells on microscopy
   - Vaginal fluid pH >4.5
   - Fishy odor with or without addition of 10% potassium hydroxide (KOH)—Whiff test

Treatment

- Metronidazole (Flagyl) 500 mg PO bid for 7 days (Category B but contraindicated in first trimester) *or*
  - Metronidazole (Flagyl) 250 mg PO tid for 7 days (Category B but contraindicated in first trimester) *or*
  - Clindamycin 300 mg PO bid for 7 days

ALERT!

Weakening of condoms and diaphragms may occur with the use of clindamycin cream for up to 5 days after intravaginal insertion of the medication. Alternative forms of birth control should be discussed with the patient.

Partner Management

According to the CDC, treating the male partners of patients with BV has not been proved beneficial because it does not prevent recurrence.

Effects on Women

BV is associated with the following effects on women:

- Increased susceptibility to HIV, if exposed to an HIV-positive partner
- Pelvic inflammatory disease (PID)
- Endometritis

During Pregnancy

During pregnancy, BV is associated with the following:

- Premature rupture of membranes
- Preterm labor
- Preterm birth
- Chorioamnionitis
- Postpartum endometritis
- Post-cesarean wound infection

While Breastfeeding

Maternal intravenous (IV) and oral (PO) metronidazole therapy has been proved in studies to cross into breast milk. Opinions vary among experts on the use of metronidazole while breastfeeding. Some sources advise that women may need to supplement and put breastfeeding on hold for 12 to 24 hours to allow for excretion of the drug. Advise the patient to discuss breastfeeding with the prescribing clinician. The mother may consider using a breast pump to maintain milk supply during this time and discard the pumped breast milk.

Effects on Fetus

Data conflict regarding whether there are effects on the fetus, but possible effects include the following:

- Preterm birth, possibly
- Low birth weight, possibly

The manufacturer of metronidazole (Flagyl) considers the drug contraindicated in the first trimester of pregnancy but acceptable in the second and third trimesters.

Effect on Infant
Infants exposed to metronidazole (Flagyl) might have a higher oral and rectal colonization of *Candida*.

Effect on Men
Although the bacteria that cause BV have been retrieved from male genitalia, men do not experience the signs and symptoms that women experience.

Chlamydia

Chlamydia is the most commonly reported STI in the United States. It is transmitted via the vaginal, anal, or oral route and affects both men and women. Chlamydia can also be transmitted vertically from an infected mother to her newborn. People diagnosed with chlamydia have a high rate of other STIs.

> **WHY IS SCREENING FOR *CHLAMYDIA* IMPORTANT?**
>
> Because women with *chlamydia* often do not become symptomatic until the infection has traveled from the cervix to the upper genital tract, screening of women at risk is recommended. Populations at risk for chlamydia include women with new partners, women who have several partners, and sexually active women 25 years or younger.

Cause
The cause of chlamydia is *Chlamydia trachomatis*.

Signs and Symptoms
About 75% of infected women and about half of men infected with chlamydia have no symptoms. If symptoms do occur, they include the following:
- Vaginal or penile discharge
- Burning on urination
- Dyspareunia
- Vaginal bleeding between periods
- Lower abdominal and back pain
- Rectal pain (Chlamydia may spread to the rectum and cause rectal pain. Pain in the rectum can be associated with a rectal infection that can manifest after participating in receptive anal intercourse for both men and women.)
- Sore throat in men and women participating in oral sex with an infected individual

Diagnosis
- Culture (gold standard but is expensive and takes several days for results)
- Nucleic acid amplification test (NAAT), using first-catch urine or vaginal swab, is the most sensitive test for chlamydia

- Direct immunofluorescence
- Enzyme immunoassays
- Nucleic hybridization

Treatment
- Azithromycin (Zithromax) 1 g PO once (Category B) *or*
- Amoxicillin 500 mg PO tid for 7 days

Partner Management
According to the CDC, sexual partners of patients diagnosed with chlamydia should be evaluated, tested, and treated. Abstinence is recommended for 7 days after both partners are treated.

Effects on Women
Effects of chlamydia infection on women include the following:
- If untreated, the infection may spread to the upper genital tract and cause PID.
- Chlamydial infection makes a woman five times more susceptible to HIV.

During Pregnancy
- Chlamydial infection may lead to preterm birth.
- Infection may be passed to the neonate during its passage through the birth canal.
- Doxycycline, ofloxacin, and levofloxacin are contraindicated in pregnancy.

Effects on Fetus/Infant
Effects of chlamydia infection on the fetus or infant include the following:
- Preterm birth
- Ophthalmic neonatorum (conjunctivitis, or "pink eye") that develops around 5 to 12 days of age
- Pneumonia may develop within 1 to 3 months after birth.

Effect on Men
Untreated chlamydia in men may spread to the epididymis and cause infertility, but this is rare.

Gonorrhea

Gonorrhea is the second most prevalent sexually transmitted bacterial disease in the United States. It is transmitted through sexual contact and childbirth. This infection can affect any part of the female reproductive tract—the cervix, fallopian tubes, and uterus—and in male individuals, it can affect the penis, urethra, and testes. It can also affect other moist mucosa of the body such as the mouth, throat, eyes, and anus.

Risks
Risks for gonorrhea in women include:
- Age ≤25 years
- Previous gonorrhea infection
- New partners and/or several partners
- Use of illicit drugs
- Prostitution
- Inconsistent use of condoms

Cause
The cause of gonorrhea is *Neisseria gonorrhoeae*.

Signs and Symptoms
- Mild or maybe asymptomatic
- White, yellow, or green vaginal discharge/yellowish penile discharge
- Burning and/or pain on urination
- Dyspareunia
- Vaginal bleeding between periods

Diagnosis
Diagnosis of gonorrhea of determined by the following:
- Culture
- NAAT
- Nucleic hybridization tests

Treatment
Ceftriaxone 250 mg IM once (Category B)
plus
Azithromycin 1 g PO once if chlamydial infection is not ruled out

Partner Management
According to the CDC, sexual partners should be evaluated, tested, and treated.

Effects on Women
Untreated infection can spread to upper genital tract and cause PID, which can cause irreversible damage to the uterus and fallopian tubes that may lead to infertility and increased risk for ectopic pregnancy.

During Pregnancy
- Gonorrhea may lead to preterm birth.
- The infection may be passed to the neonate.

Effects on Infant

Effects of gonorrhea on infants include:

- Ophthalmia neonatorum (conjunctivitis, or "pink eye") that may develop when newborn is 2 to 5 days of age
- Sepsis that may also develop and can include meningitis

Effect on Men

If left untreated, gonorrhea can cause epididymitis and lead to infertility.

Human Papillomavirus Infection

There are more than 100 known human papillomavirus (HPV) types, one-third of which can cause an infection of the genitalia in both men and women. HPV is the most common viral STI. Some types (16, 18, 31, 33, 35) are associated with an increased risk for genital cancers, particularly cervical cancer, whereas other types (commonly types 6 and 11) are associated with genital warts (see later).

HPV is transmitted primarily through sexual contact (penis in the vagina) and possibly through oral–genital and hand–genital transmission, although very unlikely. HPV can also be vertically transmitted from mother to neonate. An HPV infection is frequently self-limiting and will likely not need treatment.

Cause

The cause of HPV is usually high-risk types 16, 18, 31, 33, and 35.

Signs and Symptoms

- Usually asymptomatic
- May cause changes in cervix noted on a Papanicolaou (Pap) smear
- May cause genital warts (cervical, vulvar, penile)
- High-risk types may cause cervical, vulvar, vaginal, anogenital, and penile cancers

Diagnosis

The diagnosis of HPV is determined by the following:

- DNA test on cervical cells scraped from the cervix to detect HPV
- Colposcopy
- Biopsy
- Acetic acid application (Applying 5% acetic acid solution will cause lesions, if present, to turn white.)

Treatment

No actual treatment for HPV exists because it is a virus. Most HPV infections will resolve on their own without treatment. The following interventions are not recommended unless cervical squamous intraepithelial lesion has been detected:

- Cryotherapy
- Loop electrosurgical excision process (LEEP)
- Laser
- Cone biopsy

Effects on Women

Many high-risk types of HPV cause cervical dysplasia and have been linked to cancer. However, most females with HPV do not experience development of cancer.

During Pregnancy

Depending on severity of dysplasia, intervention is usually delayed until the postpartum period.

Effect on Fetus/Infant

High-risk HPV types have not been proved to cause problems in infants.

Effects on Men

The effects of HPV on men include the following:

- 1 in 100,000 risk for penile cancer
- Anal cancer is rare, but men having sex with men are 17 times more likely to experience development of anal cancer than heterosexual men

Genital Warts

Some types of HPV are associated with genital warts. Sometimes called *Condylomata acuminata*, the warts may be raised or flat, small or large, and sometimes occur in clusters that look like cauliflower bumps. They may occur in women in the vulva, cervix, and in and around the vagina and anus; in men, they may occur on the penis and/or scrotum.

Cause

HPV, usually low-risk types 6 and/or 11, causes genital warts; occasionally, HPV types 16, 18, 31, 33, and 35 are the cause. Commonly, genital warts are caused by multiple types of HPV.

Signs and Symptoms

- Warts may be cauliflower-like.
- Dome-shaped or flat papules that are slightly raised and may be painful
- Color varies from skin color, pink to hyperpigmented.

Diagnosis
Diagnosis of genital warts is made by the following:
- Visual inspection
- Biopsy

Treatment
Patient Applied
Patient-applied treatment of genital warts for nonpregnant women includes the following:
- **Podofilox 0.5% solution or gel:** Apply bid for 3 days and then stop for 4 days. May repeat cycle four times (Category C).
- **Imiquimod (Aldara) 5% cream:** Apply at night 3 times a week up to 16 weeks. Wash with soap and water 6 to 10 hours after application (Category C).

Provider Administered
Provider-administered treatment of genital warts includes the following:
- Cryotherapy with liquid nitrogen to lesion
- Podophyllin (Podofin) resin 10% to 25% in compound tincture of benzoin directly to lesion; wash off after 4 hours; not to be used in pregnancy
- Trichloroacetic acid to lesion
- Surgical removal

Partner Management
Counseling and examination of sexual partners for genital warts and other STIs are recommended.

⭐ BEST PRACTICES

Gardasil® and Cervarix® are vaccines against HPV types that cause most cervical cancers. They are recommended for women between 9 and 26 years old. Gardasil® is the only vaccine that can be given to male individuals between 9 and 26 years old to protect them against genital warts. The vaccine is given intramuscularly in three divided doses over a 6-month period, ideally before sexual debut. However, commencement of sexual activity does not exclude a female from receiving the vaccine. Safety in pregnancy has not been established, and Gardasil® administration should be avoided until the postpartum period.

QSEN Application

Integration of evidence-based practice includes attitudes such as:
- Appreciating strengths and weaknesses of scientific bases for practice
- Valuing the need for ethical conduct of research and quality improvement
- Valuing the concept of evidence-based practice as integral to determining best clinical practice

In this chapter, together with information about care of pregnant women and newborns, QSEN competencies assure delivery of the best nursing care.

http://qsen.org/competencies/pre-licensure-ksas/#patient-centered_care

Effects on Women
The effects of genital warts on women include the following:
- There is no evidence to associate the development of cervical cancer with untreated genital warts.
- Some patients will clear warts on their own without treatment. Recurrence may occur within 6 to 12 weeks after treatment.

During Pregnancy
Use of podofilox, imiquimod, and podophyllin should be avoided.

Effects on Fetus/Infant
The effects of genital warts on the fetus and infant include the following:
- HPV types 6 and 11 can cause respiratory papillomatosis in infants and children.
- If a child develops warts in the conjunctiva, larynx, vulva, or anus within the first 1 to 3 years of life, there is a high likelihood that the mother has an HPV infection that is the causative agent.

Effect on Men
In the United States, an estimated 1% of sexually active men have genital warts.

Hepatitis A

Replication of the hepatitis A virus (HAV) happens in the liver, and the virus is shed in high concentration via the feces; thus, hepatitis A is primarily spread through the fecal–oral route. During sexual activity, transmission may occur if fecal–oral contact occurs. Transmission may also occur if contaminated food or water is ingested. This disease does not lead to chronic liver infection and is self-limiting.

Cause
The cause of hepatitis A is HAV.

Signs and Symptoms
- Fever
- Fatigue
- Loss of appetite
- Nausea
- Vomiting
- Abdominal pain
- Dark urine
- Clay-colored bowel movements
- Joint pain
- Jaundice

Diagnosis
Serology positive for immunoglobulin M (IgM) antibody to HAV indicates acute infection.

Treatment

Treatment for HAV includes the following:
- Supportive care unless hospitalization for dehydration resulting from excessive nausea and vomiting is needed.
- Avoid medications that are metabolized by the liver.

Effects on Women

Effects of HAV on female individuals include the following:
- HAV infection is self-limited and does not cause chronic infection.
- Acute liver failure from hepatitis A is rare.

Effects on Fetus/Infant

Effects of HAV on the fetus and infant include the following:
- Vertical transmission is rare.
- Vaccine cannot be given to infant younger than 12 months.

Effect on Men

Men who have sex with other men are at a greater risk for acquiring HAV.

Hepatitis B

The transmission of the causative agent responsible for hepatitis B, the hepatitis B virus (HBV), can occur through vertical transmission (infected mother to neonate), sexual contact, use of illicit injected drugs, sharing products such as toothbrushes and razors, accidental needle sticks, or exposure to infected blood or an open sore of an infected person.

Cause

The cause of hepatitis B is HBV.

Signs and Symptoms

Signs and symptoms of hepatitis B are similar to those for hepatitis A.

Diagnosis

Diagnosis of hepatitis B is determined by the following:
- Serology positive for the surface antigen of the HBV (HBsAg) indicates acute and chronic infection.

- Positive IgM anti-HB core antigen (anti-HBc) indicates either acute or recently acquired HBV infection.
- Presence of anti-HBsAg indicates a resolved infection or immunity by vaccination.

Treatment
- No medication is available to treat acute HBV.
- People with chronic HBV should be closely monitored by an infectious disease specialist and/or gastroenterologist.

Effects on Women
Hepatitis B may lead to chronic HBV infection, premature death because of cirrhosis, or hepatocellular carcinoma.

During Pregnancy
Vertical transmission of hepatitis B is possible during pregnancy.

While Breastfeeding
Women with hepatitis B can breastfeed, but immunizations with hepatitis B vaccine and hepatitis B immunoglobulin (HBIg) are needed within 12 hours of the neonate's life. The second dose of the hepatitis B vaccine should be given at age 1 to 2 months and the third dose at age 6 months. After the completion of the vaccine series at age 9 to 18 months, the infant should be tested for hepatitis B to determine if the vaccine worked and to establish that the infant is not infected with the hepatitis B virus from exposure to the infected mother's blood during delivery.

Effects on Fetus/Infant
The effects of hepatitis B on the fetus and infant include:
- Vertical transmission from infected mother to infant
- Usually asymptomatic
- A 90% chance of development of chronic HBV

⭐ BEST PRACTICES

Vaccination is available for the prevention of hepatitis B. It is an intramuscular injection given in three doses (0, 1, and 6 months apart). Immunization against HBV is recommended for all infants (with the initial dose given at birth), all nonvaccinated persons younger than 19 years, and individuals exposed to HBsAg-positive persons in their household. The following are individuals at high risk for contracting the disease; they should be counseled to obtain the vaccine:
- Sexual partners of HBsAg-positive persons
- IV drug users
- Men who have sex with men
- Men and women who are not monogamous
- Patients receiving hemodialysis treatments
- Health-care workers

If mother is acutely infected, hepatitis B vaccine and HBIg are needed within 12 hours of the neonate's life

Effect on Men
Men who have sex with other men are at a greater risk for acquiring HBV.

Hepatitis C

Hepatitis C is likely transmitted through exposure to contaminated blood via transfusion or IV drug use. Risk for sexual transmission of hepatitis C is low; however, persons seeking STI treatment should be screened for hepatitis C exposure and risk factors. Vertical transmission (from infected mother to neonate) is another mode of transmission.

Cause
The cause of hepatitis C is hepatitis C virus (HCV).

Signs and Symptoms
The signs and symptoms of hepatitis C are similar to those for hepatitis A.

Diagnosis
Diagnosis of hepatitis C is determined by the following:
- **Screening:** anti-HCV
- If screening is positive, proceed to HCV RNA testing using reverse transcriptase (RT) polymerase chain reaction to confirm diagnosis.

Treatment
Treatment for hepatitis C includes the following:
- Combination therapy of pegylated interferon (Category C) and ribavirin (Category X)
- No vaccine is available.

Effects on Women
Women are at greater risk than men for acquiring HCV through sexual contact. If HCV is left untreated, complications may occur. These complications include:
- Chronic HCV infection
- Liver disease
- Cirrhosis
- Liver cancer
- Death

During Pregnancy
Vertical transmission of HCV is possible during pregnancy.

While Breastfeeding
Transmission of HCV via breast milk is not apparent, but if nipples are bleeding or cracked, the mother should be counseled to stop breastfeeding.

She may resume once the nipples are healed. The mother needs to consult her child's pediatrician.

Effect on Fetus/Infant
Use of ribavirin as treatment for HCV disease is teratogenic to the fetus.

Effect on Men
Male individuals may have a lower rate of spontaneous clearing of HCV than female individuals.

HIV Infection

According to the CDC, about 1.1 million persons age 13 and older are living with HIV in the United States. Women account for more than a quarter of all new HIV diagnoses.

Transmission of HIV is through sexual contact with infected body fluids; through contact with infected blood or blood products; or from an infected woman to her fetus/child during pregnancy, childbirth, or breastfeeding. The presence of a reproductive tract infection increases the chances for the transmission or acquirement of HIV. Therefore, HIV screening should be offered to persons seeking STI treatment and to any sexually active individual.

Cause
The cause of HIV infection is the human immunodeficiency virus. This is the virus that can lead to acquired immune deficiency syndrome (AIDS).

Signs and Symptoms
It may take up to 10 years to exhibit any of the following:
- Rapid weight loss
- Malaise
- Dry cough

★ BEST PRACTICES

Testing for HIV should be voluntary, and an oral and/or written consent should be obtained before testing. See individual state laws regarding HIV testing consent procedures.

The nearest testing center can be accessed in the following ways:
- Phone: Call 1-800-CDC-INFO (1-800-232-4636).
- Text: Mobile users can text their zip code to KNOWIT (566948) and a message containing information on the nearest testing center will be sent back.
- Web: Visit www.hivtest.org and type in any zip code to obtain the nearest testing center information.

- White spots in the mouth or on the throat or tongue
- Red, pink, brown, or purplish skin findings inside the nose, mouth, or eyelids
- Recurring fever
- Lymphadenopathy

Diagnosis
The diagnosis of HIV is determined by the following:
- **Screening:** serology to detect antibodies for HIV-1/2
- **Diagnosis:** Western blot or immunofluorescence assay

Treatment
Treatment of HIV includes the following:
- Nonnucleoside RT inhibitors
- RT inhibitors
- Nucleoside/nucleotide RT inhibitors
- Protease inhibitors
- Entry and fusion inhibitors
- Integrase inhibitors

See the Department of Health and Human Services Web site (http://aidsinfo.nih.gov/Guidelines/) for more detailed information on HIV treatment guidelines.

Partner Management
Encourage HIV-infected patients to inform not only their sexual partners, but also any partners with whom they may have shared needles while injecting drugs, of their possible exposure to HIV. Notification of partners allows for early diagnosis and treatment, which reduces morbidity. If HIV-infected patients are not willing to notify their partners, physicians or other health-care providers, such as nurse practitioners, may, depending on the state in which they practice, use confidential partner notification procedures.

Effects on Women
The effects of HIV on female individuals include the following:
- HIV is the sixth leading cause of death in women 25 to 34 years old.
- A woman will more likely contract HIV than a man during vaginal intercourse.

During Pregnancy
If a pregnant woman with HIV is not treated, the vertical transmission rate is 15% to 25%; if the woman is given antiretrovirals, the transmission rate decreases to less than 2%.

While Breastfeeding
Breastfeeding is contraindicated in HIV-positive women.

Effects on Fetus/Infant
The effects of HIV on the fetus and infant include:
- Positive serology for infected and noninfected infants is common due to the transfer of HIV antibodies through the placenta.
- Infants younger than 18 months need HIV nucleic acid testing for diagnosis.

Effects on Men
The effects of HIV on male individuals include:
- Among heterosexual men, injection drug use puts men at the greatest risk.
- The highest sexual risk behavior for heterosexually identified and homosexual men is to engage in unprotected anal sex with other men.

Genital Herpes

Of individuals 12 years and older, one of five has been infected by the herpes simplex virus (HSV). Two types of herpes virus—herpes simplex viruses 1 (HSV-1) and 2 (HSV-2)—are very similar, but HSV-1 is usually associated with "fever blisters" or "cold sores" on the mouth or lips, but can through oral–genital contact affect the genitalia. HSV-2—genital herpes—is usually associated with genital infection.

Herpes may be transmitted through sexual contact (vaginal, anal, and oral); kissing; sharing food, eating and drinking utensils, and cosmetics, toiletries, and bath items, including lipstick/balm, soaps, washcloths, and towels. The herpes virus may also be transmitted vertically from an infected mother to her baby. Once infected, there is no treatment to rid the body of this virus completely. The virus lays dormant in the nerve ganglion for life.

Cause
The cause of genital herpes is HSV-2 (and sometimes HSV-1).
   Triggers for the reactivation of a dormant virus include the following:
- Stress
- Fatigue
- Injury/trauma to the skin
- Lowered immune response in pregnancy
- Hormonal changes in a woman's menstrual cycle
- Medical illness
- Sun exposure
- Food allergies

Signs and Symptoms
- **Primary outbreak:** small, tender, red blisters around the genital area and/or rectum with possible flu-like symptoms such as fever, swollen glands, vaginal discharge
- **Subsequent outbreaks:** symptoms usually less severe than primary outbreak

Diagnosis
- Viral culture and type-specific serologic test
- Cannot be fully ruled out even if tests are negative given that person may not have been actively shedding the virus when specimen was obtained

Treatment
There is no treatment for herpes; however, antiviral medications may decrease the length of an outbreak and viral shedding. The safety of systemic acyclovir, valacyclovir, and famciclovir therapy in pregnant women has not been established definitively.

- **First clinical episode of genital herpes:**
  - Acyclovir (Zovirax) 400 mg PO tid for 7 to 10 days *or*
  - Acyclovir (Zovirax) 200 mg PO 5 times a day for 7 to 10 days
  - Valacyclovir (Valtrex) 1 g PO bid for 7 to 10 days
- **Episodic therapy for recurrent infection:**
  - Acyclovir (Zovirax) 400 mg PO tid for 5 days *or*
  - Valacyclovir (Valtrex) 500 mg PO bid for 3 days
- **Oral suppressive therapy:**
  - Acyclovir (Zovirax) 400 mg PO bid daily

or
  - Valacyclovir (Valtrex) 0.5 to 1 g PO daily

Partner Management
Encourage sexual partners to be evaluated and, if symptomatic, treated.

Effects on Women
Effects of HSV on female individuals include the following:
- One of four women is affected.
- Individuals with herpes are more likely to be susceptible to HIV.

During Pregnancy
Vertical transmission rate of herpes is less than 1% risk among women with recurrent herpes, and 30% to 50% for women acquiring HSV near time of delivery. If herpes lesions are present in genital area at delivery, a cesarean section is recommended. Suppression therapy may be offered by the HCP at 36 weeks for women with a history of genital HSV infection.

While Breastfeeding
Women with HSV can breastfeed as long as lesions/sores are not on nipple(s) and/or areola, and are covered. Transmission of HSV can occur if newborn comes into contact with lesions/sores. Advise patient that if lesions/sores are on nipple(s) and/or areola, do not breastfeed from that breast; pump milk from that side to maintain supply and prevent engorgement until sore clears. The pumped breast milk should be discarded. Advise patient to discuss with prescribing HCP and the newborn's pediatrician about the effects of medication, if being treated for the HSV outbreak.

Effect on Fetus/Infant

Neonatal herpes may be fatal. Prompt treatment of the neonate with IV acyclovir recommended.

Syphilis

Syphilis is an STI that can lead to serious health problems and even death. It is a reportable disease, meaning that the health department needs to be notified of every new case of syphilis. Approximately 36,000 cases of syphilis were reported in the United States in 2006. Syphilis may be transmitted through sexual contact and vertically from an infected mother to her infant.

Cause

The cause of syphilis is *Treponema pallidum,* a spirochete.

Signs and Symptoms

Primary Stage

Signs and symptoms of syphilis in the primary stage include painless, firm, round chancre on genitals or elsewhere at site of infection.

Secondary Stage

The secondary stage is 6 weeks to 6 months after the primary stage. Signs and symptoms during this stage include the following:

- Nonpruritic reddish brown skin rash appearing on the palms of the hands, the soles of the feet, and mucous membranes.
- Possible fever
- Possible sore throat
- Possible swollen glands
- Possible weight loss

Latent Stage

- Early latent stage occurs within a year after the second stage. Rash may recur but likely is not contagious.
- Late latent stage is more than 1 year after primary infection.

Tertiary Stage

- May occur up to 20 years after an untreated latency stage.
- Internal organ involvement happens in this stage and may cause dementia, paralysis, numbness, uncoordinated muscle movements, and death.

Diagnosis

Diagnosis of syphilis is determined by the following:

- Visualization of spirochete under a dark-field microscope when examining tissue or exudate from an infected chancre or sore

ALERT!

HSV-infected individuals should be advised that they could be shedding the virus even if they do not have symptoms of an outbreak. Asymptomatic viral shedding is more likely with HSV-2 than with HSV-1 and can infect the patient's partner(s). Encourage patients to inform current partners regarding the infection. Partners need to be advised of the possibility of asymptomatic infection and the need for type serologic testing. Use of latex condoms have been proved in research to provide some protection against the transmission of herpes.

- If nontreponemal serologic test—rapid plasma reagin (RPR) or Venereal Disease Research Laboratory (VDRL)—is positive, confirmatory test with treponemal test (FTA-ABS or TP-PA) is necessary.

Treatment

Penicillin (Category B) is the drug of choice for treatment of syphilis.

- **Primary and secondary syphilis**
  - Benzathine penicillin (PCN) G 2.4 million units IM in a single dose
- **Latent syphilis**
  - **Early latent:** Benzathine PCN G 2.4 million units IM in a single dose
  - **Late latent:** Benzathine PCN G 7.2 million units total, administered as 3 doses of 2.4 million units IM at 1-week intervals
- **Tertiary syphilis**
  - Benzathine PCN G 7.2 million units total, administered as 3 doses of 2.4 million units IM at 1-week intervals
- **Neurosyphilis**
  - Aqueous crystalline penicillin G 18 to 24 million units per day administered as 3 to 4 million units IV every 4 hours or continuous infusion for 10 to 14 days

Partner Management

The CDC recommends notification, evaluation, and treatment of sexual partners. Partner treatment generally depends on length of time preceding the diagnosis of the infection and nontreponemal serologic test titers.

Effects on Women

The effects of syphilis on female individuals include the following:

- Women 20 to 24 years old comprise the highest incidence of primary and secondary syphilis among women.
- The latent stage may be fatal because of internal organ damage. Syphilis may affect the brain, nerves, eyes, heart, liver, bones, and joints.

During Pregnancy

Syphilis may be transmitted vertically to the fetus during pregnancy. There is a high risk for stillbirth.

⭐ **BEST PRACTICES**

If a person is allergic to penicillin, desensitization and then treatment with penicillin is recommended. Doxycycline and tetracycline are also used as alternative treatments for those with an allergy to penicillin; however, data on their effectiveness are limited.

While Breastfeeding

Transmission of syphilis to a newborn may occur if the newborn comes into contact with an open sore. If sore is on nipple(s) and/or areola, advise mother not to breastfeed from the affected breast(s); advise patient to pump milk from that side to maintain supply and prevent engorgement until sore clears. The pumped breast milk should be discarded. Advise patient to discuss with the prescribing HCP and the newborn's pediatrician about the effects of medication, if the patient is being treated for syphilis. Also discuss with HCP to assess whether lesion is completely healed and if it is safe to resume breastfeeding.

Effects on Fetus/Infant

The effects of syphilis on the fetus and infant include the following:
* Congenital syphilis cases increased from 339 cases in 2005 to 349 cases in 2006.
* Increased risk for neonatal death
* Infant at risk for seizures and developmental delays

Effects on Men

The effects of syphilis on male individuals include the following:
* Rate of increase in primary and secondary syphilis in men is six times more than in women; this correlates with the increase in syphilis among men who have sex with men.
* 65% of syphilis cases are found among men who have sex with men.

Trichomoniasis

An estimated 7.4 million individuals are diagnosed with trichomoniasis each year. It is transmitted by sexual contact (penis in the vagina or vulva to vulva). Proper and consistent usage of latex condoms provides some protection against a trichomoniasis infection.

Cause

The cause of trichomoniasis is *Trichomonas vaginalis,* a protozoan with flagella that allows it to be motile.

Signs and Symptoms

Signs and symptoms of trichomoniasis include malodorous, yellow–green vaginal discharge.

Diagnosis

Diagnosis of trichomoniasis is determined by the following:
* Microcopy of vaginal secretion, but this is only 60% to 70% sensitive
* Immunochromatographic capillary flow dipstick technology and nucleic acid probe test are more than 83% sensitive and 97% specific and may be done in the physician's office.
* Culture is most sensitive and specific, but needs to be sent to a laboratory.

Treatment
- Metronidazole 2 g PO in a single dose (Category B)

Partner Management
Sexual partners should be treated and instructed to abstain from sexual intercourse until both (or all) partners are cured and asymptomatic.

Effect on Women
The effect of trichomoniasis on female individuals includes increased susceptibility to contraction of HIV.

During Pregnancy
Vaginal trichomoniasis has been associated with adverse outcomes such as premature rupture of membranes, preterm delivery, and low birth weight.

MEDICA-TION INSIGHT

Metronidazole was approved by the FDA in the early 1960s for the treatment of trichomoniasis. Side effects may include a metallic taste and nausea. Patients should be counseled to avoid the use of alcohol while taking metronidazole to prevent a disulfiram-like reaction.

While Breastfeeding
See text on metronidazole treatment while breastfeeding in the section on BV, page 204.

Effect on Fetus
See effects of metronidazole use on fetus in the section on BV.

Effect on Infant
See effects of metronidazole use on infant in the section on BV.

Effect on Men
Untreated trichomoniasis in men may lead to an infection of the urethra or prostate gland.

Vulvovaginal Candidiasis

Approximately one-third of women will experience at least one episode of vulvovaginal candidiasis (VVC). Sometimes called simply candidiasis, yeast infection, or monilia, VVC is not commonly transmitted via sexual contact, and partner treatment is not usually advised unless the candidiasis is of the recurrent type.

Cause
VVC is commonly caused by *Candida albicans;* sometimes other *Candida* species are the cause.

Signs and Symptoms
- Thick cottage cheese–like vaginal discharge
- Pruritus

- Dyspareunia
- Dysuria

Diagnosis

Diagnosis of VVC is determined by the following:
- Presence of yeasts or pseudohyphae on wet preparation (saline + 10% KOH) or Gram stain of vaginal discharge under microscopy
- Culture of vaginal discharge positive for a *Candida* species
- Usually vaginal pH is normal at < 4.5

Treatment

Intravaginal Therapies

Over-the-counter intravaginal therapies include:
- Clotrimazole (Mycelex, FemCare) 1% cream 5 g intravaginally for 7 to 14 days (Category B), available OTC *or*
- Miconazole (Monistat) 2% cream 5 g intravaginally for 7 days (Category C), available OTC
- Tioconazole (Vagistat) 6.5% ointment 5 g intravaginally in a single application (Category C) *or*

Prescription intravaginal therapies include:
- Nystatin (Mycostatin) 100,000-unit vaginal tablet, 1 tablet for 14 days (Category C) *or*
- Terconazole (Terazol or Zazole) 0.4% cream 5 g intravaginally × 7 days (Category C)

Oral Therapy
- Oral fluconazole 150 mg PO in a single dose (Category C)

Partner Treatment

Unless the woman has recurrent infections, treatment of sex partners is not recommended by the CDC because VVC is not transmitted through sexual intercourse. If the male partner develops balanitis, wherein his penis becomes pruritic and irritated, he may benefit from antifungal treatment.

Effects on Women

The effects of VVC on female individuals include:
- Vaginal irritation from the presence of yeast
- Dyspareunia associated with vaginal irritation

During Pregnancy

Only topical azole treatment for 7 days is recommended during pregnancy.

While Breastfeeding

Women with VVC may breastfeed.

Effect on Men

Balanitis is a possible effect on male partners (see earlier section regarding partner treatment).

Pelvic Inflammatory Disease

PID occurs when an infection travels from the vagina and/or the cervix into the uterus, fallopian tubes, ovaries, and the peritoneal membrane. The infections that cause PID, such as gonorrhea and chlamydia, are transmitted sexually. PID is a devastating disease that may lead to irreversible consequences such as infertility. Approximately 1 million women suffer from PID every year in the United States.

Cause

Typically, *Neisseria gonorrhoeae* and *Chlamydia trachomatis* cause PID.

Signs and Symptoms
- Pelvic/lower abdominal pain
- Abnormal bleeding
- Dyspareunia
- Vaginal discharge

Diagnosis

The diagnosis of PID is determined by the following:
- Cervical motion tenderness, uterine tenderness, or adnexal tenderness
- Oral temperature higher than 101°F
- Mucopurulent discharge
- Elevated erythrocyte sedimentation rate or C-reactive protein
- Presence of *N. gonorrhoeae* and *C. trachomatis*
- Endometritis on biopsy
- Magnetic resonance imaging showing thickened fluid-filled tubes

Treatment

Parenteral Treatment

Parenteral treatment is usually continued for 24 hours after clinical improvement and transitioned to oral regimen.
- Cefotetan (Cefotan) 2 g IV bid (Category B)

or
- Cefoxitin (Mefoxin) 2 g IV qid

plus
- Doxycycline (Vibramycin) 100 mg PO or IV bid (Category D)

Oral Treatment
- Ceftriaxone 250 mg IM × 1 dose

plus
- Doxycycline 100 mg PO bid × 14 days

with or without
- Metronidazole 500 mg PO bid × 14 days

Other regimens are available for the treatment of PID. Please refer to the CDC's Sexually Transmitted Disease Treatment Guidelines 2010 in *Morbidity and Mortality Weekly Report* (www.cdc.gov/mmwr/pdf/rr/rr5912.pdf) for more details.

Partner Treatment

Empirical treatment of sex partners for gonorrhea and chlamydia is recommended by the CDC.

Effects on Women

Effects of PID on female individuals include the following:

- Irreversible damage to the uterus and fallopian tubes leading to infertility and ectopic pregnancy
- The CDC estimates that 100,000 women become infertile as a result of PID each year.

During Pregnancy

A pregnant woman with PID needs to be hospitalized and treated with IV antibiotics.

While Breastfeeding

Discuss with prescribing OB-GYN practitioner and pediatrician the effects of the individual medications being used to treat PID on breast milk.

Effect on Fetus/Infant

Refer to the earlier sections on the effects of gonorrhea and chlamydia infection on newborns.

Effect on Men

Refer to the earlier sections on the effects of gonorrhea and chlamydia infections on male individuals.

> **TIP**
>
> For more complete and updated treatment guidelines for sexually transmitted diseases, refer to the CDC's Sexually Transmitted Diseases Treatment Guidelines 2010 in *Morbidity and Mortality Weekly Report* (www.cdc.gov/mmwr/pdf/rr/rr5912.pdf).

CHAPTER 9

Violence Against Women

According to the Centers for Disease Control and Prevention (CDC), an approximated 5.3 million women are abused annually in the United States, resulting in 1300 deaths and 2 million injuries. Unfortunately, the true prevalence of violent acts against women is likely much higher because of under-reporting by victims and failure of health-care practitioners (HCPs) to recognize signs of abuse.

Intimate partner violence (IPV) refers to any act of physical, sexual, economic, or psychological abuse, whether actual or threatened, inflicted by a person who is a family member or spouse/boyfriend/partner. Although the term **IPV** is sometimes used interchangeably with the term ***domestic violence***, domestic abuse is a broader term, including, in addition to victims of IPV, child abuse and elder abuse.

Populations at Risk for Domestic Violence

Although IPV and domestic violence may be seen across the life span and are found in all racial, ethnic, religious, and socioeconomic groups, vulnerable populations that are at increased risk include:

- Children
- Adolescents
- Pregnant women
- Women with disabilities
- Immigrants and refugee women
- Lesbian, gay, bisexual, and transgendered (LGBT) women
- Elderly

Incidence and Effects of Violence Against Women

The incidence of violence against women varies among the different at-risk populations. So, too, do the effects of the abuse. Many factors, including age, health status, and socioeconomic conditions, play a role.

In this section, we focus particularly on violence against vulnerable female populations: women who are pregnant, female immigrants, women who have disabilities, and women who identify as lesbians.

Pregnant Women

Violence inflicted on a pregnant woman affects not only the woman, but also the fetus. It is recommended that all pregnant women be screened at the first prenatal visit, during every trimester, and at the postpartum check-up. In addition, it would be wise to screen for abuse when a woman is admitted to the labor and delivery unit, and during her postpartum recovery at the hospital/birth center before discharge.

Incidence

The incidence of abuse during pregnancy and factors that contribute to it include:

- 50% to 75% of women abused before pregnancy also are abused during pregnancy.
- Approximately 20% of pregnant women report being victims of domestic violence during pregnancy.
- Pregnant adolescents between the ages of 13 and 17 have an increased risk for IPV compared with pregnant adults 18 years and older.

Maternal Complications Linked to Violence During Pregnancy

The following are maternal complications linked to violence during pregnancy:

- Second- and third-trimester bleeding
- Poor weight gain and nutrition, often resulting in anemia
- Infection

- Spleen and liver injury
- Placental abruption
- Premature rupture of the membranes
- Preterm labor

Fetal/Neonatal Complications Linked to Violence During Pregnancy

The following are fetal/neonatal complications linked to violence during pregnancy:

- Intrauterine fetal demise
- Neonatal death
- Preterm delivery
- Low birth weight
- Direct injury to neonate

Women With Disabilities

- According to the National Women's Health Information Center, 10% to 13% of women with disabilities have been the victim of abuse.
- The dilemma of reporting an abuser who may also be the caregiver contributes to the under-reporting of abuse in women with disabilities. Caregivers can withhold medications and assistive devices such as wheelchairs, or refuse to assist with activities of daily living such as eating and bathing.

Immigrants and Refugee Women

- Studies on Latina, South Asian, and Korean immigrants report a 30% to 50% incidence of IPV.
- Abusers may inhibit the woman from learning English; thus, the woman becomes further isolated from the general population. A woman who lacks English proficiency will struggle to find employment and thus may remain financially dependent on the abuser.
- A woman who is not a legal resident may not seek help for fear of being reported to the authorities and deported to her country of origin.

Women Who Identify as Lesbians

- A National Institute of Justice survey conducted in 2000 found that 39.2% of women in same-sex relationships reported being victims of rape, physical abuse, and/or stalking by their partner.
- LGBT individuals are likely to stay in an abusive relationship longer because of denial of the existence of IPV in LGBT communities and fear of being "outed" by their partner to family, friends, and employer.
- It is important that HCPs universally screen for abuse regardless of the client's sexual orientation.

Signs of Abuse

Because there are many forms of abuse, victims of IPV and domestic violence may have differing clinical presentations. The American College of Obstetrics and Gynecology (ACOG) lists these clinical manifestations of possible abuse:
- Unexplained physical injuries (possibly seeing injuries at different stages of healing)
- Complaints of chronic pelvic pain, urinary problems, and sexual dysfunction with unknown cause
- Sexually transmitted diseases that are recurrent and persistent despite adequate/repeated treatment
- Somatization of stress presenting as generalized aches and pains, backache, sleeping difficulties, and eating disorders
- Unintended pregnancy
- Post-traumatic stress disorder symptoms, including depression; anxiety; phobia; panic attacks; feelings of shame, worthlessness, and suicidal ideation

TIPS

Use Your "RADAR"
R—Remember to ask.
A—Ask directly.
D—Document findings.
A—Assess safety.
R—Review options.

From Alpert, EJ: The RADAR model of the physician's approach to domestic violence. In Intimate Partner Violence: The Clinician's Guide to Identification, Assessment, Intervention, and Prevention, ed. 5. Waltham, MA: Massachusetts Medical Society, 2010. Used with permission.

What You Should Do

The nurse or other HCPs should screen all patients for signs/symptoms of domestic abuse and should report the abuse to authorities, based on pertinent laws and/or the victim's age and/or wishes.

Screening

- Screen everyone. It is important that the screening be done apart from the patient's partner, family, or friends (see the Best Practice box on page 232).
- ACOG recommends this opening question, "Because violence is so common in many women's lives and because there is help available for women being abused, I now ask every patient about domestic violence," followed by these three simple, but direct questions:
  1. Within the past year—or since you have been pregnant—have you been hit, slapped, kicked, or otherwise physically hurt by someone?
  2. Are you in a relationship with a person who threatens or physically hurts you?
  3. Has anyone forced you to have sexual activities that made you feel uncomfortable?
- Once abuse is suspected or recognized, you will need to intervene by involving the whole health-care team, including the physician, nurse practitioner, midwife, and/or physician assistant, social worker, psychiatrist (if needed), and pastoral care (if requested).
- Provide support for the patient. The patient needs to know that you are concerned for her health and well-being. You may want to say, "I am worried about you and your safety."
- Refer patient to a case manager, community shelter, court advocacy, domestic violence agency, and/or legal counsel.
- Make sure to schedule the patient for a follow-up appointment.

Documenting Your Findings

Recording the abuse using the patient's own words is vital; use direct quotations whenever possible. When describing the extent and severity of the abuse, the name of the person who caused the injury should also be documented. Use statements such as "Patient reports being hit in the . . ." Use a body map to record the injuries and bruises. If possible, offer to photograph injuries with the patient's consent.

Reporting

Reporting cases of abuse is meant to identify these acts and prevent future incidents of abuse. Because it has not been proved in research that mandatory reporting is beneficial to a victim's safety and confidentiality, it is argued that women should still have the power to veto reporting.

Reporting laws vary by state, except for suspected child abuse, which is reportable across all states. In some states, IPV and domestic violence injuries, and the involvement of a gun, knife, or deadly weapon need to be reported as well. Knowing the reporting laws in your state and hospital/office protocols is crucial to properly intervening in suspected

"HITS" DOMESTIC VIOLENCE SCREENING TOOL

HITS Tool for Intimate Partner Violence Screening: Please read each of the following descriptors and put a check in the column that best indicates the frequency with which your partner acts in the way depicted.

HOW OFTEN DOES YOUR PARTNER?	NEVER (1)	RARELY (2)	SOMETIMES (3)	FAIRLY OFTEN (4)	FREQUENTLY (5)
1. Physically Hurt you					
2. Insult or talk down to you					
3. Threaten you with harm					
4. Scream or curse at you					

Each item is scored from 1 to 5. Thus, scores for this inventory range from 4 to 20. A score greater than 10 is considered positive for abuse.

From Sherin KM, Sinacore JM, Li X-Q, Zitter RE, Shakil A. HITS: A short domestic violence screening tool for use in a family practice setting. *Fam Med*. 1998;30:508–512.

or confirmed abuse cases. It is also important to be informed of domestic violence agencies and help lines in your area (see Box 9–1).

The National Domestic Violence Hotline provides anonymous and confidential help 24 hours a day, 7 days a week: 1-800-799-SAFE (7233) or www.thehotline.org.

EVIDENCE FOR PRACTICE BOX 9–1

According to the Violence Against Women Act (VAWA), which was passed in Congress in 1994, immigrants involved in an abusive marriage to a legal U.S. resident may self-petition for lawful residency without the knowledge of the spouse/abuser to obtain safety and independence for themselves and their child/children. In 2013, VAWA extended protection from abuse to lesbians, gays, the transgendered, and Native Americans.

10 Multicultural Nursing

CHAPTER 10

Multicultural Nursing

As the world's population reached 6.8 billion people in 2008, America's population also continued to grow—to an estimated 306 million people. The makeup of America's population continues to become more ethnically and culturally diverse (see Box 10–1). It is the responsibility of health-care providers (HCPs) to identify and educate themselves on their patients' cultural/ethnic beliefs, practices, and values. The application of this knowledge in clinical practice will enhance communication between the patient and nurse, and will increase the nurse's understanding and sensitivity to different cultural/religious/ethnic populations. We must remember, however, that although a patient may be of a particular culture, race, or ethnicity, she is an individual and we cannot generalize and assume she accepts or applies the popular/dominant beliefs, practices, and values of her culture (see Box 10–2).

The intent of this chapter is to give the nurse an overview of the different populations in America; it does not take the place of an extensive curriculum on cultural competence. We provide some general information (e.g., religion, language) concerning the different ethnic groups; list some of the widespread beliefs, ideas, and practices of different ethnic groups (*in italics*); and then suggest ways in which the nurse can provide culturally sensitive care to ensure the well-being of the patient, newborn, and family unit. See Box 10–3 for resources for pregnancy, postpartum, and newborn care available in different languages.

Women of African Heritage

Dominant Language
The dominant language of people of African heritage is English.

Major Religions
The major religions of people of African heritage are Christianity, Islam, and Judaism.

QSEN Application

Patient-centered care includes attitudes such as:
- Valuing seeing health-care situations "through patients' eyes"
- Respecting and encouraging individual expression of patient values, preferences, and expressed needs
- Valuing the patient's expertise with her health and symptoms
- Seeking learning opportunities with patients who represent all aspects of human diversity
- Recognizing personally held attitudes about working with patients from different ethnic, cultural, and social backgrounds
- Willingly supporting patient-centered care for individuals and groups whose values differ from own

In this chapter, together with information about care of pregnant women and newborns, Quality and Safety Education for Nurses (QSEN) competencies assure delivery of the best nursing care.

http://qsen.org/competencies/pre-licensure-ksas/#patient-centered_care

---

Box 10–1 Countries of Origin for The Top Five Largest Immigrant Groups Obtaining Permanent Legal Residence in the United States in 2008

1. Mexico
2. China
3. India
4. Philippines
5. Cuba

Brookings Metropolitan Policy Program (2008).

Box 10–2 Definitions

1. Race: A group of people with similar physical characteristics that are genetically inherited
2. Ethnicity: Learned characteristics of a group or individual such as language and religion based on cultural heritage.
3. Culture: Integrated system of ideas, values, and beliefs that are transmitted to succeeding generations
4. Family: Two or more individuals who live in the same household and/or belong to the same ancestry
5. Community: A social group

Data from Willis W. Culturally competent nursing care during the perinatal period. *J Perinat Neonat Nurs*. 1999;13:46.

Pregnancy and Childbearing Beliefs and Practices

- *Pica, a disorder in which non-nutritive substances such as clay or paint chips are ingested, is a common practice among women of African heritage.* When assessing the patient's nutritional status, the nurse should ask the patient whether she eats substances such as cornstarch, dirt, tissue paper, or paint chips. If she does, the nurse needs to provide more extensive nutrition counseling. (Refer to the "Nutrition" section in Chapter One "Normal Pregnancy.")

- **Labor:** *Eating a heavy meal, drinking castor oil, or sniffing pepper may induce labor.* The nurse should counsel the woman that such eating/drinking/sniffing will not induce labor. Also, remind the woman scheduled for a cesarean section that she should not eat after midnight the day of the scheduled surgery.
- **Postpartum:** *It is important to avoid cold air after birth.* If the postpartum woman believes this, offer to turn off air-conditioning or to close the windows and doors to keep cold air from entering the room.
- **Infant:** *A bellyband should be used on top of the newborn's umbilical area to prevent the protrusion of the belly button.* The nurse should educate the mother that keeping the umbilical clean, dry, and open to air is best to prevent infection.

Women of Arabic Heritage

Dominant Language
The dominant language of people of Arabic heritage is Arabic.

Major Religion
The major religion of people of Arabic heritage is Islam.

Pregnancy and Childbearing Beliefs and Practices
- Permanent, irreversible forms of birth control, such as a tubal ligation, vasectomy, and abortion (except when the mother's health is threatened) are considered unlawful. Reversible forms of birth control are not outlawed, but they are frowned upon. If the patient desires, the nurse should give comprehensive contraceptive counseling regarding options such as long-term reversible methods like the Nexplanon, ParaGard intrauterine device (IUD), or Mirena intrauterine system (IUS).
- Pregnant women are excused from fasting during Ramadan.
- **Labor:** *Verbal and nonverbal expression of pain is encouraged.*
- **Postpartum:** *Once she gives birth, the woman may be hesitant to bathe because of a fear that air may enter her body, causing an illness.* Offer the woman a washcloth, a basin of tepid water, and warm towels.

- **Breastfeeding:** *Washing the breasts may "thin the milk." It is believed that colostrum will "make the baby dumb"; thus, breastfeeding is delayed until the second or third day postpartum. Lentil soup is eaten to increase breast milk production.* The nurse should educate the patient regarding the benefits of colostrum and initiating breast-feeding as early as possible after delivery.

Women of Chinese Heritage

Official Language
The official language of people of Chinese heritage is Mandarin.

Major Religions
The major religions of people of Chinese heritage are Buddhism, Catholicism, Protestantism, Taoism, and Islam.

Pregnancy and Childbearing Beliefs and Practices
- In China, where a one-child law is in effect, the IUD is the most popular method of birth control; sterilization and abortion are also common, and all contraception is free.
- *A balance of yin and yang is important for good health.*
- Use of traditional Chinese medicine is common.
- **Labor:** *Female obstetrician or midwife is preferred.*
- **Postpartum:** *Mother is encouraged to eat warm foods (yang) to decrease the cold (yin) energy and to increase meals to five or six meals a day. Typical "hot" foods contain ginger, eggs, chicken, and pork.* When counseling regarding nutrition, the nurse should focus on reviewing food sources for iron and increasing caloric intake for breastfeeding mothers. *Mothers may be seen in layered clothing, even during warm temperatures, to keep cold air from entering their bodies.* Offer warm blankets and extra patient gowns.
- **Breastfeeding:** *Drinking rice wine is believed to increase milk production.* Discuss with patient that rice wine contains about 16% to 20% alcohol. Refer to Chapter 11 "Substance Abuse" for more information.

⭐ **BEST PRACTICES**

Common methods used in traditional Chinese medicine include:
- Herbal therapy
  - Ginseng, believed to enhance male fertility
  - Ginger, believed to ease morning sickness
  - Cranberry for the prevention of urinary tract infections
  - Blue/black cohosh, believed to induce or augment labor
  - Milk thistle, believed to increase the milk supply
- Acupuncture and acupressure, which are used to relieve nausea and vomiting in pregnancy, augment and induce labor, and relieve pain
- Moxibustion in which burning of the herb *moxa*, or mugwort, near the tip of the fifth toe is believed to correct fetal malpresentation

---

Women of Filipino Heritage

Official Language
The official language of people of Filipino heritage is Filipino, which is primarily Tagalog and inclusive of English- and Spanish-derived words; however, more than 100 other dialects are spoken in different regions of the Philippines, including Ilocano and Cebuano.

Major Religion
The major religion of people of Filipino heritage is Roman Catholicism.

Pregnancy and Childbearing Beliefs and Practices
- The Roman Catholic Church has a strong influence on child-bearing and fertility beliefs and practices in the Philippines. *Abortion is considered a sin. The rhythm method is the only acceptable contraception.* The nurse, however, must not assume every Filipino patient is Catholic. If the patient is Catholic, the nurse should never assume the Roman Catholic Church influences her health-care practices.
- *Vitamins are avoided because of a fear that they may cause birth defects.* The nurse should explain the benefits of folic acid in preventing neural tube defects and discuss the importance of supplementing the diet with calcium, iron, and other vitamins and minerals during pregnancy.
- **Labor:** *Instead of their husbands, some women choose their mothers to be their labor coach.* Respect the patient and family's decision on who the support person is going to be during the labor and delivery process. However, encourage the father's involvement before, during, and after labor and delivery to facilitate paternal bonding.
- **Postpartum:** *Help from relatives to care for the new baby and pamper the mother is common.* The nurse may interpret the family members' eagerness to help as a lack of motivation on the part of the mother to care for herself and her baby. The nurse should not assume this but should educate the mother on how to care for herself and her infant. If the mother desires, incorporate the family members and teach them how to best assist the patient in the hospital and at home. Answer any questions and give evidence-based information regarding the mother's postpartum recovery and the infant's needs.
- **Breastfeeding:** *There is a high incidence of breastfeeding, but often, foods are introduced and supplemented as early as 2 months.* The nurse should educate the new mother regarding the recommendations of the American Academy of Family Physicians, the American Academy of Pediatrics, and the World Health Organization; advise her to breastfeed exclusively for 6 months to provide continued protection against many diseases; and encourage breastfeeding for a year postpartum.

Women of Indian Heritage

Dominant Language
There are 15 national languages in India and 1600 dialects, but the most popular is Hindi.

Major Religions
The major religions of people of Indian heritage are Hinduism, Christianity, and Buddhism.

Pregnancy and Childbearing Beliefs and Practices

- *Pregnancy is considered a normal experience that does not necessitate medical intervention; therefore, a woman of Indian heritage may not seek prenatal care until late in the pregnancy. Pregnancy rituals performed during certain times throughout gestation are believed to ward off evil spirits.* Preconception counseling regarding the reasons for prenatal surveillance should be discussed with the patient.
- *Foods are often categorized as "hot" or "cold"; this categorization varies in different regions of India and does not depend on the temperature of the foods. "Cold foods," such as milk and rice, are generally believed to be beneficial during the early stages of pregnancy. "Hot foods," such as beans and garlic, are encouraged toward the end of pregnancy to initiate labor.* Ask the patient which types of foods she considers "hot" and "cold" and then, taking into account her preferences, proceed with nutrition counseling.
- **Labor:** *A female HCP is preferred. Verbalization of pain is encouraged by female relatives present during the delivery.*
- **Postpartum:** *A confinement period of 40 days is generally observed.* The mother is assisted by family members who nourish her back to health and help care for her infant.
- **Breastfeeding:** *Colostrum is typically withheld. According to ancient Indian scriptures, breastfeeding should begin on the fifth day.* Wide variation on initiation of breastfeeding exists depending on the socioeconomic and educational levels of the woman. Educate the patient regarding the benefits of colostrum and initiating breastfeeding as early as possible after delivery.

ALERT!

Toxins produced by *Clostridium botulinum* may colonize the infant gut and may be life-threatening. Spores of this organism can be found in honey and contaminated soil.

- **Newborn:** *Giving the infant honey as its first food in the first 24 hours of life is an accepted practice.* Educate the mother regarding the risk for infant botulism with the ingestion of honey.

Women of Korean Heritage

Dominant Language
The dominant language of people of Korean heritage is Korean (Hangul).

Major Religions

The major religions of people of Korean heritage are Buddhism, Confucianism, Christianity, and Cheondogyo.

Pregnancy and Childbearing Beliefs and Practices

- Birth control is covered by health insurance, and abortion is legal and widely used in Korea.
- *High incidence of lactose intolerance, resulting in the avoidance of dairy products.* Provide nutrition counseling regarding the importance of calcium during pregnancy and the need for nondairy sources of calcium such as fortified cereals, tofu, and spinach.
- **Labor:** *Labor is usually in the supine position, but the woman may walk, squat, or crawl.* Offer the patient information on the different positions for labor. *The Korean woman is expected to be stoic during labor.* Ask the woman, "How do you want your labor to be?" and encourage an open line of communication between yourself and the patient. *A female HCP is preferred.*
- **Postpartum:** *Eating or drinking cold substances, showering, and bathing are discouraged to avoid illness. Bed rest for up to 90 days is encouraged to promote emotional and physical health.* Offer warm food and liquids and additional blankets. Encourage increasing physical activity as tolerated and desired by the patient.
- **Breastfeeding:** *Women are served seaweed soup, which is believed to increase milk production. Some Korean women believe that breastfeeding should not be initiated until the third day postpartum.* Educate on the benefits of colostrum and initiating breastfeeding as soon as possible after birth.
- **Newborn:** *The newborn is usually wrapped in warm blankets to prevent harm from the cold.* The nurse should instruct the parents to use light sleep clothing for the infant, avoid the use of blankets, and keep the room temperature at a comfortable level. Overheating is linked to sudden infant death syndrome (SIDS).

Women of Jewish Heritage and/or Religion

Official Language in Israel

Hebrew is the official language in Israel.

Major Religion

Judaism is the major religion of people of Jewish heritage.

Pregnancy and Childbearing Beliefs and Practices

- *Prevention of pregnancy is believed to go against the commandment to be fruitful and multiply; therefore, birth control is frowned upon by some Orthodox Jews. Permission from a rabbi to use contraception may be sought. Condoms, barrier methods, and withdrawal go against the biblical instruction of releasing sperm in the uterus only.* Education on nonbarrier forms of contraception, such as oral contraceptive pills, hormonal patch and ring, IUD, and Nexplanon should be discussed with the patient.

- **Labor:** *The Jewish Orthodox patient may want to be completely covered, and the husband may excuse himself from the delivery. If he remains during the birth, he is not allowed to touch his wife or look at the infant emerging from the birth canal and may only provide verbal coaching. A Jewish woman who is in the hospital during Shabbat, or "day of rest," may refrain from performing certain activities such as signing consent forms and turning electricity on and off.* The health-care team must try to assist as much as possible by performing some of the tasks, such as turning the lights on and off for the patient.

- **Postpartum:** *A female provider is preferred. The family is very involved in caring for the woman and her newborn. Some Jews only eat "kosher" food and will avoid pork or shellfish.* Request kosher meals from the hospital's food services department for the patient who wants them. If this is not available, encourage the patient to bring kosher food from home. If possible, use gelatin-free medications because gelatin is made from non-kosher animals.

- **Breastfeeding:** *Breastfeeding is highly encouraged. During Shabbat, the use of an electric breast pump is not allowed unless medically necessary.*

- **Newborn:** Circumcision is a religious rite performed on the eighth day of life by a mohel.

Native American Women

Most Popular Language

The most popular language for Native American people is the Navajo language. Although hundreds of different Native American languages are no longer used, close to 300 languages are spoken today (see Box 10–4).

Major Religion

Instead of a formal religion, most Native Americans believe in a Creator or "Master Spirit," an afterlife, and the human soul's immortality (see Box 10–5).

Pregnancy and Childbearing Beliefs and Practices

- *Prenatal care is thought unnecessary, because pregnancy is considered a normal event and not viewed as a physical state requiring surveillance*

Box 10–4 Nursing Resources in Caring for Native American Women

- Indian Health Services (IHS): www.ihs.gov
- IHS Maternal Child Health: www.ihs.gov
- Breastfeeding Guide for American Indian and Alaskan Native Families: http://www.womenshealth.gov/publications/our-publications/breastfeeding-guide/BreastfeedingGuide-NativeAmerican-English.pdf

---

⭐ **BEST PRACTICES**

Native Americans are at high risk for diabetes. Breastfeeding may help reduce the infant's risk of developing diabetes and may help the mother by possibly decreasing blood sugar level and encouraging weight loss.

by a HCP. This viewpoint may be misinterpreted by the Western HCP as the mother not caring about her pregnancy.

- **Labor:** *Touch is avoided unless necessary. Pregnant women avoid being around the dead; thus, they may avoid hospitals and prefer delivery at home.*
- **Postpartum:** *Placentas are taken home to be buried under a juniper tree and become one with the land.* If the patient expresses the desire to take the placenta home, check your hospital's policy and determine where the placenta should be stored while the patient is recovering in the hospital.
- **Breastfeeding:** *There is a belief that nursing passes on traditional values to the child.*
- **Newborn:** *When the umbilical cord falls off, it is not thrown away. It is believed to affect the child's destiny and is buried where the family believes the child's future will most benefit. For example, the parents will bury the cord on farm land if they wish their child to become a farmer.*

ALERT!

According to a 2004 study by the Bureau of Justice Statistics, Native Americans are twice as likely as other women to experience sexual assault crimes. The National Institute of Justice reports that one in three Native American women admits to having been raped. It is highly important to screen for intimate partner violence (IPV) and risk for abuse at each prenatal visit, on admission to hospital, and before discharge from the hospital, as well as at the postpartum follow-up visit. Refer to Chapter Nine "Violence Against Women" for further resources.

Latina or Hispanic Women

Dominant Language

The dominant language of people of Latin or Hispanic heritage is Spanish.

Major Religion

Catholicism is the major religion of people of Latin or Hispanic heritage (see Box 10–6).

Pregnancy and Childbearing Beliefs and Practices

Because of the strong influence of the Catholic Church, *birth control is widely unaccepted, and abortion is considered a sin.* However, the nurse should not assume that the patient is not seeking contraceptive education despite general beliefs.

- **Labor:** *The mother is encouraged to cry out in order for God to hear her suffering. The father is not supposed to be present during the delivery and should avoid seeing the mother and the infant until they are cleaned.* The nurse should encourage the involvement of the father as soon as possible to facilitate family bonding.
- **Postpartum:** *A warm environment is encouraged. Showering for up to 40 days is discouraged to avoid the cold.* Offer warm sponge baths and use of sitz baths for the perineum.
- **Breastfeeding:** *Extending the breastfeeding period is seen as a form of birth control.* Discuss with the patient the effectiveness of the lactation amenorrhea method. Refer to Chapter Seven "Contraceptive Counseling" for further details.
- **Newborn:** *Newborns are believed to be vulnerable to evil spirits and are bundled tightly.* Educate regarding the link between SIDS and infant overheating caused by excessive swaddling (see Box 10–7).

Women Who Identify as Lesbians

- Obtaining a comprehensive history is an essential element of excellent medical care. The sexual history should be taken without bias and without assuming the patient's sexual orientation.
- The nurse should not assume that a woman who identifies herself as heterosexual does not engage in sex with other women. It also cannot be assumed that a woman who identifies herself as a lesbian has or has had sex only with women.

- Women having sex with women are still at risk for sexually transmitted infections (STIs) though oral sex, mutual masturbation, and sharing of sex toys.
- Among teenagers aged 12 to 19 years, the rate of pregnancy is higher in lesbians (12%) than in their heterosexual peers (6%). A woman or teenager identifying herself as a lesbian still needs contraceptive counseling, because many lesbians also have sex with men.
- Assisted reproductive technology, often using donor sperm, may be used by a lesbian woman to become pregnant. Adoption is also another option explored by many same-sex couples.
- Same-sex marriage is legal in only a handful of states. A lesbian who is not legally married to her partner may not be able to obtain health insurance as a spouse, have visitation rights at the hospital if visits are restricted to only immediate family, or have automatic guardianship over their children.
- According to 2007 data from the Federal Bureau of Investigation, 15.9% of hate crime victims were targeted because of their sexual orientation. Ask the patient about a history of threat and abuse (see Box 10–8).

Women of Advanced Maternal Age

Women of advanced maternal age are women who are 35 years or older at the time of delivery. (Some authorities set the cutoff age as 40 years.)

QSEN Application

Patient-centered care includes attitudes such as:
- Acknowledging the tension that may exist between patient rights and the organizational responsibility for professional, ethical care
- Appreciating shared decision making with empowered patients and families, even when conflicts occur
- Respecting patient preferences for degree of active engagement in care process
- Respecting patient's right to access to personal health records

In this chapter, together with information about care of pregnant women and newborns, QSEN competencies assure delivery of the best nursing care.

http://qsen.org/competencies/pre-licensure-ksas/#patient-centered_care

---

Box 10–8 Resources for Lesbian Health

- Health-care professional training designed to educate and raise awareness of lesbian health issues: www.mautnerproject.org
- Gay and Lesbian Medical Association: www.glma.org
- The National Coalition for LGBT Health: www.lgbthealth.net

There are increased risks associated with pregnancy in women of advanced maternal age, including:

- Miscarriage
- Sterility
- Unsuccessful in vitro fertilization
- Pre-existing comorbidities such as hypertension and diabetes. Thorough history-taking is needed to address the implications of these comorbidities on pregnancy.
- Leiomyomata (fibroids), which may increase the risk for postpartum hemorrhage. Strict monitoring for signs of hemodynamic instability in the intrapartum and postpartum periods is necessary.
- Congenital anomalies such as trisomy 21 (Down syndrome; see Table 10–1)
- Pre-eclampsia
- Placental abruption and placenta previa
- Birth of baby that is large for gestational age, which may increase risk for shoulder dystocia at delivery, injury to the brachial nerve plexus, increased levels of insulin, and hypoglycemia. Close monitoring of the newborn is warranted.
- Fetal malpresentation
- Cesarean delivery

Adolescent Girls

When managing the care of adolescent girls, usage of developmentally appropriate teaching methods is essential.

The nurse should address the following topics.

- **Nutrition**
  - Screen for eating disorders.
  - Address increased nutritional needs to support both the adolescent's continuing growth and the needs of the fetus.

Table 10–1 Down Syndrome Risk Related to Maternal Age

AGE AT DELIVERY DATE	RISK FOR DOWN SYNDROME	RISK FOR ANY CHROMOSOMAL ABNORMALITIES
20	1/1667	1/526
25	1/1250	1/476
30	1/952	1/384
35	1/385	1/204
40	1/106	1/65
45	1/30	1/20

From Gabbe SG, Neibyl JR, Simpsons JL. Cytogenic disorders. In *Obstetrics: Normal and Problem Pregnancies.* 5th ed. New York: Elsevier;2007:138. Used with permission.

- Address increased needs for calcium, magnesium, and phosphorus.
- Discuss the components of a well-balanced diet and the importance of prenatal vitamins.
- Discourage skipping meals and eating "fast foods," which are high in calories and fat.
- Refer patient to the Women, Infants, and Children (WIC) program and local community resources.

- **Substance abuse:** Educate the adolescent on the effects of alcohol, tobacco, and illegal drugs on her growing body and on the fetus. Offer support and community resources for cessation/treatment. Consult the social worker for treatment facilities for pregnant adolescents.
- **Interpersonal violence and other domestic abuse:** Screen the patient at each visit. If positive, offer resources to get help.
- **STI prevention:** Instruct the adolescent to use condoms with every sexual encounter, even during pregnancy, to help prevent an STI.
- **Risk prevention:** Adolescents often are involved in high-risk, impulsive behavior. Ascertain use of safety measures such as seat belts and bike helmets.
- **Immunizations:** Assess the adolescent's immunization status. A pregnant adolescent may need to wait until the postpartum period to receive vaccines such as the quadrivalent HPV vaccine (Gardasil) and the rubella vaccine.
- **Support**
  - Determine whether the father of the baby is involved and if friends and family are supportive of the pregnancy.
  - Screen for depression.
- **Supplies**
  - Ask the patient whether she has heat, water, and electricity at home.
  - Determine whether she has infant supplies, including an infant car seat, diapers, and formula (if choosing this method of feeding; see Box 10–9).
- **School**
  - Collaborate with the school nurse, guidance counselor, and social worker regarding scheduling prenatal visits after

---

Box 10–9 Limitations to Teen Care

Teens generally have limited access to care because of factors such as health insurance coverage, parental consent (refer to individual state laws), availability of low-cost health services, fear of lack of confidentiality (refer to individual state laws), access to transportation, school and work schedules, and fear of HCPs.

school hours and arranging transportation to and from the clinic.

- If the adolescent is to miss school during the hospitalization and postpartum recovery period, ascertain whether tutors are available.

- **Breastfeeding:** Educate the adolescent on the health benefits to mother and baby as well as other advantages, such as the convenience and inexpensiveness of breastfeeding.

Box 10–10 Adolescent Resources

U.S. Department of Health and Human Services
- Office of Adolescent Health: http://www.hhs.gov/ash/oah/
- Women's Health: http://womenshealth.gov

CDC
- Adolescent and School Health: www.cdc.gov/healthyyouth
- Teen Pregnancy and Sexual Health: www.cdc.gov/TeenPregnancy/HealthCareProviders.htm

- Society for Adolescent Health and Medicine: www.adolescenthealth.org

---

11 Substance Abuse

CHAPTER 11

Substance Abuse

Substance abuse and dependence in women has numerous implications for the mother and the fetus/neonate. Education for the prevention of substance use is a key role for nurses. Another role is to screen all patients for substance use, because this behavioral disorder may occur regardless of age, ethnicity, religion, or sexual orientation. Some patients may try to deny substance abuse, whereas others may abuse not just one substance, but several. Thus, a thorough screening is necessary. The nurse also plays a vital role in implementing interventions to care for the recovering mother and withdrawing neonate.

Rather than vague questioning, direct, matter-of-fact, nonjudgmental questioning of patients, using a valid screening tool, is the preferred approach. Many different screening tools are available; copies of several general screening tools are provided in this chapter. See Box 11–1 for one of the tools for screening substance abuse.

The nurse should refer patients thought to have a substance-abuse problem to physicians, nurse practitioners, midwives, or physician assistants trained and experienced in dealing with substance abuse, so the patient may be properly diagnosed, managed, and treated. The nurse should know resources available in the community and seek the help of social workers to determine whether inpatient and outpatient facilities for addiction detoxification and treatment and self-help programs, such as Narcotics Anonymous and Alcoholics Anonymous, are available. Support groups, such as Al-Anon, are also available for family and friends of people suffering from alcoholism.

Substance abuse has wide-ranging effects not only on a woman and her young children, but on the entire family unit. This chapter discusses commonly abused substances, concentrating on the effects of each on women, pregnant women, breastfeeding women, and the fetus/neonate. Treatment options, if available, are also discussed.

LABORATORY TESTING TO DETECT ILLICIT DRUGS MAY BE PERFORMED ON:

- Urine (most common)
- Hair
- Saliva
- Sweat
- Blood
- Nails

FIVE P'S SUBSTANCE ABUSE SCREENING QUESTIONS

Did any of your PARENTS have a problem with using alcohol or drugs?

| YES* | NO | NO ANSWER |

Do any of your friends (PEERS) have a problem with drug or alcohol use?

| YES* | NO | NO ANSWER |

Does your PARTNER have a problem with drug or alcohol use?

| YES* | NO | NO ANSWER |

Before you knew you were pregnant, how often did you drink beer, wine, wine coolers, or liquor?

| NOT AT ALL | RARELY* | SOMETIMES* | FREQUENTLY* |

In the past month (PRESENT), how often did you drink beer, wine, wine coolers, or liquor?

| NOT AT ALL | RARELY* | SOMETIMES* | FREQUENTLY* |

*Considered positive responses.
From Kennedy C, Frankelstein N, Hutchins E, Maloney J. Improving screening for alcohol use during pregnancy: the Massachusetts ASAP program. *Matern Child Health J*. 2004;8:137–147. Used with permission by Kluwer Academic Publishers.

SPEAKING OUT

The professional nurse upholds the patient's confidentiality. A patient's right to privacy should be respected. Drug test results should be treated as confidential medical information unless reporting is specifically required by law. Some states mandate reporting of positive drug tests in pregnancy.

Alcohol (Ethanol)

There is no established safe level of alcohol use in pregnancy. Exposing the fetus to alcohol is associated with a wide range of birth defects that fall under the umbrella of fetal alcohol spectrum disorders (FASD). Therefore, alcohol consumption is contraindicated in pregnancy, and its use during breastfeeding is controversial. Screening tools for alcohol abuse specific to pregnant women should be used, such as the TWEAK (see Box 11–2) and T-ACE (see Box 11–3).

Effects on Women

- After consuming the same amount of alcohol as a man, a woman reaches higher blood alcohol levels and is at more of a risk for alcohol-induced liver disease and cirrhosis than a man.
- Estrogen may play a role in increasing the liver's sensitivity to ethanol.

Box 11–2 TWEAK

TWEAK SUBSTANCE ABUSE SCREENING FOR PREGNANT WOMEN

T—TOLERANCE: How many drinks can you hold? If five or more drinks, score 2 points.

W—Have close friends or relatives WORRIED or complained about your drinking in the past year? If "Yes," 2 points.

E—EYE OPENER: Do you sometimes take a drink in the morning when you get up? If "Yes," 1 point.

A—AMNESIA: Has a friend or family member told you about things you said or did while you were drinking that you could not remember? If "Yes," 1 point.

K(C)—Do you sometimes feel the need to CUT DOWN on your drinking? If "Yes," score 1 point.

A positive screening test for drinking risk in pregnancy is indicated by a total score of 2 or more points.

From Chan AW, Pristach EA, Welte JW, Rusell M. Use of the TWEAK test in screening for alcoholism/heavy drinking in three populations. *Alcohol Clin Exp Res.* 1993;17:1188–1192. Used with permission.

Box 11–3 T-ACE

T-ACE PREGNANCY RISK SCREENING

T—TOLERANCE: How many drinks does it take to make you feel high? More than 2 drinks is a positive response; score 2 points.

A—Have people ANNOYED you by criticizing your drinking? If "Yes," score 1 point.

C—Have you ever felt you ought to CUT DOWN on your drinking? If "Yes," score 1 point.

E—EYE OPENER: Have you ever had a drink first thing in the morning to steady your nerves or get rid of your hangover? If "Yes," score 1 point.

A positive screening test for drinking risk in pregnancy is indicated by a total score of 2 or more points.
From Sokol RJ, Martier SS, Ager JW. The T-ACE questions: practical prenatal detection of risk drinking. *Am J Obstet Gynecol.* 1989;160:863–870. Used with permission.

- Risk for malnutrition includes deficiency in thiamine, riboflavin, pyridoxine, niacin, and vitamin C.
- Alcohol increases risk for breast cancer.

Effects on Pregnant Woman
- One in 12 women report drinking during pregnancy, and 1 in 30 report binge drinking (which is defined as having ≥5 drinks during any one occasion).
- Ethanol crosses the placenta and fetal blood–brain barrier.
- There is no safe level of alcohol during pregnancy.
- An intoxicated pregnant woman is at an increased risk for pulmonary aspiration during labor.
- Malnutrition is a concern for women who abuse alcohol.

Effects on Breastfeeding
- Although the American Academy of Pediatrics (AAP) classifies ethanol as compatible with breastfeeding, it also recognizes ethanol as having detrimental effects on the newborn.
- No more than 0.5 g/kg ethanol may be consumed while lactating, according to the Institute of Medicine.
- There is no sure way to determine what minimum amount of alcohol can be guaranteed not to affect the infant *and* exactly how long alcohol remains in the body before it is completely cleared. Careful counseling of breastfeeding women by the obstetrician, pediatrician, and nurse is needed if a patient is considering alcohol use while nursing.

Effects on the Fetus, Neonate, and Beyond
- Alcohol is broken down at a slower rate in a fetus's body compared with an adult's; thus, the alcohol level remains higher and stays in the bloodstream longer.
- FASDs refer to a range of effects on a fetus who was exposed to alcohol in utero.
  - **Types of FASDs**
    - Fetal alcohol syndrome (FAS) is at the severe end of the spectrum of FASDs. Commonly, people with FAS have distinct abnormal facial features such as a smooth philtrum, low nasal bridge, and thin upper lip, and they may also suffer from problems with memory, communication, vision, and hearing (see Fig. 11–1).
    - Alcohol-related neurodevelopmental disorder is associated with poor motor skills, functional impairments, and mental impairments.
    - Alcohol-related birth defects describe skeletal and organ malformations and defects that affect the heart, bones, and kidneys.

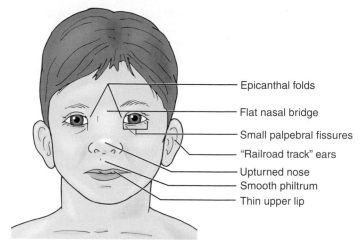

Epicanthal folds
Flat nasal bridge
Small palpebral fissures
"Railroad track" ears
Upturned nose
Smooth philtrum
Thin upper lip

FIGURE 11-1: Fetal alcohol syndrome features.

Treatment

Treatment should involve personal intervention and assessment; referral to other health-care professionals, groups, and agencies that are trained and experienced in dealing with substance abuse; and the use of drugs, if available, to help treat the problem.

Nonpharmacological Treatment

- Brief interventions: *You*, the nurse, can make a difference by providing counseling on the negative effects of alcohol. Studies by Fleming and Manwell and DiClemente have shown that counseling from primary care physicians and nursing staff is effective in reducing alcohol consumption.
- Programs, such as 12-step self-help programs like Alcoholics Anonymous, have been designed to combat alcohol abuse.
- Psychosocial and motivational therapy are effective treatment methods.

Pharmacological Treatment

There are only three U.S. Food and Drug Administration–approved drugs for treating alcohol dependence.

- Disulfiram (Antabuse): Causes unpleasant symptoms such as nausea, throbbing headache, and flushing when alcohol is ingested.
- Naltrexone: This is an opioid receptor antagonist that may cause gastrointestinal side effects such as stomach cramps and constipation.

ALERT!

Alcohol withdrawal in adults usually occurs 6 to 48 hours after consumption.
  Sign and symptoms include:

- Cardiac failure
- Seizures
- Hypertension
- Tachycardia
- Delirium
- Nausea

- Acamprosate (Campral): This is thought to affect the brain pathways related to alcohol abuse. It is generally well tolerated, with the most common negative side effects being headache and gastrointestinal complaints; however, some serious adverse effects, including allergic reactions, irregular heartbeat, and changes in blood pressure, can occur.

Heroin

Heroin is a synthetic opioid drug derived from morphine extracted from the Asian opium poppy plant (*Papaver somniferum*). Heroin is usually injected but can also be snorted, sniffed, or smoked.

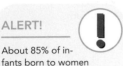

ALERT!

About 85% of infants born to women using heroin may be born physically dependent on heroin and suffer from withdrawal after birth. Withdrawal symptoms usually occur within 48 hours, but they may be exhibited up to 6 days after birth. The neonate/infant usually requires hospitalization.
  Symptoms include:

- Hyperactivity
- Respiratory distress
- Fever
- Diarrhea
- Mucous secretion
- Sweating
- Convulsions
- Yawning
- Face scratching

Effects on Women
- May cause drowsiness, dry mouth, skin flushing, and constipation
- May result in respiratory depression, which may be fatal
- Increases risk for contracting HIV and hepatitis C with needle sharing

Effects on Pregnant Women
- Drug rapidly crosses the placenta and thus can affect the fetus
- Increases risk for spontaneous abortion

Effects on Fetus and Neonate
- Within 1 hour of use, heroin may be found in fetal tissues
- Meconium staining of amniotic fluid
- Increased perinatal mortality risk
- Low birth weight and lower weight at age 3 to 6 years
- Developmental delays

Effect on Breastfeeding
Because heroin crosses into breast milk, the AAP considers heroin use to be contraindicated in breastfeeding.

Treatment
Nonpharmacological
Nonpharmacological treatment includes behavioral therapy on an outpatient or in-hospital basis.
Pharmacological
Pharmacological treatment may be used to help prevent relapse. Several medications may be used to treat heroin addiction.
- Methadone, which binds to the same receptors as heroin, is prescribed to be taken orally to gradually decrease the desire for

heroin and alleviate withdrawal symptoms. Methadone treatment is dispensed only through treatment programs. It is the drug of choice for treating heroin abuse in pregnancy.

- Buprenorphine is a narcotic antagonist that works in the same way as methadone but with reduced risk for overdose. A patient may obtain a prescription for this drug and does not need to be in a specialized treatment program.
- Naltrexone is a narcotic antagonist. There is a problem with compliance, and it is not as popular as the other two drugs.

Neonatal Abstinence Syndrome

Infants withdrawing from substances on which they have become physically dependent because of exposure while in utero suffer from neonatal abstinence syndrome (NAS). Newborns who suffer the severest withdrawal symptoms are those exposed to opioids such as heroin, morphine, and methadone. Common symptoms of NAS include high-pitched cry, irritability, hyper-reflexia, tremors, diarrhea, vomiting, tachypnea, apnea, flaring, retractions, and skin excoriations. Time of onset and severity of symptoms vary depending on drug(s) used. Methadone may be used antenatally with a low-maintenance dosage as substitution therapy for women who are addicted to heroin. Methadone might put the neonate at greater risk for NAS than heroin; however, methadone maintenance therapy is related to increased antenatal care, leading to better maternal outcomes such as a reduced risk for preterm delivery (PTD) and low-birth weight infants.

Treatment
NAS is commonly treated with morphine and methadone.

Recommended Nursing Interventions
The following are recommended nursing interventions for newborns suffering from NAS.

- Minimize tactile stimuli.
- Provide a quiet, dimly lit environment.
- Gently rock the infant.
- Swaddle infant with a blanket.
- Offer a pacifier.
- Provide small, frequent feedings.
- As per order, obtain toxicology screen (usually via urine) on neonate.
- Monitor the newborn closely for any signs of NAS.
- Use a neonatal abstinence scoring tool to objectively assess for signs of withdrawal and report abnormal results to the physician, nurse practitioner, or physician's assistant.

- Educate the mother and her family and/or foster mother and her family on common symptoms exhibited by infants suffering from withdrawal, and prepare them for the anticipated length of hospital stay while the infant is being treated.
- Facilitate mother–infant bonding by providing a calm environment for the couplet, and teach the mother or foster mother techniques for soothing the infant.
- Ensure follow-up care for both mother and infant before discharge from the hospital.

Marijuana

A hallucinogen, marijuana is the most commonly abused drug in the United States. More than 94 million Americans aged 12 years and older have tried marijuana at least once. Also known as weed, pot, grass, reefer, or Mary Jane, marijuana comes from the flowers, stems, seeds, and leaves of the *Cannabis sativa* plant. Its main psychoactive agent is delta-9-tetrahydrocannabinol (THC). Marijuana usually is smoked as a cigarette (called a "joint") or in a pipe. An oral formulation of marijuana is available and can be used legally in some states as an antiemetic agent.

Effects on Women
The effects of marijuana use on women include:
- Distorted perception
- Impaired coordination and balance
- Suboptimal learning and memory
- Increased rates of anxiety, depression, suicidal ideation, and schizophrenia
- Four times the risk for myocardial infarction (MI) in the first hour after smoking marijuana
- Increased risk for lung infections

Effects on Pregnant Women
- THC crosses the placenta to the fetus at term.
- Meconium-stained amniotic fluid
- Precipitous labor

Effects on Fetus and Neonate
- Intrauterine growth restriction (IUGR) leading to low birth weight and length
- Cognitive deficits in children: difficulty applying skills and sustaining attention
- Increased tremors*
- Exaggerated startles*
- Increase in irritability*
- Decreased visual responses*

---

*According to the Ottawa Prenatal Prospective Study of infants exposed to marijuana in utero

Effects on Breastfeeding
THC is excreted in breast milk. The AAP strongly discourages the use of marijuana while breastfeeding.

Treatment
Currently, there is no pharmacological regimen available for treating marijuana addiction. Cognitive-behavioral therapy has been shown to be effective in treating marijuana addiction.

Methamphetamine

Methamphetamine is an inexpensive central nervous system stimulant that is also known as meth, ice, and crystal meth. Methamphetamine can be ingested orally, injected, smoked, or sniffed.

Effects on Women
- Changes in blood pressure
- Tachycardia and arrhythmias
- Insomnia
- Nausea, vomiting, and anorexia
- Stroke
- Psychiatric symptoms such as anxiety, panic, hallucinations, depression, self-mutilation, and psychosis

Effects on Pregnant Women
- Rapidly crosses the placenta to the fetus
- IUGR
- PTD

Effects on Fetus and Neonate
- Accumulates in fetal tissues
- Shrill cries
- Marked drowsiness
- Irritability

Effect on Breastfeeding
Methamphetamine crosses into the breast milk and can be found in the urine of breastfed infants. Effects on breastfed infants are unknown. The AAP classifies amphetamine use as a contraindication to breastfeeding.

ALERT!

Methampheta-mine withdrawal in newborns is character-ized by:

- Abnormal sleep patterns
- Tremor
- Hypertonia
- Poor feeding

Treatment
Currently, no pharmacological regimen is available for treating methamphetamine addiction. Behavioral therapy has been shown to be an effective treatment approach when combined with family education and family counseling.

Tobacco

Despite the fact that tobacco use is related to 500,000 deaths in the United States each year, the National Survey on Drug Use and Health reports that 70.3 million Americans aged 12 years or older use tobacco. Tobacco may be smoked as cigarettes, cigars, or in a pipe; it can also be chewed.

Effects on Women

- According to the U.S. Department of Health and Human Services (USDHHS), 90% of lung cancer deaths in women are due to smoking; lung cancer deaths in the United States in women have increased 600% in the past 50 years
- 60% increased risk for infertility in women
- **Increased risk for many types of cancers:** mouth, pharynx, larynx, esophagus, lung, stomach, pancreas, cervix, kidney, ureter, and bladder
- Increased risk for lung diseases, including pneumonia, chronic bronchitis, and emphysema
- Increased risk for exacerbation of asthma
- Increase in blood glucose level
- Increase in blood pressure, heart rate, and respiratory rate
- Increased risk for heart disease leading to stroke, MI, vascular disease, and aneurysm

Effects on Pregnant Women

- Cigarette smoking is contraindicated in pregnancy.
- Nicotine crosses the placenta to reach the fetus.
- There is an increased risk for spontaneous abortion, PTD, premature rupture of the membranes, ectopic pregnancy, placental abruption, placenta previa, and stillbirth.

Effects on Breastfeeding

- Nicotine can be found in breast milk.
- Infants are exposed to nicotine through ingestion of breast milk and inhalation of cigarette smoke.
- Nicotine may decrease the volume of breast milk.
- Duration of breastfeeding is shorter (in number of days) in mothers who smoke.

WHY ARE CIGARETTE CONTENTS IMPORTANT?

Nicotine is one of the main addictive components of tobacco; however, there are more than 3000 different compounds found in cigarette smoke, such as carbon monoxide, hydrogen cyanide, and ammonia, that may contribute to adverse health outcomes.

HOW DOES NICOTINE INCREASE A SMOKER'S BLOOD PRESSURE, HEART RATE, AND RESPIRATION RATE?

Nicotine stimulates the adrenal glands that then produce more epinephrine (adrenaline). Adrenaline stimulates the body to increase blood pressure, heart rate, and respiratory rate.

There is insufficient data regarding the use of nicotine replacement therapy (NRT; patches, gum, inhaler, nasal sprays) during breastfeeding. Although the AAP encourages smoking cessation during the period of lactation, no position is made regarding breastfeeding and use of nicotine replacement products.

Effects on Fetus and Neonate

- Nicotine may accumulate in fetal blood and amniotic fluid; fetus may have 15% greater concentration of nicotine than the mother
- Intrauterine growth restriction leading to low birth weight
- Increased risk for sudden infant death syndrome (SIDS)
- Increased risk for oral clefts
- Learning and behavioral problems in children
- Children exposed to secondhand smoke have an increased risk for development of otitis media and respiratory diseases, including asthma.

Additional studies are needed to ascertain the risk for NRT to the embryo/fetus.

Treatment

Refer to Box 11–4 for smoking guidelines for clinicians from the USDHHS.

Box 11–4 Smoking Cessation

SMOKING CESSATION GUIDELINES FOR CLINICIANS

THE FIVE A'S APPROACH

ASK about tobacco use.

Identify and document tobacco use status for every patient at every visit.

ADVISE to quit.

In a clear, strong, and personalized manner, urge every tobacco user to quit.

ASSESS willingness to make an attempt at quitting.

Is the tobacco user willing to make a quit attempt at this time?

ASSIST in quit attempt.

For the patient willing to make a quit attempt, use counseling and pharmacotherapy (prescribed by a physician, nurse practitioner, Certified Nurse-Midwife, or physician's assistant) to help her quit:

1. Suggest and encourage the use of problem-solving methods and skills for smoking cessation (e.g., identify "trigger" situations).
2. Provide social support as part of the treatment (e.g., "we can help you quit").
3. Arrange social support in the smoker's environment (e.g., identify "quit buddy" and smoke-free space).
4. Provide self-help smoking cessation materials.

ARRANGE follow-up.

Schedule follow-up contact, preferably within the first week after quit date.

From Agency for Healthcare Research and Quality. Treating tobacco use and dependence: 2008 update. Available at: www.ahrq.gov/clinic/tobacco/treating_tobacco_use08.pdf. Accessed September 6, 2012.

Nonpharmacological

Nonpharmacological approaches include counseling (in-person, telephone, or web-based), social support (through family and friends), and community resources.

Pharmacological

Medications for smoking cessation include:

- bupropion (Wellbutrin-SR; Category B)
- nicotine gum (Category C)
- nicotine patch (NicoDerm CQ; Category D)
- nicotine inhaler and spray (Category D)
- nicotine lozenge (Category D)

Resources for Patients

- Alcoholics Anonymous: www.aa.org
- Centers for Disease Control and Prevention: www.cdc.gov
- March of Dimes: www.marchofdimes.com
- Narcotics Anonymous: www.na.org
- Smoking cessation: www.smokefree.gov and www.cdc.gov/tobacco

---

★ BEST PRACTICE

Once you have recognized that your patient is a tobacco user, you should warn her about its use and if she is pregnant or breastfeeding, about its possible effects on the fetus/neonate/infant. There is no such thing as a safe tobacco product. Whether the tobacco product is a cigarette, cigar, tobacco in a pipe, or chewing (smokeless) tobacco and whether it is advertised as "light," "ultra light," "low tar," "mild," "additive free," or "naturally grown," it is still detrimental to a person's health and may cause many forms of cancer.

QSEN Application

Patient-centered care includes skills such as:

- Recognizing the boundaries of therapeutic relationships
- Facilitating informed patient consent for care
- Removing barriers to presence of families and other designated surrogates based on patient preferences
- Assessing level of patient's decisional conflict and providing access to resources
- Engaging patients or designated surrogates in active partnerships that promote health, safety, well-being, and self-care management

In this chapter, together with information about care of pregnant women and newborns, QSEN competencies assure delivery of the best nursing care.

http://qsen.org/competencies/pre-licensure-ksas/#patient-centered_care

12 Tools

CHAPTER 12

Tools

Table 12–1 Metric Conversions

WEIGHT		TEMPERATURE		HEIGHT		
LBS	KG	°F	°C	CM	IN	FT/IN
300	136.4	212	100 boil	142	56	4′ 8″
275	125.0	107	42.2	145	57	4′ 9″
250	113.6	106	41.6	147	58	4′ 10″
225	102.3	105	40.6	150	59	4′ 11″
210	95.5	104	40.0	152	60	5′ 0″
200	90.9	103	39.4	155	61	5′ 1″
190	86.4	102	38.9	157	62	5′ 2″
180	81.8	101	38.3	160	63	5′ 3″
170	77.3	100	37.8	163	64	5′ 4″
160	72.7	99	37.2	165	65	5′ 5″
150	68.2	98.6	37.0	168	66	5′ 6″
140	63.6	98	36.7	170	67	5′ 7″
130	59.1	97	36.1	173	68	5′ 8″
120	54.5	96	35.6	175	69	5′ 9″
110	50.0	95	35.0	178	70	5 ′10″
100	45.5	94	34.4	180	71	5 ′11″
90	40.9	93	34.0	183	72	6′ 0″

Continued

Table 12-1 Metric Conversions—cont'd

WEIGHT		TEMPERATURE		HEIGHT		
LBS	KG	°F	°C	CM	IN	FT/IN
80	36.4	92	33.3	185	73	6' 1"
70	31.8	91	32.8	188	74	6' 2"
60	27.3	90	32.1	191	75	6' 3"
50	22.7	**32**	**0** freeze	193	76	6' 4"
40	18.2			196	77	6' 5"
30	13.6					
20	9.1					
10	4.5					
5	2.3					
2.2	**1**					
2	0.9					
1	**0.45**					
lb = kg x 2.2		*or*	kg = lb x 0.45			
°F = (°C x 1.8) + 32			*or*	°C = (°F – 32) x 0.556		
inches = cm x 0.394			*or*	cm = inches x 2.54		

From Litwack K. *Clinical Coach for Effective Nursing Care*. Philadelphia, PA: FA Davis Company; 2009.

Table 12–2 Basic English-to-Spanish Translation

ENGLISH PHRASE	PRONUNCIATION	SPANISH PHRASE
INTRODUCTIONS—GREETINGS		
Hello.	**oh**-lah	Hola
Good morning.	**bweh**-nohs **dee**-ahs	Buenos días
Good afternoon.	**bweh**-nohs **tahr**-dehs	Buenos tardes
Good evening.	**bweh**-nahs **noh**-chehs	Buenas noches
My name is...	*meh* **yah**-*moh*	Me llamo
I am a nurse.	soy lah oon en-fehr-**meh**-ra	Soy la enfermera
What is your name?	koh-moh seh yah-mah oo-sted?	¿ Cómo se llama usted?
How are you?	**koh-moh eh-stah oo-stehd?**	¿Como esta usted?
Very well.	*mwee b' yehn*	Muy bien
Thank you.	grah-s'yahs	Gracias
Yes, No.	sce, noh	Sí, No
Please.	pohr fah-vohr	Por favor
You're welcome.	deh **nah**-dah	De nada
ASSESSMENT—AREAS OF THE BODY		
Head	kah-beh-sah	Cabeza
Eye	oh-hoh	Ojo
Ear	oh-ee-doh	Oído
Nose	nah-reez	Nariz
Throat	gahr-gahn-tah	Garganta
Neck	kweh-yoh	Cuello
Chest, Heart	peh-choh, kah-rah-sohn	Pecho, corazón
Back	eh-spahl-dah	Espalda
Abdomen	ahb-doh-mehn	Abdomen

Continued

Table 12–2 Basic English-to-Spanish Translation—cont'd

ENGLISH PHRASE	PRONUNCIATION	SPANISH PHRASE
Stomach	eh-stoh-mah-goh	Estómago
Rectum	rehk-toh	Recto
Penis	peh-neh	Pene
Vagina	vah-hee-nah	Vagina
Arm, Hand	brah-soh, mah-noh	Brazo, Mano
Leg, Foot	p'yehr-nah, p'yeh	Pierna, Pie
ASSESSMENT—HISTORY		
Do you have...	T'yeh-neh oo-stehd...	¿Tiene usted...
• Difficulty breathing?	di-fi-kul-thad	¿Dificultad para respirar?
• Chest pain?	doh-lorh hen lh peh-chow	¿Dolor en el pecho?
• Abdominal pain?	doh-lorh ab-do-minl	¿Dolor abdominal?
• Diabetes?	dee-ah-beh-tehs	¿Diabetes?
Are you...	ehs-tah	¿Esta...
• Dizzy?	ma:r-eh-a-dho(dha)	¿Mareado(a)?
• Nauseated?	ka:n now-she-as	¿Con nauseas?
• Pregnant?	¿ehm-bah-rah-sah-dah?	¿Embarazada?
Are you allergic to any medications?	¿ehs ah-lehr-hee-koh ah ahl-goo-nah meh-dee-see-nah?	¿Es alergico a alguna medicina?
ASSESSMENT—PAIN		
Do you have pain?	T'yeh-neh oo-stehd doh-lorh?	¿Tiene usted dolor?
Where does it hurt?	dohn-deh leh dweh-leh?	¿Donde le duele?
Is the pain...	es oon doh-lor...	¿Es un dolor...
• Dull?	Leh-veh	¿Leve?
• Aching?	ka:ns-tan-the	¿constante?
• Crushing?	ah-plahs-than-teh?	¿Aplastante?

Table 12–2 **Basic English-to-Spanish Translation—cont'd**

ENGLISH PHRASE	PRONUNCIATION	SPANISH PHRASE
• Sharp?	ah-goo-doh?	¿Agudo?
• Stabbing?	ah-poo-neo-lawn-teh	¿Apuñalante?
• Burning?	Ahr-d'yen-the?	¿Ardiente?
Does it hurt when I press here?	Leh dweh-leh kwahn-doh ah-pree-eh-toh ah-kee?	¿Le duele cuando le aprieto aqui?
Does it hurt to breathe deeply?	S'yen-teh oo-sted doh-lor kwahn-doh reh-spee-rah pro-foon-dah-men-teh?	¿Siente usted dolor cuando respira profundamente?
Does it move to another area?	Lh doh-lor zeh moo-eh-veh a oh-thra ah-ri-ah	¿El dolor se mueve a otra area?
Is the pain better now?	c-n-the al-goo-nah me-horr-i-ah	¿Siente alguna mejoria?

From Litwack K. *Clinical Coach for Effective Nursing Care.* Philadelphia, PA: FA Davis Company; 2009.

Table 12-3 Newborn Weight Conversions Pounds and Ounces to Grams

OUNCES	POUNDS												
	0	1	2	3	4	5	6	7	8	9	10	11	12
0	0	454	907	1361	1814	2268	2722	3175	3629	4082	4536	4990	5443
1	28	482	936	1389	1843	2296	2750	3203	3657	4111	4564	5019	5471
2	57	510	964	1417	1871	2325	2778	3232	3685	4139	4593	5046	5500
3	85	539	992	1446	1899	2353	2807	3260	3714	4167	4621	5075	5528
4	113	567	1021	1474	1928	2381	2835	3289	3742	4196	4649	5103	5557
5	142	595	1049	1503	1956	2410	2863	3317	3770	4224	4678	5131	5585
6	170	624	1077	1531	1984	2438	2892	3345	3799	4252	4706	5160	5613
7	198	652	1106	1559	2013	2466	2920	3374	3827	4281	4734	5188	5642

8	227	680	1134	1588	2041	2495	2949	3402	3856	4309	4763	5216	5670
9	255	709	1162	1616	2070	2523	2977	3430	3884	4337	4791	5245	5698
10	284	737	1191	1644	2098	2551	3005	3459	3912	4366	4819	5273	5727
11	312	765	1219	1673	2126	2580	3034	3487	3941	4394	4848	5301	5755
12	340	794	1247	1701	2155	2608	3062	3515	3969	4423	4876	5330	5783
13	369	822	1276	1729	2183	2637	3091	3544	3997	4451	4904	5358	5812
14	397	850	1304	1758	2211	2665	3119	3572	4026	4479	4933	5386	5840
15	425	879	1332	1786	2240	2693	3147	3600	4054	4508	4961	5415	5868

Important Websites

American Academy of Pediatrics: www.aap.org
American Congress of Obstetricians and Gynecologists: www.acog.org
Association of Women's Health, Obstetric and Neonatal Nurses: www.awhonn.org
Centers for Disease Control and Prevention: www.cdc.gov
- Adolescent and School Health: www.cdc.gov/healthyyouth
- Teen Pregnancy and Sexual Health: www.cdc.gov/TeenPregnancy/HealthCareProviders.htm
- Sexually Transmitted Disease Treatment Guidelines: www.cdc.gov/std/treatment/
National Institutes of Health: www.nih.gov
- LactMed: lactmed.nlm.nih.gov
- National Institute on Minority Health and Health Disparities: www.nimhd.nih.gov
Society for Adolescent Health and Medicine: www.adolescenthealth.org
U.S. Department of Agriculture: Food and Nutrition Service: www.fns.usda.gov/
- Nutrition Education: www.choosemyplate.gov
- Women, Infants, and Children (WIC) Program: www.fns.usda.gov/wic
U.S. Department of Health and Human Services: http://www.hhs.gov/
- Office of Adolescent Health: www.hhs.gov/ash/oah/
- Women's Health: http://womenshealth.gov

Figure Credits

Figures 1-1, 2-3, 3-1, 3-2, 3-3, 3-5, 3-6, 4-1, 4-3, 6-8, 6-9, 6-10, 6-16, and 7-2 are from Ward S and Hisley S (2011). Maternal-Child Nursing Care: Optimizing Outcomes for Mothers, Children, and Families, Enhanced Revised Reprint. Philadelphia: F. A. Davis Company.

Figures 1-2, 1-3, 1-4, 6-1, 6-3, 6-4, 6-5, 6-6, 6-11, 6-12, 6-13, and 6-14A and B are from Dillon P (2007). Nursing Health Assessment: A Critical Thinking, Case Studies Approach, Second Edition. Philadelphia: F.A. Davis Company.

Figures 1-5, 1-6, 1-7, 1-8, 2-1, 2-2, 3-4, 3-7, 3-8, 3-9, 4-2 are from Holloway B, Moredich C, Aduddell K (2006). OB Peds Women's Health Notes: Nurse's Clinical Pocket Guide. Philadelphia: F.A. Davis Company.

Figures 6-2 and 6-17 and unnumbered figures 6-1, 6-2, 6-3, and 6-4 are from Chapman L and Durham RF (2009). Maternal-Newborn Nursing: The Critical Components of Nursing Care. Philadelphia: F.A. Davis Company.

Figure 6-7 is courtesy of Kimm Sun, CNM; Dalia Alvarenga; and Baby Aren.

References

Academy of Breastfeeding Medicine. Clinical protocols. Available at: www.bfmed.org/Resources/Protocols.aspx. Accessed December 7, 2012.

American Academy of Family Physicians. Labor, delivery, and post-partum issues. *Ameri Fami Physician J.* Available at: www.aafp.org/afp/topicModules/viewTopicModule.htm?topicModuleId=16. Updated July 30, 2012.

American Academy of Pediatrics. Breastfeeding education for health professionals. *Health Professionals Resource Guide.* Available at: www2.aap.org/breastfeeding/healthProfessionaIsResourceGuide. html#breastfeedingEducationForHealthProfessionals.

American Academy of Pediatrics Policy Statement. Breastfeeding and the use of human milk. *Pediatr.* 2005;115(2):496-506.

American Association of Diabetes Educators. Guidelines for the practice of diabetes education. 2011. Available at: www.diabeteseducator.org/export/sites/aade/_resources/pdf/general/PracticeGuidelines2011.pdf

American Bar Association. Domestic violence statistics. Available at: www.americanbar.org/groups/domestic_violence/resources/statistics.html.

American College of Obstetricians and Gynecologists. ACOG Practice Bulletin No. 106: Intrapartum fetal heart rate monitoring: nomenclature, interpretation, and general management principles. *Obstet Gynecol.* 2009;114:192–202. Available at: www.ohsu.edu/academic/som/obgyn/programs/ACOG%20Practice%20Bulletin%20106,%20July%202009.pdf.

American College of Obstetricians and Gynecologists. If your baby is breech. Available at: www.acog.org/~/media/For%20Patients/faq079.pdf?dmc=1&ts=20121201T2209072052. Published August 2011.

American College of Obstetricians and Gynecologists Committee on Practice Bulletins-Obstetrics; Society for Maternal-Fetal Medicine; ACOG Joint Editorial Committee. ACOG Practice Bulletin #56: Multiple gestation: complicated twin, triplet, and high-order multifetal pregnancy. *Obstet Gynecol.* 2004;104:869-883.

American College of Obstetricians and Gynecologists Committee on Practice Bulletins—Obstetrics. ACOG Practice Bulletin. Clinical management guidelines for obstetrician-gynecologists. Number 30, September 2001 (replaces Technical Bulletin Number 200, December 1994). Gestational diabetes. *Obstet Gynecol.* 2001; 98:525-538.

American Society for Colposcopy and Cervical Pathology. 2006 Consensus Guidelines for the Management of Women With Abnormal Cervical Screening Tests. Available at: www.asccp.org/ConsensusGuidelines/AbnormalCervicalScreeningTests/tabid/5958/Default.aspx.

Anderson FWJ, Johnson CT. Complementary and alternative medicine in obstetrics. *Int J Gynecol Obstet.* 2005;91(2):116-124. doi:10.1016/j.ijgo.2005.07.009.

Association of Reproductive Health Professionals. Postpartum counseling: quick reference guide for physicians. 2006. Available at: www.arhp.org/uploadDocs/QRGpostpartum.pdf

Ballard JL, Khoury JC, Wedig K,Wang L, Eilers-Walsman BL, Lipp R. New Ballard Score, expanded to include extremely premature infants. *J Pediatr.* 1991;119(3):417-423.

Berkowitz B. Cultural aspects in the care of the Orthodox Jewish woman. *J Midwifery Womens Health.* 2008;53(1):62-66.

Berry T. *Religions of India.* 2nd ed. New York, NY: Columbia University Press; 1992.

Bullock L, Bloom T, Davis J, Kilburn E, Curry MA. Abuse disclosure in privately and medicaid-funded pregnant women. *J Midwifery Womens Health* 2006;51(5):361-369.

Buz Harlor AD Jr, Bower C. Hearing assessment in infants and children: recommendations beyond neonatal screening. *Pediatr.* 2009;124(4):1252-1263.

Centers for Disease Control and Prevention. Basic statistics. Atlanta, GA: U.S. Department of Health and Human Services; 2011. Available at: www.cdcnpin.org/scripts/population/men.asp.

Centers for Disease Control and Prevention. Diethylstilbestrol (DES) information. Available at: www.cdc.gov/DES.

Centers for Disease Control and Prevention. New estimates of U.S. HIV prevalence, 2006. Available at: www.cdc.gov/hiv/topics/surveillance/resources/factsheets/prevalence.htm.

Centers for Disease Control and Prevention. Proper handling and storage of human milk. Available at: www.cdc.gov/breastfeeding/recommendations/handling_breastmilk.htm.

Centers for Disease Control and Prevention. Smoking and tobacco use: how to quit. Available at: www.cdc.gov/tobacco/quit_smoking/how_to_quit/index.htm.

Centers for Disease Control and Prevention. Vaccines and immunizations. Available at: www.cdc.gov/vaccines.

Chapman L, Durham R. *Maternal-newborn nursing: the critical components of nursing care.* Philadelphia, PA: FA Davis Company; 2009.

Choudhry UK. Traditional practices of women from India: pregnancy, childbirth and newborn care. *J Obstet Gynecol Neonat Nurs.* 1997;26(5):533-539.

Darby SB. Traditional Chinese medicine: a complement to conventional. *Nurs Womens Health.* 2009;13(3):200-206.

Dombrowski MP. Asthma and pregnancy. *Obstet Gynecol.* 2006;108(3):667-681.

Dombrowski MP, Schatz M; ACOG Committee on Practice Bulletins-Obstetrics. ACOG practice bulletin: clinical management guidelines for obstetrician-gynecologists number 90, February 2008: asthma in pregnancy. *Obstet Gynecol.* 2008;111(2, pt 1):457-464.

Dutton MA, Orloff L, Hass GA. Characteristics of help-seeking behaviors, resources and service needs of battered immigrant Latinas: legal and policy implications. *Georgetown J Poverty Law Policy.* 2000:7:245-305.

EBSCO MegaFILE database. Gay youth have higher pregnancy rates than straight youth. *Contemporary Sexuality.* 2009. Available at: search.ebscohost.com.

Futures Without Violence. *Health.* Available at: www. futureswithoutviolence.org/section/our_work/health.

Gabbe SG, Niebyl JR, Simpson JL, et al., eds. *Obstetrics: Normal and Problem Pregnancies.* 5th ed. Philadelphia, PA: Churchill Livingstone; 2007:138.

Ganley AL: The health impact of domestic violence. In: Warshaw C, Ganley AL, eds. *Improving the Healthcare Response to Domestic Violence: A Resource Manual for Health Care Providers* 2nd ed. San Francisco, CA: Family Violence Prevention Fund; 1996:15-16.

George MS, Rahangdale L. Domestic violence and South Asian women. *N C Med J.* 1999;60(3):157-159.

Henneman T. Birth control for lesbian teens. *Advocate.* 2008; (1008):12.

Holloway BW, Moredich C, Aduddell K. *Ob Peds Women's Health Notes: Nurse's Clinical Pocket Guide.* Philadelphia, PA: FA Davis Company; 2006.

Huntley AL, Coon JT, Ernst E. Complementary and alternative medicine for labor pain: a systematic review. *Am J Obstet Gynecol.* 2004;191(1):36-44.

Krulewitch C, Pierre-Louis ML, deLeon-Gome R, Guy R, Green R: Hidden from view: violent deaths among pregnant women in the District of Columbia, 1988–1996. *J Midwifery Women's Health* 2001;46(1):4-10.

Ladewig PW, London ML, Davidson M. *Clinical Handbook for Contemporary Maternal-Newborn Nursing Care.* 6th ed. Upper Saddle River, NJ: Pearson Prentice Hall; 2006.

Margulies R, Miller L. Fruit size as a model for teaching first trimester uterine sizing in bimanual examination. *Obstet Gynecol.* 2001;98(2):341-344.

Mao LC, Pan X, Que F. Antioxidant activities of five Chinese rice wines and the involvement of phenolic compounds. *Food Res Int.* 2006;39:581-587.

Mattson S. Caring for Latino women. *AWHONN Lifelines.* 2003;7(3): 258-260.

Mayeaux EJ: *Optimizing the Papanicolaou smear.* Louisiana State University Shreveport Health and Sciences Center. Available at: www.sh.lsuhsc.edu/fammed/OutpatientManual/PapSmear.htm.

Midura TF, Snowden S, Wood RM, Arnon SS. Isolation of Clostridium botulinum from honey. *J Clin Microbiol.* 1979;9(2):282-283.

National Center on Birth Defects and Developmental Disabilities. Fetal alcohol syndrome: guidelines for referral and diagnosis. May 2005.

National Diabetes Information Clearinghouse. What I need to know about gestational diabetes. Available at: http://diabetes.niddk.nih. gov/dm/pubs/gestational. Accessed December 6, 2011.

National Heart Lung and Blood Institute. Lung diseases information. Available at: www.nhlbi.nih.gov/health/public/lung/index. htm#asthma

O'Connor M. The breastfeeding couple: Initiation—nursing immediately after birth. Available at: www.breastfeedingbasics.org/cgi-bin/ deliver.cgi/content/Normal/firstfeed.html.

Parsons L, Goodwin MM, Petersen R. Violence against women and reproductive health: toward defining a role for reproductive health care services. *Matern Child Health J.* 2000;4(2):135-140.

Que F, Linchun M, Xin P: Isolation of Clostridium botulinum from honey. *Food Res Int* 2006;89:581-587.

Raj A, Silverman JG. Immigrant South Asian women at greater risk for injury from intimate partner violence. *Am J Public Health.* 2003;93(3):435-437.

Rodriguez R. Evaluation of the MSN domestic violence assessment form and pilot prevalence study. *Clin Suppl Migr Clin Netw.* 1995;1-2.

Rubin R. Maternal tasks in pregnancy. *Matern Child Nurs J.* 1975;4(3): 143-153.

Saltzman LE, Johnson CH, Gilbert BC, Goodwin MM. Physical abuse around the time of pregnancy: an examination of prevalence and risk factors in 16 states. *Matern Child Health J.* 2003;7(1): 31-43.

Sanfilippo JS, Lara-Torre E. Adolescent gynecology. *Obstet Gynecol.* 2009;113(4):935-947. Retrieved from EBSCO MegaFILE database: search.ebscohost.com.

Schatz M, Dombrowski MP, Wise R, et al. Asthma morbidity during pregnancy can be predicted by severity classification. *J Allergy Clin Immunol.* 2003;112(2):283-288.

Song YI. *Battered Women in Korean Immigrant Families: The Silent Scream.* New York, NY: Garland; 1996.

Tjaden P, Thoennes N. *Extent, nature and consequences of intimate partner violence: Findings from the national violence against women survey.* Philadelphia, PA: U.S. Department of Justice; 2000:36.

Trudelle Schwarz M. *Navajo Lifeways: Contemporary Issues, Ancient Knowledge.* Norman, OK: University of Oklahoma Press; 2001.

University of Utah Healthcare. Pediatric neurologic exam. Available at: http://library.med.utah.edu/pedineurologicexam/html/ newborn_n.html#23.

University of Washington. Hepatitis web study. Available at: http://depts.washington.edu/hepstudy/index.html.

U.S. Department of Agriculture. Protect your baby and yourself from listeriosis. Available at: www.fsis.usda.gov/PDF/Protect_Your_Baby.pdf.

U.S. Department of Health and Human Services. Women's health: an easy guide to breastfeeding for American Indian and Alaska Native families. Available at: www.womenshealth.gov/publications/our-publications/breastfeeding-guide/BreastfeedingGuide-Native American-English.pdf

U.S. Department of Transportation, National Highway Traffic Safety Administration (NHTSA). *Traffic Safety Facts 2006: Alcohol-Impaired Driving.* Washington DC: NHTSA; 2008. www-nrd. nhtsa.dot.gov/Pubs/810801.PDF.

Usta IM, Nassar AH. Advanced maternal age. Part I: obstetric complications. *Am J Perinatol.* 2008;25(8):521-534.

Werner C, Westerst_hl A. Donor insemination and parenting: concerns and strategies of lesbian couples. A review of international studies. *Acta Obstet Gynecol Scand.* 2008;87(7):697-701. doi:10.1080/00016340802011603

Willis WO. Culturally competent nursing care during the perinatal period. *J Perinat Neonatal Nurs.* 1999;13(3):45-59.

Medications*

High Alert

oxytocin (ox-i-**toe**-sin)
Pitocin

Classification

Therapeutic: hormones

Pharmacologic: oxytocics

Pregnancy Category X

Indications

IV: Induction of labor at term. **IV:** Facilitation of threatened abortion.
IV, IM: Postpartum control of bleeding after expulsion of the placenta.

Action

Stimulates uterine smooth muscle, producing uterine contractions similar to those in spontaneous labor. Has vasopressor and antidiuretic effects. **Therapeutic Effects:** Induction of labor. Control of postpartum bleeding.

Pharmacokinetics

Absorption: IV administration results in 100% bioavailability.

Distribution: Widely distributed in extracellular fluid. Small amounts reach fetal circulation.

Metabolism and Excretion: Rapidly metabolized by liver and kidneys.

Half-life: 3–9 min.

Time/Action Profile (reduction in uterine contractions)

ROUTE	ONSET	PEAK	DURATION
IV	Immediate	Unknown	1 hr
IM	3–5 min	Unknown	30–60 min

Contraindications/Precautions

Contraindicated in: Hypersensitivity; anticipated nonvaginal delivery.

Use Cautiously in: OB: First and second stages of labor; slow infusion over 24 hr has caused water intoxication with seizure and coma or maternal death caused by oxytocin's antidiuretic effect.

---

*Data from Vallerand AH, Sanoski C. Davis's Drug Guide for Nurses. 13th ed. Philadelphia, PA: F.A. Davis Company; 2013.

Adverse Reactions/Side Effects (CAPITALS indicate life-threatening; underlines indicate most frequent.)
Maternal adverse reactions are noted for IV use only.

> **CNS: maternal:** COMA, SEIZURES; **fetal:** INTRACRANIAL HEMORRHAGE.
> **Resp: fetal:** ASPHYXIA, hypoxia. **CV: maternal:** hypotension; **fetal:**
> arrhythmias. **F and E: maternal:** hypochloremia, hyponatremia, water
> intoxication. **Misc: maternal:** ↑ uterine motility, painful contractions,
> abruptio placentae, ↓ uterine blood flow, hypersensitivity.

Interactions

> **Drug–Drug:** Severe hypertension may occur if oxytocin follows administra-
> tion of **vasopressors**. Concurrent use with **cyclopropane** anesthesia may
> result in excessive hypotension.

Route/Dosage

Induction/Stimulation of Labor

> **IV (adults):** 0.5–2 mU/min; ↑ by 1–2 mU/min q15–60min until pattern
> established (usually 5–6 mU/min; maximum 20 mU/min), then ↓ dose

Postpartum Hemorrhage

> **IV (adults):** 10 U infused at 20–40 mU/min
>
> **IM (adults):** 10 U after delivery of placenta

Incomplete/Inevitable Abortion

> **IV (adults):** 10 U at a rate of 20–40 mU/min

Availability (generic available)

> **Solution for injection:** 10 units/mL

Nursing Implications

Assessment

- Fetal maturity, presentation, and pelvic adequacy should be assessed
  before administration of oxytocin for induction of labor.

- Assess character, frequency, and duration of uterine contractions; resting
  uterine tone; and fetal heart rate frequently throughout administration. If
  contractions occur < 2 min apart and are > 50–65 mm Hg on monitor, if
  they last ≥60–90 sec, or if a significant change in fetal heart rate develops,
  stop infusion and turn patient on her left side to prevent fetal anoxia.
  Notify health-care professional immediately.

- Monitor maternal BP and pulse frequently and fetal heart rate continuously
  throughout administration.

- This drug occasionally causes water intoxication. Monitor patient for signs
  and symptoms (drowsiness, listlessness, confusion, headache, anuria), and
  notify physician or other health-care professional if they occur.

- *Laboratory Test Considerations:* Monitor maternal electrolytes. Water
  retention may result in hypochloremia or hyponatremia.

Potential Nursing Diagnoses
Deficient knowledge, related to medication regimen (Patient/Family Teaching).

Implementation

- Do not administer oxytocin simultaneously by more than one route.

IV Administration

- **pH:** 3.0–5.0.

- **Continuous Infusion:** Rotate infusion container to ensure thorough
  mixing. Store solution in refrigerator, but do not freeze.

- Infuse via infusion pump for accurate dose. Oxytocin should be connected via Y-site injection to an IV of 0.9% NaCl for use during adverse
  reactions.

- Magnesium sulfate should be available if needed for relaxation of the myometrium.

- **Induction of Labor:** *Diluent:* Dilute 1 mL (10 U) in 1 L compatible infusion fluid (0.9% NaCl, D5W, or LR). *Concentration:* 10 mU/mL. *Rate:* Begin infusion at 0.5–2 mU/min (0.05–0.2 mL); increase in increments of 1–2 mU/min at 15- to 30-min intervals until contractions simulate normal labor.

- **Postpartum Bleeding:** *Diluent:* For control of postpartum bleeding, dilute 1–4 mL (10–40 units) in 1 L compatible infusion fluid. *Concentration:* 10–40 mU/mL. *Rate:* Begin infusion at a rate of 20–40 mU/min to control uterine atony. Adjust rate as indicated.

- **Incomplete or Inevitable Abortion:** *Diluent:* For incomplete or inevitable abortion, dilute 1 mL (10 units) in 500 mL of 0.9% NaCl or D5W. *Concentration:* 20 mU/mL. *Rate:* Infuse at a rate of 20–40 mU/min.

- **Y-Site Compatibility:** acyclovir, alfentanil, allopurinol, amikacin, aminocaproic acid, aminophylline, amphotericin B liposome, anidulafungin, argatroban, ascorbic acid, atracurium, atropine, azathioprine, azithromycin, aztreonam, benztropine, bivalirudin, bumetanide, buprenorphine, butorphanol, calcium chloride, calcium gluconate, capreomycin, caspofungin, cefazolin, cefepime, cefoperazone, cefotaxime, cefotetan, cefoxitin, ceftazidime, ceftriaxone, cefuroxime, chloramphenicol, ciprofloxacin, cisatracurium, clindamycin, cyanocobalamin, cyclosporine, daptomycin, dexamethasone, dexmedetomidine, digoxin, digoxin, diphenhydramine, dobutamine, dolasetron, dopamine, doxycycline, droperidol, enalaprilat, ephedrine, epinephrine, epoetin alfa, eptifibatide, ertapenem, erythromycin, esmolol, famotidine, fenoldopam, fentanyl, fluconazole, folic acid, foscarnet, fosphenytoin, furosemide, ganciclovir, gentamicin, glycopyrrolate, granisetron, heparin, hydrocortisone sodium succinate, hydromorphone, imipenem/cilastatin, isoproterenol, ketamine, ketorolac, labetalol, leucovorin calcium, levofloxacin, lidocaine, linezolid, lorazepam, magnesium sulfate, mannitol, meperidine, meropenem, metaraminol, methoxamine, methyldopate, methylprednisolone, metoclopramide, metoprolol, metronidazole, midazolam, milrinone, morphine, moxifloxacin, multivitamins, mycophenolate, nafcillin, nalbuphine, naloxone, nesiritide, nicardipine, nitroglycerin, nitroprusside, norepinephrine, ondansetron, oxacillin, palonosetron, pamidronate, pantoprazole, papaverine, penicillin G pentamidine, pentazocine, pentobarbital, phenobarbital, phentolamine, phenylephrine, phytonadione, piperacillin/tazobactam, potassium acetate, potassium chloride, potassium phosphates, procainamide, prochlorperazine, promethazine, propranolol, protamine, pyridoxine, quinupristin/dalfopristin, ranitidine, sodium acetate, sodium bicarbonate, sodium phosphates, streptokinase, succinylcholine, sufentanil, tacrolimus, theophylline, thiamine, ticarcillin/clavulanate, tigecycline, tirofiban, tobramycin, tolazoline, trimetaphan, vancomycin, vasopressin, verapamil, vitamin B complex with C, voriconazole, warfarin, zidovudine, zoledronic acid

- **Y-Site Incompatibility:** dantrolene, diazepam, diazoxide, indomethacin, phenytoin, remifentanil, trimethoprim/sulfamethoxazole

- **Solution Compatibility:** dextrose/Ringer's or lactated Ringer's combinations, dextrose/saline combinations, Ringer's or lactated Ringer's injection, D5W, D10W, 0.45% NaCl, 0.9% NaCl

Patient/Family Teaching
- Advise patient to expect contractions similar to menstrual cramps after administration has started.

- Onset of effective contractions
- Increase in uterine tone
- Reduction in postpartum bleeding

methylergonovine (meth-ill-er-goe-**noe**-veen)
Methergine

Classification
Therapeutic:

Pharmacologic: ergot alkaloids

Pregnancy Category C

Indications
Prevention and treatment of postpartum or postabortion hemorrhage caused by uterine atony or subinvolution.

Action
Directly stimulates uterine and vascular smooth muscle. **Therapeutic Effects:** Uterine contraction.

Pharmacokinetics
Absorption: Well absorbed after oral or IM administration.

Distribution: Unknown. Enters breast milk in small quantities.

Metabolism and Excretion: Probably metabolized by the liver.

Half-life: 30–120 min.

Time/Action Profile (effects on uterine contractions)

ROUTE	ONSET	PEAK	DURATION
PO	5–15 min	Unknown	3 hr
IM	2–5 min	Unknown	3 hr
IV	Immediate	Unknown	45 min–3 hr

Contraindications/Precautions
Contraindicated in: Hypersensitivity; OB: Should not be used to induce labor.

Use Cautiously in: Patients with hypertension or eclampsia (more susceptible to hypertensive and arrhythmogenic side effects); severe hepatic or renal disease; sepsis.

Exercise Extreme Caution in: OB: Third stage of labor.

Adverse Reactions/Side Effects (CAPITALS indicate life-threatening; underlines indicate most frequent.)
CNS: dizziness, headache. **EENT:** tinnitus. **Resp:** dyspnea. **CV:** HYPERTENSION, arrhythmias, chest pain, palpitations. **GI:** nausea, vomiting. **GU:** cramps. **Derm:** diaphoresis. **Misc:** allergic reactions.

Interactions
Drug–Drug: Excessive vasoconstriction may result when used with heavy cigarette smoking (**nicotine**) or other **vasopressors**, such as **dopamine**.

Route/Dosage
PO (adults): 200–400 mcg (0.4–0.6 mg) q6–12h for 2–7 days

IM, IV (adults): 200 mcg (0.2 mg) q2–4h for up to 5 doses

Tablets: 200 mcg (0.2 mg). **Injection:** 200 mcg (0.2 mg)/mL

Nursing Implications

Assessment

- Monitor BP, heart rate, and uterine response frequently during medication administration. Notify health-care professional promptly if uterine relaxation becomes prolonged or if character of vaginal bleeding changes.

- Assess for signs of ergotism (cold, numb fingers and toes, chest pain, nausea, vomiting, headache, muscle pain, weakness).

- *Laboratory Test Considerations:* If no response to methylergonovine, calcium levels may need to be assessed. Effectiveness of medication is ↓ with hypocalcemia.

- May cause ↓ serum prolactin levels.

Potential Nursing Diagnoses

Acute pain (Adverse Reactions/Side Effects)

Implementation

IV Administration

- **pH:** 2.7–3.5.

- **IV:** IV administration is used for emergencies only. Oral and IM routes are preferred.

- **Direct IV:** *Diluent:* May be given undiluted or diluted in 5 mL of 0.9% NaCl and administered through Y-site. Do not add to IV solutions. Do not mix in syringe with any other drug. Refrigerate; stable for storage at room temperature for 60 days; deteriorates with age. Use only solution that is clear and colorless, and that contains no precipitate. *Concentration:* 0.2 mg/mL. *Rate:* Administer at a rate of 0.2 mg over at least 1 min.

- **Y-Site Compatibility:** heparin, hydrocortisone sodium succinate, potassium chloride, vitamin B complex with C

Patient/Family Teaching

- Instruct patient to take medication as directed; do not skip or double up on missed doses. If a dose is missed, omit it and return to regular dose schedule.

- Advise patient that medication may cause menstrual-like cramps.

- Caution patient to avoid smoking, because nicotine constricts blood vessels.

- Instruct patient to notify health-care professional if infection develops, because this may cause increased sensitivity to the medication.

Evaluation/Desired Outcomes

- Contractions that maintain uterine tone and prevent postpartum hemorrhage.

dinoprostone (dye-noe-**prost**-one)

Cervidil Vaginal Insert, Prepidil Endocervical Gel, Prostin E Vaginal Suppository

Classification

Therapeutic: cervical ripening agent

Pharmacologic: oxytocics, prostaglandins

Pregnancy Category C

Indications

Endocervical Gel, Vaginal Insert: Used to "ripen" the cervix in pregnancy at or near term when induction of labor is indicated. Vaginal Suppository: Induction of midtrimester abortion, management of missed abortion up to 28 wk, management of nonmetastatic gestational trophoblastic disease (benign hydatidiform mole).

Action
Produces contractions similar to those occurring during labor at term by stimulating the myometrium (oxytocic effect). Initiates softening, effacement, and dilation of the cervix ("ripening"). Also stimulates GI smooth muscle. **Therapeutic Effects:** Initiation of labor. Expulsion of fetus.

Pharmacokinetics

Absorption: Rapidly absorbed.

Distribution: Unknown. Action is mostly local.

Metabolism and Excretion: Metabolized by enzymes in lung, kidneys, spleen, and liver tissue.

Half-life: Unknown.

Time/Action Profile

ROUTE	ONSET	PEAK	DURATION
Cervical ripening (gel)	Rapid	30–45 min	Unknown
Cervical ripening (insert)	Rapid	Unknown	12 hr
Abortion time (suppository)	10 min	12–24 hr	2–3 hr

Contraindications/Precautions

Contraindicated in: Hypersensitivity to prostaglandins or additives in the gel or suppository. The gel/insert should be avoided in situations in which prolonged uterine contractions should be avoided, including previous cesarean section or uterine surgery, cephalopelvic disproportion, traumatic delivery or difficult labor, multiparity (≥6 term pregnancies), hyperactive or hypertonic uterus, fetal distress (if delivery is not imminent), unexplained vaginal bleeding, placenta previa, vasa previa, active herpes genitalis, obstetric emergency requiring surgical intervention, situations in which vaginal delivery is contraindicated; presence of acute pelvic inflammatory disease or ruptured membranes; concurrent oxytocic therapy (wait for 30 min after removing insert before using oxytocin).

Use Cautiously in: Uterine scarring; asthma; hypotension; cardiac disease; adrenal disorders; anemia; jaundice; diabetes mellitus; epilepsy; glaucoma; pulmonary, renal, or hepatic disease; multiparity (up to 5 previous term pregnancies); women >30 yr old, those with complications during pregnancy, and those with a gestational age >40 wk (↑ risk for disseminated intravascular coagulation).

Adverse Reactions/Side Effects (CAPITALS indicate life-threatening; underlines indicate most frequent.)

Endocervical Gel, Vaginal Insert

GU: uterine contractile abnormalities, warm feeling in vagina. **MS:** back pain. **Misc:** AMNIOTIC FLUID EMBOLISM, fever

Suppository

CNS: headache, drowsiness, syncope. **Resp:** coughing, dyspnea, wheezing. **CV:** hypotension, hypertension. **GI:** diarrhea, nausea, vomiting. **GU:** UTERINE RUPTURE, urinary tract infection, uterine hyperstimulation, vaginal/uterine pain. **Misc:** ALLERGIC REACTIONS INCLUDING ANAPHYLAXIS, chills, fever.

Interactions

Drug–Drug: Augments the effects of other **oxytocics**.

Route/Dosage

Cervical Ripening

Vag (adults, cervical): *Endocervical gel*—0.5 mg; if response is unfavorable, may repeat in 6 hr (not to exceed 1.5 mg/24 hr). *Vaginal insert*—one 10-mg insert.

Abortifacient

Vag (adults): One 20-mg suppository, repeat q3–5h (not to exceed 240 mg total or >48 hr).

Availability

Endocervical gel (Prepidil): 0.5 mg dinoprostone in 3 g gel vehicle in a prefilled syringe with catheters. **Vaginal insert (Cervidil):** 10 mg. **Vaginal suppository (Prostin E Vaginal):** 20 mg.

Nursing Implications

Assessment

- **Abortifacient:** Monitor frequency, duration, and force of contractions and uterine resting tone. Opioid analgesics may be administered for uterine pain.

- Monitor temperature, pulse, and BP periodically throughout therapy. Dinoprostone-induced fever (elevation >1.1°C or 2°F) usually occurs within 15–45 min after insertion of suppository. This returns to normal 2–6 hr after discontinuation or removal of suppository from vagina.

- Auscultate breath sounds. Wheezing and sensation of chest tightness may indicate hypersensitivity reaction.

- Assess for nausea, vomiting, and diarrhea in patients receiving suppository. Vomiting and diarrhea occur frequently. Patient should be premedicated with antiemetic and antidiarrheal.

- Monitor amount and type of vaginal discharge. Notify health-care professional immediately if symptoms of hemorrhage (increased bleeding, hypotension, pallor, tachycardia) occur.

- **Cervical Ripening:** Monitor uterine activity, fetal status, and dilation and effacement of cervix continuously throughout therapy. Assess for hypertonus, sustained uterine contractility, and fetal distress. Insert should be removed at the onset of active labor.

Potential Nursing Diagnoses

Deficient knowledge, related to medication regimen (Patient/Family Teaching)

Implementation

- **Abortifacient:** Warm the suppository to room temperature just before use.

- Wear gloves when handling unwrapped suppository to prevent absorption through skin.

- Patient should remain supine for 10 min after insertion of suppository; then she may be ambulatory.

- **Vaginal Insert:** Place vaginal insert transversely in the posterior vaginal fornix immediately after removing from foil package. Warming of insert and sterile conditions are not required. Use vaginal insert only with a retrieval system. Use minimal amount of water-soluble lubricant during insertion; avoid excess because it may hamper release of dinoprostone from insert. Patient should remain supine for 2 hr after insertion, then may ambulate.

- Vaginal insert delivers 0.3 mg/hr dinoprostone over 12 hr. Remove insert at the onset of active labor, before amniotomy, or after 12 hr.

- Oxytocin should not be used during or <30 min after removal of insert.

- **Endocervical Gel:** Determine degree of effacement before insertion of the endocervical catheter. Do not administer above the level of the internal os. Use a 20-mm endocervical catheter if no effacement is present and a 10-mm catheter if the cervix is 50% effaced.

- Use caution to prevent contact of dinoprostone gel with skin. Wash hands thoroughly with soap and water after administration.

- Bring gel to room temperature just before administration. Do not force warming with external sources (water bath, microwave). Remove peel-off seal from end of syringe; then remove the protective end cap and insert end cap into plunger stopper assembly in barrel of syringe. Aseptically remove catheter from package. Firmly attach catheter hub to syringe tip; click is evidence of attachment. Fill catheter with sterile gel by pushing plunger to expel air from catheter before administration to patient. Gel is stable for 24 mo if refrigerated.

- Patient should be in dorsal position with cervix visualized using a speculum. Introduce gel with catheter into cervical canal using sterile technique. Administer gel by gentle expulsion from syringe and then remove catheter. Do not attempt to administer small amount of gel remaining in syringe. Use syringe for only one patient; discard syringe, catheter, and unused package contents after using.

- Patient should remain supine for 15–30 min after administration to minimize leakage from cervical canal.

- Oxytocin may be administered 6–12 hr after desired response from dinoprostone gel. If no cervical/uterine response to initial dose of dinoprostone is obtained, repeat dose may be administered in 6 hr.

Patient/Family Teaching

- Explain purpose of medication and vaginal examinations.

- **Abortifacient:** Instruct patient to notify health-care professional immediately if fever and chills, foul-smelling vaginal discharge, lower abdominal pain, or increased bleeding occurs.

- Provide emotional support throughout therapy.

- **Cervical Ripening:** Inform patient that she may experience a warm feeling in her vagina during administration.

- Advise patient to notify health-care professional if contractions become prolonged.

Evaluation/Desired Outcomes

- Complete abortion. Continuous administration for >2 days is not usually recommended.

- Cervical ripening and induction of labor.

misoprostol (mye-soe-**prost**-ole)

Cytotec

Classification

Therapeutic: antiulcer agents cytoprotective agents

Pharmacologic: prostaglandins

Pregnancy Category X

Indications

Prevention of gastric mucosal injury from NSAIDs, including aspirin, in high-risk patients (geriatric patients, debilitated patients, or those with a history of ulcers).

With mifepristone for termination of pregnancy. **Unlabeled Use:** Treatment of duodenal ulcers. Cervical ripening and labor induction.

Action

Acts as a prostaglandin analogue, decreasing gastric acid secretion (antisecretory effect) and increasing the production of protective mucus (cytoprotective effect). Causes uterine contractions. **Therapeutic Effects:** Prevention of gastric ulceration from NSAIDs. With mifepristone, terminates pregnancy of < 49 days.

Pharmacokinetics

Absorption: Well absorbed after oral administration and rapidly converted to its active form (misoprostol acid).

Distribution: Unknown.

Protein Binding: 85%.

Metabolism and Excretion: Undergoes some metabolism and is then excreted by the kidneys.

Half-life: 20–40 min.

Time/Action Profile (effect on gastric acid secretion)

ROUTE	ONSET	PEAK	DURATION
PO	30 min	Unknown	3–6 hr

Contraindications/Precautions

Contraindicated in: Hypersensitivity to prostaglandins. OB: Should not be used to prevent NSAID-induced gastric injury because of potential for fetal harm or death. Lactation: May cause severe diarrhea in the nursing infant.

Use Cautiously in: OB: Patients with childbearing potential should be counseled to avoid pregnancy during misoprostol therapy for prevention of NSAID-induced gastric injury. Pregnancy status should be determined before initiating therapy. Pedi: Safety not established.

Exercise Extreme Caution in: When used for cervical ripening (unlabeled use), may cause uterine rupture (risk factors are late trimester pregnancy, previous cesarean section or uterine surgery, or ≥5 previous pregnancies).

Adverse Reactions/Side Effects (CAPITALS indicate life-threatening; underlines indicate most frequent.)

CNS: headache. **GI:** <u>abdominal pain</u>, <u>diarrhea</u>, constipation, dyspepsia, flatulence, nausea, vomiting. **GU:** <u>miscarriage</u>, menstrual disorders.

Interactions

Drug–Drug: ↑ risk for diarrhea with **magnesium-containing antacids**.

Route/Dosage

PO (adults): *Antiulcer*—200 mcg 4 times daily with or after meals and at bedtime, *or* 400 mcg twice daily, with the last dose at bedtime. If intolerance occurs, dose may be ↓ to 100 mcg 4 times daily. *Termination of pregnancy*—400 mcg single dose 2 days after mifepristone if abortion has not occurred.

Intravaginally (adults): 25 mcg (1/4 of 100-mcg tablet); may repeat q3–6h, if needed.

Availability (generic available)

Tablets: 100 mcg (0.1 mg), 200 mcg (0.2 mg). *In combination with:* diclofenac (Arthrotec).

Nursing Implications

Assessment

- Assess patient routinely for epigastric or abdominal pain, and for frank or occult blood in the stool, emesis, or gastric aspirate.
- Assess women of childbearing age for pregnancy. Misoprostol is usually begun on second or third day of menstrual period after a negative pregnancy test result.
- **Termination of pregnancy:** Monitor uterine cramping and bleeding during therapy.
- **Cervical Ripening:** Assess dilation of cervix periodically during therapy.

Potential Nursing Diagnoses

Acute pain (Indications)

Implementation

- Do not confuse Cytotec (misoprostol) with Mifeprex (mifepristone).
- Misoprostol therapy should be started at the onset of treatment with NSAIDs.
- **PO:** Administer medication with meals and at bedtime to reduce severity of diarrhea.
- Antacids may be administered before or after misoprostol for relief of pain. Avoid those containing magnesium, because of increased diarrhea with misoprostol.

Patient/Family Teaching

- Instruct patient to take medication as directed for the full course of therapy, even if she is feeling better. Take missed doses as soon as possible unless next dose is due within 2 hr; do not double doses.
- Advise patient not to share misoprostol with others, even if they have similar symptoms; may be dangerous.
- Inform patient that misoprostol will cause spontaneous abortion. Women of childbearing age must be informed of this effect through verbal and written information, and must use contraception throughout therapy. If pregnancy is suspected, the woman should stop taking misoprostol and immediately notify her health-care professional.
- Inform patient that diarrhea may occur. Health-care professional should be notified if diarrhea persists for >1 wk. Also advise patient to report onset of black, tarry stools or severe abdominal pain.
- Advise patient to avoid alcohol and foods that may cause an increase in GI irritation.

Evaluation/Desired Outcomes

- Prevention of gastric ulcers in patients receiving chronic NSAID therapy
- Termination of pregnancy
- Cervical ripening and induction of labor

High Alert

magnesium sulfate (IV, parenteral) (9.9% Mg; 8.1 mEq Mg/g) (mag-**nee**-zee-um **sul**-fate)

Classification

Therapeutic: mineral and electrolyte replacements/supplements

Pharmacologic: minerals/electrolytes

Pregnancy Category A

Indications
Treatment/prevention of hypomagnesemia. Treatment of hypertension. Anticonvulsant associated with severe eclampsia, pre-eclampsia, or acute nephritis. **Unlabeled Use:** Preterm labor. Treatment of torsade de pointes. Adjunctive treatment for bronchodilation in moderate-to-severe acute asthma.

Action
Essential for the activity of many enzymes. Plays an important role in neurotransmission and muscular excitability. **Therapeutic Effects:** Replacement in deficiency states. Resolution of eclampsia.

Pharmacokinetics
Absorption: IV administration results in complete bioavailability; well absorbed from IM sites.

Distribution: Widely distributed. Crosses the placenta and is present in breast milk.

Metabolism and Excretion: Excreted primarily by the kidneys.

Half-life: Unknown.

Time/Action Profile (anticonvulsant effect)

ROUTE	ONSET	PEAK	DURATION
IM	60 min	Unknown	3–4 hr
IV	Immediate	Unknown	30 min

Contraindications/Precautions
Contraindicated in: Hypermagnesemia; hypocalcemia; anuria; heart block. OB: Unless used for preterm labor, avoid continuous use during active labor or within 2 hr of delivery because of potential for magnesium toxicity in newborn.

Use Cautiously in: Any degree of renal insufficiency. Geri: May require ↓ dosage because of age-related ↓ in renal function.

Adverse Reactions/Side Effects (CAPITALS indicate life-threatening; <u>underlines</u> indicate most frequent.)
CNS: drowsiness. **Resp:** ↓ respiratory rate. **CV:** arrhythmias, bradycardia, hypotension. **GI:** <u>diarrhea</u>. **MS:** muscle weakness. **Derm:** flushing, sweating. **Metab:** hypothermia.

Interactions
Drug–Drug: May potentiate **calcium channel blockers** and **neuromuscular blocking agents**.

Route/Dosage
Treatment of Deficiency (expressed as milligrams of magnesium)
IM, IV (adults): *Severe deficiency—*8–12 g/day in divided doses; *mild deficiency—*1 g q6h for 4 doses or 250 mg/kg over 4 hr

IM, IV (children > 1 mo): 25–50 mg/kg/dose q4–6h for 3–4 doses, maximum single dose: 2 g

IV (neonates): 25–50 mg/kg/dose q8–12h for 2–3 doses

Seizures/Hypertension

IM, IV (adults): 1 g q6h for 4 doses as needed

IM, IV (children): 20–100 mg/kg/dose q4–6h as needed; may use up to 200 mg/kg/dose in severe cases

Torsade de Pointes

IV (infants and children): 25–50 mg/kg/dose, maximum dose: 2 g

Bronchodilation

IV (adults): 2 g single dose

IV (children): 25 mg/kg/dose, maximum dose: 2 g

Eclampsia/Pre-eclampsia

IV, IM (adults): 4–5 g by IV infusion, concurrently with up to 5 g IM in each buttock; then 4–5 g IM q4h *or* 4 g by IV infusion followed by 1–2 g/hr continuous infusion (not to exceed 40 g/day or 20 g/48 hr in the presence of severe renal insufficiency)

Part of Parenteral Nutrition

IV (adults): 4–24 mEq/day

IV (children): 0.25–0.5 mEq/kg/day

Availability (generic available)

Injection: 500 mg/mL (50%). **Premixed infusion:** 1 g/100 mL, 2 g/100 mL, 4 g/50 mL, 4 g/100 mL, 20 g/500 mL, 40 g/1000 mL

Nursing Implications

Assessment

- **Hypomagnesemia/Anticonvulsant:** Monitor pulse, BP, respirations, and ECG frequently throughout administration of parenteral magnesium sulfate. Respirations should be at least 16/min before each dose.

- Monitor neurological status before and throughout therapy. Institute seizure precautions. Patellar reflex (knee jerk) should be tested before each parenteral dose of magnesium sulfate. If response is absent, no additional doses should be administered until positive response is obtained.

- Monitor newborn for hypotension, hyporeflexia, and respiratory depression if mother has received magnesium sulfate.

- Monitor intake and output ratios. Urine output should be maintained at a level of at least 100 mL/4 hr.

- *Laboratory Test Considerations:* Monitor serum magnesium levels and renal function periodically throughout administration of parenteral magnesium sulfate.

Potential Nursing Diagnoses

Risk for injury (Indications, Side Effects)

Implementation

- *High Alert:* Accidental overdosage of IV magnesium has resulted in serious patient harm and death. Have second practitioner independently double-check original order, dose calculations, and infusion pump settings. Do not confuse milligram (mg), gram (g), or milliequivalent (mEq) dosages.

- **IM:** Administer deep IM into gluteal sites. Administer subsequent injections in alternate sides. Dilute to a concentration of 200 mg/mL before injection.

IV Administration

- **pH:** 5.5–7.0.

- **Direct IV:** *Diluent:* 50% solution must be diluted in 0.9% NaCl or D5W to a concentration of ≤20% before administration. *Concentration:* ≤20%. *Rate:* Administer at a rate not to exceed 150 mg/min.

- **Continuous Infusion:** *Diluent:* Dilute in D5W, 0.9% NaCl, or LR. *Concentration:* 0.5 mEq/mL (60 mg/mL; may use maximum concentration of 1.6 mEq/mL [200 mg/mL] in fluid-restricted patients). *Rate:* Infuse over 2–4 hr. Do not exceed a rate of 1 mEq/kg/hr (125 mg/kg/hr). When rapid infusions are needed (severe asthma or torsade de pointes), may infuse over 10–20 min.

- **Y-Site Compatibility:** acyclovir, aldesleukin, alfentanil, amifostine, amikacin, argatroban, ascorbic acid, atracurium, atropine, aztreonam, benztropine, bivalirudin, bleomycin, bumetanide, buprenorphine, butorphanol, calcium gluconate, carboplatin, carmustine, caspofungin, cefazolin, cefotaxime, cefoxitin, ceftazidime, chloramphenicol, chlorpromazine, cisatracurium, cisplatin, clindamycin, clonidine, cyanocobalamin, cyclophosphamide, cytarabine, dactinomycin, daptomycin, dexmedetomidine, digoxin, diltiazem, diphenhydramine, dobutamine, docetaxel, dopamine, doripenem, doxacurium, doxorubicin liposome, doxycycline, enalaprilat, epinephrine, epoetin alfa, eptifibatide, ertapenem, esmolol, etoposide, etoposide phosphate, famotidine, fenoldopam, fentanyl, fluconazole, fludarabine, fluorouracil, folic acid, gemcitabine, gentamicin, glycopyrrolate, granisetron, heparin, hetastarch, hydromorphone, idarubicin, ifosfamide, imipenem/cilastatin, insulin, irinotecan, isoproterenol, kanamycin, ketamine, ketorolac, labetalol, lidocaine, linezolid, lorazepam, mannitol, mechlorethamine, metaraminol, methotrexate, methyldopate, metoclopramide, metoprolol, metronidazole, micafungin, midazolam, milrinone, mitoxantrone, morphine, multivitamins, mycophenolate, nafcillin, nalbuphine, nesiritide, nicardipine, nitroglycerin, nitroprusside, norepinephrine, octreotide, ondansetron, oxaliplatin, oxytocin, paclitaxel, palonosetron, pamidronate, pancuronium, pantoprazole, papaverine, penicillin G potassium, pentobarbital, phenobarbital, phentolamine, phenylephrine, piperacillin/tazobactam, potassium acetate, potassium chloride, procainamide, prochlorperazine, promethazine, propofol, propranolol, protamine, pyridoxine, quinupristin/dalfopristin, ranitidine, remifentanil, rituximab, rocuronium, sargramostim, sodium acetate, sodium bicarbonate, streptokinase, succinylcholine, sufentanil, tacrolimus, telavancin, teniposide, theophylline, thiamine, thiotepa, ticarcillin/clavulanate, tigecycline, tirofiban, tobramycin, tolazoline, trastuzumab, trimetaphan, vancomycin, vasopressin, vecuronium, verapamil, vincristine, vinorelbine, vitamin B complex with C, voriconazole, zoledronic acid

- **Y-Site Incompatibility:** aminophylline, amphotericin B cholesteryl sulfate, amphotericin B lipid complex, amphotericin B liposome, anidulafungin, azathioprine, calcium chloride, cefepime, ceftriaxone, cefuroxime, ciprofloxacin, dantrolene, dexamethasone sodium phosphate, diazepam, doxorubicin hydrochloride, epirubicin, haloperidol, indomethacin, methylprednisolone sodium succinate, pentamidine, phenytoin, phytonadione

Patient/Family Teaching
- Explain purpose of medication to patient and family.

Evaluation/Desired Outcomes
- Normal serum magnesium concentrations
- Control of seizures associated with toxemias of pregnancy

terbutaline (ter-**byoo**-ta-leen)

Bricanyl

Classification

Therapeutic: bronchodilators

Pharmacologic: adrenergics

Pregnancy Category B

Indications

Management of reversible airway disease because of asthma or chronic obstructive pulmonary disease; inhalation and subcutaneous used for short-term control and oral agent as long-term control. **Unlabeled Use:** Management of preterm labor (tocolytic; the U.S. Food and Drug Administration has recommended that injectable terbutaline should not be used in pregnancy for the prevention or prolonged treatment [> 48–72 hr] of preterm labor in either the inpatient or outpatient settings because of the potential for serious maternal heart problems and death; oral terbutaline should not be used for the prevention or any treatment of preterm labor because of a lack of efficacy and the potential for serious material heart problems and death).

Action

Results in the accumulation of cyclic adenosine monophosphate (cAMP) at β-adrenergic receptors. Produces bronchodilation. Inhibits the release of mediators of immediate hypersensitivity reactions from mast cells. Relatively selective for $β_2$ (pulmonary)-adrenergic receptor sites, with less effect on $β_1$(cardiac)-adrenergic receptors. **Therapeutic Effects:** Bronchodilation.

Pharmacokinetics

Absorption: 35%–50% absorbed after oral administration but rapidly undergoes first-pass metabolism. Well absorbed after SC administration.

Distribution: Enters breast milk.

Metabolism and Excretion: Partially metabolized by the liver; 60% excreted unchanged by the kidneys after SC administration.

Half-life: Unknown.

Time/Action Profile (bronchodilation)

ROUTE	ONSET	PEAK	DURATION
PO	Within 60–120 min	Within 2–3 hr	4–8 hr
SC	Within 15 min	Within 0.5–1 hr	1.5–4 hr

Contraindications/Precautions

Contraindicated in: Hypersensitivity to adrenergic amines.

Use Cautiously in: Cardiac disease; hypertension; hyperthyroidism; diabetes; glaucoma. Geri: More susceptible to adverse reactions; may require dose ↓. Excessive use may lead to tolerance and paradoxical bronchospasm (inhaler). OB/Lactation: Pregnancy (near term) and lactation.

Adverse Reactions/Side Effects (CAPITALS indicate life-threatening; underlines indicate most frequent.)

CNS: <u>nervousness</u>, <u>restlessness</u>, <u>tremor</u>, headache, insomnia. **Resp:** pulmonary edema. **CV:** angina, arrhythmias, hypertension, myocardial ischemia, tachycardia. **GI:** nausea, vomiting. **Endo:** hyperglycemia. **F and E:** hypokalemia.

Interactions

Drug–Drug: Concurrent use with other **adrenergics** (sympathomimetic) will have additive adrenergic side effects. Use with **MAO inhibitors** may lead to hypertensive crisis. **β-Blockers** may negate therapeutic effect.

Drug–Natural: Use with caffeine-containing herbs (**cola nut**, **guarana**, **mate**, **tea**, **coffee**) ↑ stimulant effect.

Route/Dosage

PO (adults and children > 15 yr): *Bronchodilation*—2.5–5 mg 3 times daily, given q6h (not to exceed 15 mg/24 hr).

PO (children 12–15 yr): *Bronchodilation*—2.5 mg 3 times daily (given q6h; not to exceed 7.5 mg/24 hr).

PO (children < 12 yr): *Bronchodilation*—0.05 mg/kg 3 times daily; may ↑ gradually (not to exceed 0.15 mg/kg 3–4 times daily or 5 mg/24 hr).

SC (adults and children ≥12 yr): *Bronchodilation*—250 mcg; may repeat in 15–30 min (not to exceed 500 mcg/4 hr).

SC (children < 12 yr): *Bronchodilation*—0.005–0.01 mg/kg; may repeat in 15–20 min.

IV (adults): *Tocolysis*—2.5–10 mcg/min infusion; ↑ by 5 mcg/min q10min until contractions stop (not to exceed 30 mcg/min). After contractions have stopped for 30 min, ↓ infusion rate to lowest effective amount and maintain for 4–8 hr (unlabeled).

Availability (generic available)
Tablets: 2.5 mg, 5 mg. **Injection:** 1 mg/mL.

Nursing Implications

Assessment

- **Bronchodilator:** Assess lung sounds, respiratory pattern, pulse, and BP before administration and during peak of medication. Note amount, color, and character of sputum produced, and notify health-care professional of abnormal findings.

- Monitor pulmonary function tests before initiating therapy and periodically throughout therapy to determine effectiveness of medication.

- **Preterm Labor:** Monitor maternal pulse and BP, frequency and duration of contractions, and fetal heart rate. Notify health-care professional if contractions persist or increase in frequency or duration, or if symptoms of maternal or fetal distress occur. Maternal side effects include tachycardia, palpitations, tremor, anxiety, and headache.

- Assess maternal respiratory status for symptoms of pulmonary edema (increased rate, dyspnea, rales/crackles, frothy sputum).

- Monitor mother and neonate for symptoms of hypoglycemia (anxiety; chills; cold sweats; confusion; cool, pale skin; difficulty in concentration; drowsiness; excessive hunger; headache; irritability; nausea; nervousness; rapid pulse; shakiness; unusual tiredness; or weakness) and mother for hypokalemia (weakness, fatigue, U wave on ECG, arrhythmias).

- *Laboratory Test Considerations:* May cause transient ↓ in serum potassium concentrations with higher than recommended doses.

- Monitor maternal serum glucose and electrolytes. May cause hypokalemia and hypoglycemia. Monitor neonate's serum glucose, because hypoglycemia may also occur in neonates.

- *Toxicity and Overdose:* Symptoms of overdose include persistent agitation, chest pain or discomfort, decreased BP, dizziness, hyperglycemia, hypokalemia, seizures, tachyarrhythmias, persistent trembling, and vomiting.

- Treatment includes discontinuing β-adrenergic agonists and symptomatic, supportive therapy. Cardioselective β-blockers are used with caution, because they may induce bronchospasm.

Potential Nursing Diagnoses
Ineffective airway clearance (Indications)

Implementation
- Do not confuse Brethine (terbutaline) with Methergine (methylergonovine).
- **PO:** Administer with meals to minimize gastric irritation.
- Tablet may be crushed and mixed with food or fluids for patients with difficulty swallowing.
- **SC:** Administer SC injections in lateral deltoid area. Do not use solution if discolored.

IV Administration
- **pH:** 3.0–5.0.
- **Continuous Infusion:** *Diluent:* May be diluted in D5W, 0.9% NaCl, or 0.45% NaCl. *Concentration:* 1 mg/mL (undiluted).
  Rate: Use infusion pump to ensure accurate dose. Begin infusion at 10 mcg/min. Increase dosage by 5 mcg every 10 min until contractions cease. Maximum dose is 80 mcg/min. Begin to taper dose in 5-mcg decrements after a 30- to 60-min contraction-free period is attained. Switch to oral dose form after patient is contraction-free 4–8 hr on the lowest effective dose.
- **Y-Site Compatibility:** insulin

Patient/Family Teaching
- Instruct patient to take medication as directed. If on a scheduled dosing regimen, take a missed dose as soon as possible; space remaining doses at regular intervals. Do not double doses. Caution patient not to exceed recommended dose; may cause adverse effects, paradoxical bronchospasm, or loss of effectiveness of medication.
- Instruct patient to contact health-care professional immediately if shortness of breath is not relieved by medication or is accompanied by diaphoresis, dizziness, palpitations, or chest pain.
- Advise patient to consult health-care professional before taking any OTC medications or alcoholic beverages concurrently with this therapy. Caution patient also to avoid smoking and other respiratory irritants.
- **Preterm Labor:** Notify health-care professional immediately if labor resumes or if significant side effects occur.

Evaluation/Desired Outcomes
- Prevention or relief of bronchospasm
- Increase in ease of breathing
- 5 of preterm labor in a fetus of 20–36 wk gestational age

NIFEdipine (nye-**fed**-i-peen)
Adalat CC, Adalat XL, Afeditab CR, Nifedical XL, Procardia, Procardia XL

Classification
Therapeutic: antianginals, antihypertensives

Pharmacologic: calcium channel blockers

Pregnancy Category C

Indications

Management of hypertension (extended-release only), angina pectoris, vasospastic (Prinzmetal's) angina. **Unlabeled Use:** Prevention of migraine headache. Management of HF or cardiomyopathy.

Action

Inhibits calcium transport into myocardial and vascular smooth muscle cells, resulting in inhibition of excitation-contraction coupling and subsequent contraction. **Therapeutic Effects:** Systemic vasodilation, resulting in decreased BP. Coronary vasodilation, resulting in decreased frequency and severity of attacks of angina.

Pharmacokinetics

Absorption: Well absorbed after oral administration, but large amounts are rapidly metabolized (primarily by CYP3A4 enzyme system), resulting in ↓ bioavailability (45%–70%); bioavailability is ↑ (80%) with long-acting (CC, PA, XL) forms.

Distribution: Unknown.

Protein Binding: 92%–98%.

Metabolism and Excretion: Mostly metabolized by the liver.

Half-life: 2–5 hr.

Time/Action Profile

ROUTE	ONSET	PEAK	DURATION
PO	20 min	Unknown	6–8 hr
PO–PA	Unknown	4 hr	12 hr
PO–CC, PA, XL	Unknown	6 hr	24 hr

Contraindications/Precautions

Contraindicated in: Hypersensitivity; sick sinus syndrome; second- or third-degree AV block (unless an artificial pacemaker is in place); systolic BP <90 mm Hg; coadministration with grapefruit juice, rifampin, rifabutin, phenobarbital, phenytoin, carbamazepine, or St. John's wort.

Use Cautiously in: Severe hepatic impairment (↓ dose recommended); history of porphyria; severe renal impairment (↓ dose may be necessary); history of serious ventricular arrhythmias or HF. OB/Lactation/Pedi: Safety not established. Geri: Short-acting forms appear on Beers list because of ↑ risk for hypotension and constipation (↓ dose recommended); also associated with ↑ incidence of falls.

Adverse Reactions/Side Effects (CAPITALS indicate life-threatening; underlines indicate most frequent.)

CNS: headache, abnormal dreams, anxiety, confusion, dizziness, drowsiness, jitteriness, nervousness, psychiatric disturbances, weakness. **EENT:** blurred vision, disturbed equilibrium, epistaxis, tinnitus. **Resp:** cough, dyspnea, shortness of breath. **CV:** ARRHYTHMIAS, HF, peripheral edema, bradycardia, chest pain, hypotension, palpitations, syncope, tachycardia. **GI:** ↑ liver enzymes, anorexia, constipation, diarrhea, dry mouth, dysgeusia, dyspepsia, GI obstruction, nausea, ulcer, vomiting. **GU:** dysuria, nocturia, polyuria, sexual dysfunction, urinary frequency. **Derm:** flushing, dermatitis, erythema multiforme, ↑ sweating, photosensitivity, pruritus/ urticaria, rash. **Endo:** gynecomastia, hyperglycemia. **Hemat:** anemia, leukopenia, thrombocytopenia. **Metab:** weight gain. **MS:** joint stiffness, muscle cramps. **Neuro:** paresthesia, tremor. **Misc:** STEVENS–JOHNSON SYNDROME, gingival hyperplasia.

Interactions

Drug–Drug: Rifampin, rifabutin, phenobarbital, phenytoin, or **carbamazepine** may significantly ↓ levels and effects; concurrent use is contraindicated. **Ketoconazole, fluconazole, itraconazole, clarithromycin, erythromycin, nefazodone, saquinavir, indinavir, nelfinavir,** or **ritonavir** may ↑ levels and effects; consider initiating nifedipine at lowest dose. Additive hypotension may occur when used concurrently with **fentanyl,** other **antihypertensives, nitrates,** acute ingestion of **alcohol,** or **quinidine.** Antihypertensive effects may be ↓ by concurrent use of **NSAIDs.** May ↑ serum levels and risk for toxicity from **digoxin.** Concurrent use with **β-blockers, digoxin, disopyramide,** or **phenytoin** may result in bradycardia, conduction defects, or HF. **Cimetidine** and **propranolol** may ↓ metabolism and ↑ risk of toxicity. May ↓ metabolism of and ↑ risk for toxicity from **cyclosporine, tacrolimus, prazosin, quinidine,** or **carbamazepine.** ↑ risk for GI obstruction when used concurrently with **H₂ blockers, opioids, NSAIDS, laxatives, anticholinergic drugs, levothyroxine,** or **neuromuscular blockers.**

Drug–Natural: St. John's wort may significantly ↓ levels and effects; concurrent use is contraindicated.

Drug–Food: Grapefruit and **grapefruit juice** ↑ serum levels and effect.

Route/Dosage

PO (Adults): 10–30 mg 3 times daily (not to exceed 180 mg/day), *or* 10–20 mg twice daily as immediate-release form, *or* 30–90 mg once daily as sustained-release (CC, XL) form (not to exceed 90–120 mg/day).

Availability (generic available)

Capsules: 5 mg, 10 mg, 20 mg. **Tablets:** 10 mg. **Extended-release tablets (Adalat CC, Afeditab CR, Nifedical XL, Procardia XL):** 10 mg, 20 mg, 30 mg, 60 mg, 90 mg

Nursing Implications

Assessment

- Monitor BP and pulse before therapy, during dose titration, and periodically during therapy. Monitor ECG periodically during prolonged therapy.

- Monitor intake and output ratios and daily weight. Assess for signs of HF (peripheral edema, rales/crackles, dyspnea, weight gain, jugular venous distention).

- Patients receiving digoxin concurrently with nifedipine should have routine tests of serum digoxin levels and be monitored for signs and symptoms of digoxin toxicity.

- Assess for rash periodically during therapy. May cause Stevens–Johnson syndrome. Discontinue therapy if severe or if accompanied with fever, general malaise, fatigue, muscle or joint aches, blisters, oral lesions, conjunctivitis, hepatitis, and/or eosinophilia.

- **Angina:** Assess location, duration, intensity, and precipitating factors of patient's anginal pain.

- *Laboratory Test Considerations:* Total serum calcium concentrations are not affected by calcium channel blockers.

- Monitor serum potassium periodically. Hypokalemia increases risk for arrhythmias; should be corrected.

- Monitor renal and hepatic functions periodically during long-term therapy. Several days of therapy may cause ↑ hepatic enzymes, which return to normal upon discontinuation of therapy.

- Nifedipine may cause positive antinuclear antibody and direct Coombs test results.

Potential Nursing Diagnoses

Decreased cardiac output (Indications)

Acute pain (Indications)

Implementation

- Do not confuse with nicardipine or nimodipine.

- **PO:** May be administered without regard to meals. May be administered with meals if GI irritation becomes a problem.

- Do not open, break, crush, or chew extended-release tablets. Empty tablets that appear in stool are not significant.

- Avoid administration with grapefruit juice.

- Sublingual use is not recommended because of serious adverse drug reactions.

Patient/Family Teaching

- Advise patient to take medication as directed, even if feeling well. Take missed doses as soon as possible unless almost time for next dose; do not double doses. May need to be discontinued gradually.

- Instruct patient on technique for monitoring pulse. Instruct patient to contact health-care professional if heart rate is < 50 bpm.

- Advise patient to avoid grapefruit or grapefruit juice during therapy.

- Caution patient to change positions slowly to minimize orthostatic hypotension.

- May cause drowsiness or dizziness. Advise patient to avoid driving or other activities requiring alertness until response to the medication is known.

- Geri: Teach patients and family about risk for falls and how to reduce risk in the home.

- Instruct patient on importance of maintaining good dental hygiene and seeing dentist frequently for teeth cleaning to prevent tenderness, bleeding, and gingival hyperplasia (gum enlargement).

- Instruct patient to notify health-care professional of all Rx or OTC medications, vitamins, or herbal products being taken and to avoid concurrent use of alcohol or OTC medications and herbal products, especially cold preparations, without consulting health-care professional.

- Advise patient to notify health-care professional if rash, irregular heartbeat, dyspnea, swelling of hands and feet, pronounced dizziness, nausea, constipation, or hypotension occurs, or if headache is severe or persistent.

- Caution patient to wear protective clothing and use sunscreen to prevent photosensitivity reactions.

- **Angina:** Instruct patient on concurrent nitrate or β-blocker therapy to continue taking both medications as directed and use SL nitroglycerin as needed for anginal attacks.

- Inform patient that anginal attacks may occur 30 min after administration because of reflex tachycardia. This is usually temporary and is not an indication for discontinuation.

- Advise patient to contact health-care professional if chest pain does not improve, worsens after therapy, or occurs with diaphoresis; if shortness of breath occurs; or if persistent headache occurs.

- Caution patient to discuss exercise restrictions with health-care professional before exertion.

- **Hypertension:** Encourage patient to comply with other interventions for hypertension (weight reduction, low-sodium diet, smoking cessation, moderation of alcohol consumption, regular exercise, and stress management). Medication controls but does not cure hypertension.

- Instruct patient and family in proper technique for monitoring BP. Advise patient to take BP weekly and to report significant changes to health-care professional.

Evaluation/Desired Outcomes
- Decrease in BP
- Decrease in frequency and severity of anginal attacks
- Decrease in need for nitrate therapy
- Increase in activity tolerance and sense of well-being

indomethacin (in-doe-**meth**-a-sin)

Classification
Therapeutic: antirheumatics ductus arteriosus patency adjuncts (IV only) nonsteroidal anti-inflammatory agents

Pregnancy Category B (first trimester)

Indications
PO: Inflammatory disorders, including rheumatoid arthritis, gouty arthritis, osteoarthritis, ankylosing spondylitis. Generally reserved for patients who do not respond to less toxic agents. **IV:** Alternative to surgery in the management of patent ductus arteriosus (PDA) in premature neonates.

Action
Inhibits prostaglandin synthesis. In the treatment of PDA, decreased prostaglandin production allows the ductus to close. **Therapeutic Effects: PO:** Suppression of pain and inflammation. **IV:** Closure of PDA.

Pharmacokinetics
Absorption: Well absorbed after oral administration in adults, incomplete oral absorption in neonates.

Distribution: Crosses the blood–brain barrier and the placenta. Enters breast milk.

Protein Binding: 99%.

Metabolism and Excretion: Mostly metabolized by the liver.

Half-life: Neonates <2 weeks: 20 hr; >2 weeks: 11 hr. Adults: 2.6–11 hr.

Time/Action Profile

ROUTE	ONSET	PEAK	DURATION
PO (analgesic)	30 min	0.5–2 hr	4–6 hr
PO-ER (analgesic)	30 min	Unknown	4–6 hr
PO (anti-inflammatory)	Up to 7 days	1–2 wk	4–6 hr
PO-ER (anti-inflammatory)	Up to 7 days	1–2 wk	4–6 hr
IV (closure of PDA)	Up to 48 hr	unknown	unknown

Contraindicated in: Hypersensitivity; known alcohol intolerance (suspension); cross-sensitivity may exist with other NSAIDs, including aspirin; active GI bleeding; ulcer disease; proctitis or recent history of rectal bleeding; intraventricular hemorrhage; thrombocytopenia. Pedi: ↑ risk for necrotizing enterocolitis and bowel perforation in premature infants with PDA.

Use Cautiously in: Severe cardiovascular, renal, or hepatic disease; history of ulcer disease; epilepsy; hypertension. OB: Not recommended during second half of pregnancy (potential for causing premature closure of ductus arteriosus). Lactation: Usually compatible with breastfeeding (AAP). Geri: ↑ risk for adverse reactions.

Adverse Reactions/Side Effects (CAPITALS indicate life-threatening; <u>underlines</u> indicate most frequent.)

CNS: <u>dizziness</u>, <u>drowsiness</u>, <u>headache</u>, <u>psychic disturbances</u>. **EENT:** blurred vision, tinnitus. **CV:** hypertension, edema. **GI: PO:** DRUG-INDUCED HEPATITIS, GI BLEEDING, <u>constipation</u>, <u>dyspepsia</u>, <u>nausea</u>, <u>vomiting</u>, discomfort, necrotizing enterocolitis. **GU:** cystitis, hematuria, renal failure. **Derm:** rashes. **F and E** hyperkalemia. **IV:** dilutional hyponatremia. **IV:** hypoglycemia. **Hemat:** thrombocytopenia, blood dyscrasias, prolonged bleeding time. **Local:** phlebitis at IV site. **Misc:** ALLERGIC REACTIONS INCLUDING ANAPHYLAXIS.

Interactions

Drug–Drug: Concurrent use with **aspirin** may ↓ effectiveness. Additive adverse GI effects with **aspirin**, other **NSAIDs**, **corticosteroids**, or **alcohol**. Chronic use of **acetaminophen** ↑ risk for adverse renal reactions. May ↓ effectiveness of **diuretics** or **antihypertensives**. May ↑ hypoglycemia from **insulins** or **oral hypoglycemic agents**. May ↑ risk for toxicity from **lithium** or **zidovudine** (avoid concurrent use with zidovudine). ↑ risk for toxicity from **methotrexate**. **Probenecid** ↑ risk for toxicity from indomethacin. ↑ risk for bleeding with **cefotetan**, **cefoperazone**, **valproic acid**, **thrombolytics**, **warfarin**, and **drugs affecting platelet function** including **clopidogrel**, **ticlopidine**, **abciximab**, **eptifibatide**, or **tirofiban**. ↑ risk for adverse hematologic reactions with **antineoplastics** or **radiation therapy**. ↑ risk for nephrotoxicity with **cyclosporine**. Concurrent use with **potassium-sparing diuretics** may result in hyperkalemia. May ↑ levels of **digitalis glycosides**, **methotrexate**, **lithium**, and **aminoglycosides** when used IV in neonates.

Drug–Natural: ↑ bleeding risk with **anise**, **arnica**, **chamomile**, **clove**, **dong quai**, **feverfew**, **garlic**, **ginger**, **ginkgo**, **Panax ginseng**.

Route/Dosage

Anti-inflammatory

PO (adults): *Antiarthritic*—25–50 mg 2–4 times daily *or* 75-mg extended-release capsule once or twice daily (not to exceed 200 mg or 150 mg SR/day). A single bedtime dose of 100 mg may be used. *Antigout*—100 mg initially, followed by 50 mg 3 times daily for relief of pain, then ↓ further.

PO (children >2 yr): 1–2 mg/kg/day in 2–4 divided doses (not to exceed 4 mg/kg/day or 150–200 mg/day).

PDA Closure

IV (Neonates): *Treatment*—0.2 mg/kg initially, then 2 subsequent doses at 12- to 24-hr intervals of 0.1 mg/kg if age <48 hr at time of initial dose; 0.2 mg/kg if 2–7 days at initial dose; 0.25 mg/kg if age >7 days at initial dose. *Prophylaxis*—0.1–0.2 mg/kg initially, then 0.1 mg/kg q12–24h for 2 doses.

Availability (generic available)

Capsules: 25 mg, 50 mg. **Sustained-release capsules:** 75 mg. **Oral suspension (fruit mint, pineapple coconut mint flavors):** 25 mg/5 mL. **Rectal suppository:** 50 mg. **Powder for injection:** 1 mg/vial.

Nursing Implications

Assessment

- Patients who have asthma, aspirin-induced allergy, and nasal polyps are at increased risk for development of hypersensitivity reactions. Monitor for rhinitis, asthma, and urticaria.

- **Arthritis:** Assess limitation of movement and pain—note type, location, and intensity before and 1–2 hr after administration.

- **PDA:** Monitor respiratory status, heart rate, BP, echocardiogram, and heart sounds routinely throughout therapy.

- Monitor intake and output. Fluid restriction is usually instituted throughout therapy.

- ***Laboratory Test Considerations:*** Evaluate BUN, serum creatinine, CBC, serum potassium levels, and liver function tests periodically in patients receiving prolonged therapy.

- Serum potassium, BUN, serum creatinine, AST, and ALT tests may show ↑ levels. Blood glucose concentrations may be altered. Hemoglobin and hematocrit concentrations, leukocyte and platelet counts, and CCr may be ↓.

- Urine glucose and urine protein concentrations may be ↑.

- Leukocyte and platelet count may be ↓. Bleeding time may be prolonged for several days after discontinuation.

Potential Nursing Diagnoses

Acute pain (Indications)

Impaired physical mobility (Indications)

Implementation

- If prolonged therapy is used, dose should be reduced to the lowest level that controls symptoms.

- **PO:** Administer after meals, with food, or with antacids to decrease GI irritation. Do not break, crush, or chew sustained-release capsules.

- Shake suspension before administration. Do not mix with antacid or any other liquid.

IV Administration

- **pH:** 6.0–7.5.

- **Direct IV:** *Diluent:* Preservative-free 0.9% NaCl or preservative-free sterile water. Reconstitute with 1 or 2 mL diluent. *Concentration:* 0.5–1 mg/mL. Reconstitute immediately before use and discard any unused solution. Do not dilute further or admix. Do not administer via umbilical catheter into vessels near the superior mesenteric artery, because these can cause vasoconstriction and compromise blood flow to the intestines. Do not administer intra-arterially.
  Rate: Administer over 20–30 min. Avoid extravasation, because solution is irritating to tissues.

- **Y-Site Compatibility:** furosemide, insulin, nitroprusside, potassium chloride, sodium bicarbonate

- **Y-Site Incompatibility:** calcium gluconate, cimetidine, dobutamine, dopamine, gentamicin, levofloxacin, tobramycin, tolazoline

Patient/Family Teaching

- Advise patient to take this medication with a full glass of water and to remain in an upright position for 15–30 min after administration.

- Instruct patient to take medication exactly as directed. Take missed doses as soon as remembered if not almost time for next dose. Do not double doses.

- May cause drowsiness or dizziness. Advise patient to avoid driving or other activities requiring alertness until response to medication is known.

- Caution patient to avoid the concurrent use of alcohol, aspirin, other NSAIDs, acetaminophen, or other OTC medications without consulting health-care professional.

- Caution patient to wear sunscreen and protective clothing to prevent photosensitivity reactions.

- Advise patient to inform health-care professional of medication regimen before treatment or surgery.

- Instruct patient to notify health-care professional if rash, itching, chills, fever, muscle aches, visual disturbances, weight gain, edema, abdominal pain, black stools, or persistent headache occurs.

- **PDA:** Explain to parents the purpose of medication and the need for frequent monitoring.

Evaluation/Desired Outcomes
- Decrease in severity of moderate pain.

- Improved joint mobility. Partial arthritic relief is usually seen within 2 wk, but maximum effectiveness may require up to 1 mo of continuous therapy. Patients who do not respond to one NSAID may respond to another.

- Successful PDA closure.

High Alert
butorphanol (byoo-**tor**-fa-nole)
Stadol
Classification
Therapeutic: opioid analgesics

Pharmacologic: opioid agonists/antagonists

Schedule IV

Pregnancy Category C

Indications
Management of moderate-to-severe pain. Analgesia during labor. Sedation before surgery. Supplement in balanced anesthesia.

Action
Binds to opiate receptors in the CNS. Alters the perception of and response to painful stimuli while producing generalized CNS depression. Has partial antagonist properties that may result in opioid withdrawal in physically dependent patients.
Therapeutic Effects: Decreased severity of pain.

Pharmacokinetics
Absorption: Well absorbed from IM sites and nasal mucosa.

Distribution: Crosses the placenta and enters breast milk.

Metabolism and Excretion: Mostly metabolized by the liver; 11%–14% excreted in the feces. Minimal renal excretion.

Half-life: 3–4 hr.

Time/Action Profile (analgesia)

ROUTE	ONSET	PEAK	DURATION
IM	Within 15 min	30–60 min	3–4 hr
IV	Within min	4–5 min	2–4 hr
Intranasal	Within 15 min	1–2 hr	4–5 hr

Contraindications/Precautions

Contraindicated in: Hypersensitivity; patients physically dependent on opioids (may precipitate withdrawal).

Use Cautiously in: Head trauma; ↑ intracranial pressure; severe renal, hepatic, or pulmonary disease (↑ interval to q6–8h initially in hepatic/renal impairment); hypothyroidism; adrenal insufficiency; alcoholism; undiagnosed abdominal pain; prostatic hyperplasia. OB/Lactation/Pedi: Safety not established but has been used during labor (may cause respiratory depression in the newborn). Geri: ↓ usual dose by 50%; give at twice the usual interval initially.

Adverse Reactions/Side Effects (CAPITALS indicate life-threatening; <u>underlines</u> indicate most frequent.)

CNS: <u>confusion</u>, <u>dysphoria</u>, <u>hallucinations</u>, <u>sedation</u>, euphoria, floating feeling, headache, unusual dreams. **EENT:** blurred vision, diplopia, miosis (high doses). **Resp:** respiratory depression. **CV:** hypertension, hypotension, palpitations. **GI:** <u>nausea</u>, constipation, dry mouth, ileus, vomiting. **GU:** urinary retention. **Derm:** <u>sweating</u>, clammy feeling. **Misc:** physical dependence, psychological dependence, tolerance.

Interactions

Drug–Drug: Use with extreme caution in patients receiving **MAO inhibitors** (may produce severe, potentially fatal reactions—reduce initial dose of butorphanol to 25% of usual dose). Additive CNS depression with **alcohol**, **antidepressants**, **antihistamines**, and **sedative/hypnotics**. May precipitate withdrawal in patients who are physically dependent on **opioids** and have not been detoxified. May ↓ effects of concurrently administered **opioids**.

Drug–Natural: Concomitant use of **kava-kava**, **valerian**, **chamomile**, or **hops** can ↑ CNS depression.

Route/Dosage

IM (adults): 2 mg q3–4h as needed (range 1–4 mg).

IV (adults): 1 mg q3–4h as needed (range 0.5–2 mg).

IM, IV (geriatric patients): 1 mg q4–6h, ↑ as necessary.

Intranasal (adults): 1 mg (1 spray in 1 nostril) initially. An additional dose may be given 60–90 min later. This sequence may be repeated in 3–4 hr. If pain is severe, an initial dose of 2 mg (1 spray in each nostril) may be given. May be repeated in 3–4 hr.

Intranasal (geriatric patients): 1 mg (1 spray in 1 nostril) initially. An additional dose may be given 90–120 min later. This sequence may be repeated in 3–4 hr.

Availability (generic available)

Injection: 1 mg/mL 2 mg/mL. **Intranasal solution:** 10 mg/mL, in 2.5-mL metered-dose spray pump (14–15 doses; 1 mg/spray).

Nursing Implications

Assessment

- Assess type, location, and intensity of pain before and 30–60 min after IM, 5 min after IV, and 60–90 min after intranasal administration. When titrating opioid doses, increases of 25%–50% should be administered until there is either a 50% reduction in the patient's pain rating on a numerical or visual analogue scale or the patient reports satisfactory pain relief. A repeat dose can be safely administered at the time of the peak if previous dose is ineffective and side effects are minimal. Patients requiring doses >4 mg should be converted to an opioid agonist. Butorphanol is not recommended for prolonged use or as first-line therapy for acute or cancer pain.

- An equianalgesic chart should be used when changing routes or when changing from one opioid to another.

- Assess BP, pulse, and respirations before and periodically during administration. If respiratory rate is <10/min, assess level of sedation. Dose may need to be decreased by 25%–50%. Respiratory depression does not increase in severity, only in duration, with increased dosage.

- Assess previous analgesic history. Antagonistic properties may induce withdrawal symptoms (vomiting, restlessness, abdominal cramps, increased BP, and temperature) in patients who are physically dependent on opioid agonists.

- Butorphanol has a lower potential for dependence than other opioids; however, prolonged use may lead to physical and psychological dependence and tolerance. This should not prevent the patient from receiving adequate analgesia. Most patients receiving butorphanol for pain do not develop psychological dependence. If tolerance develops, changing to an opioid agonist may be required to relieve pain.

- *Laboratory Test Considerations:* May cause ↑ serum amylase and lipase levels.

- *Toxicity and Overdose:* If an opioid antagonist is required to reverse respiratory depression or coma, naloxone (Narcan) is the antidote. Dilute the 0.4 mg ampule of naloxone in 10 mL of 0.9% NaCl and administer 0.5 mL (0.02 mg) by direct IV push every 2 min. For children and patients weighing <40 kg, dilute 0.1 mg naloxone in 10 mL of 0.9% NaCl for a concentration of 10 mcg/mL and administer 0.5 mcg/kg every 1–2 min. Titrate dose to avoid withdrawal, seizures, and severe pain.

Potential Nursing Diagnoses

Acute pain (Indications)

Risk for injury (Side Effects)

Disturbed sensory perception (visual, auditory) (Side Effects)

Implementation

- **High Alert:** Accidental overdosage of opioid analgesics has resulted in fatalities. Before administering, clarify all ambiguous orders; have second practitioner independently check original order, dose calculations, route of administration, and infusion pump programming.

- Explain therapeutic value of medication before administration to enhance the analgesic effect.

- Regularly administered doses may be more effective than prn administration. Analgesic is more effective if given before pain becomes severe.

- Coadministration with nonopioid analgesics may have additive analgesic effects and permit lower opioid doses.

- **IM:** Administer IM injections deep into well-developed muscle. Rotate sites of injections.

IV Administration

- **pH:** 3.0–5.5.
- **Direct IV:** *Diluent:* May give IV undiluted.
- *Concentration:* 1–2 mg/mL.
  Rate: Administer over 3–5 min. **High Alert:** Rapid administration may cause respiratory depression, hypotension, and cardiac arrest.
- **Y-Site Compatibility:** acyclovir, alemtuzumab, allopurinol, amifostine, amikacin, aminocaproic acid, aminophylline, amphotericin B lipid complex, amphotericin B liposome, anidulafungin, argatroban, ascorbic acid, atracurium, atropine, aztreonam, benztropine, bivalirudin, bleomycin, bumetanide, buprenorphine, calcium chloride, calcium gluconate, carboplatin, carmustine, caspofungin, cefazolin, cefepime, cefoperazone, cefotaxime, cefotetan, ceftazidime, ceftriaxone, cefuroxime, chlorpromazine, cisatracurium, cladribine, clindamycin, cyanocobalamin, cyclophosphamide, cyclosporine, cytarabine, dexamethasone, dexmedetomidine, digoxin, diltiazem, diphenhydramine, dobutamine, docetaxel, dopamine, doxacurium, doxorubicin hydrochloride, doxorubicin liposome, doxycycline, enalaprilat, ephedrine, epinephrine, epirubicin, epoetin alfa, eptifibatide, ertapenem, erythromycin, esmolol, etoposide, etoposide phosphate, famotidine, fenoldopam, fentanyl, filgrastim, fluconazole, fludarabine, fluorouracil, gemcita bine, gentamicin, glycopyrrolate, granisetron, heparin, hydrocortisone, idarubicin, ifosfamide, imipenem/cilastatin, irinotecan, isoproterenol, ketorolac, labetalol, levofloxacin, lidocaine, linezolid, lorazepam, magnesium sulfate, mannitol, mechlorethamine, melphalan, meperidine, metaraminol, methotrexate, methoxamine, methyldopate, methylprednisolone, metoclopramide, metoprolol, metronidazole, milrinone, mitoxantrone, morphine, multivitamins, mycophenolate, nafcillin, nalbuphine, naloxone, nesiritide, nicardipine, nitroglycerin, nitroprusside, norepinephrine, octreotide, ondansetron, oxacillin, oxaliplatin, oxytocin, paclitaxel, palonosetron, pamidronate, pancuronium, papaverine, pemetrexed, penicillin G, pentazocine, phenobarbital, phentolamine, phenylephrine, phytonadione, piperacillin/tazobactam, potassium acetate, potassium chloride, procainamide, prochlorperazine, promethazine, propofol, propranolol, protamine, pyridoxine, quinupristin/dalfopristin, ranitidine, remifentanil, rituximab, rocuronium, sargramostim, sodium acetate, streptokinase, succinylcholine, sufentanil, tacrolimus, teniposide, theophylline, thiamine, thiotepa, ticarcillin/clavulanate, tigecycline, tirofiban, tobramycin, tolazoline, trastuzumab, trimethaphan, vancomycin, vasopressin, vecuronium, verapamil, vincristine, vinorelbine, voriconazole, zoledronic acid
- **Y-Site Incompatibility:** amphotericin B cholesteryl , amphotericin B colloidal, azathioprine, chloramphenicol, dantrolene, diazepam, diazoxide, furosemide, ganciclovir, indomethacin, insulin, pantoprazole, pentamidine, pentobarbital, phenytoin, sodium bicarbonate, trimethoprim/sulfamethoxazole
- **Intranasal:** Administer 1 spray in 1 nostril.

Patient/Family Teaching

- Instruct patient on how and when to ask for pain medication.
- Medication may cause drowsiness or dizziness. Advise patient to call for assistance when ambulating and to avoid driving or other activities requiring alertness until response to the medication is known.
- Encourage patients on bedrest to turn, cough, and deep-breathe every 2 hr to prevent atelectasis.
- Instruct patient to change positions slowly to minimize orthostatic hypotension.

- Caution patient to avoid concurrent use of alcohol or other CNS depressants with this medication.

- Advise patient that good oral hygiene, frequent mouth rinses, and sugarless gum or candy may decrease dry mouth.

- **Intranasal:** Instruct patient on proper use of nasal spray. See package insert for detailed instructions. Instruct patient to replace protective clip and clear cover after use, and to store the unit in the child-resistant container. Caution patient that medication should not be used by anyone other than the person for whom it was prescribed. Excess medication should be disposed of as soon as it is no longer needed. To dispose of, unscrew cap, rinse bottle and pump with water, and dispose of in waste can.

  - If 2-mg dose is prescribed, administer additional spray in other nostril. May cause dizziness and dysphoria. Patient should remain recumbent after administration of 2-mg dose until response to medication is known.

Evaluation/Desired Outcomes
Decrease in severity of pain without a significant alteration in level of consciousness or respiratory status.

High Alert
nalbuphine (nal-byoo-feen)
Nubain
Classification
>Therapeutic: opioid analgesics
>
>Pharmacologic: opioid agonists/analgesics

Pregnancy Category C

Indications
Moderate-to-severe pain. Also provides analgesia during labor, sedation before surgery, supplement to balanced anesthesia. Prevention or treatment of opioid-induced pruritus.

Action
Binds to opiate receptors in the CNS. Alters the perception of and response to painful stimuli while producing generalized CNS depression. In addition, has partial antagonist properties, which may result in opioid withdrawal in physically dependent patients.
Therapeutic Effects: Decreased pain.

Pharmacokinetics
>**Absorption:** Well absorbed after IM and SC administration.
>
>**Distribution:** Probably crosses the placenta and enters breast milk.
>
>**Protein Binding:** 50%.
>
>**Metabolism and Excretion:** Mostly metabolized by the liver and eliminated in the feces via biliary excretion. Minimal amounts excreted unchanged by the kidneys.
>
>**Half-life:** Children 1–8 yr: 0.9 hr. Adults: 3.5–5 hr.

Time/Action Profile (analgesia)

ROUTE	ONSET	PEAK	DURATION
IM	<15 min	60 min	3–6 hr
SC	<15 min	Unknown	3–6 hr
IV	2–3 min	30 min	3–6 hr

Contraindicated in: Hypersensitivity to nalbuphine or bisulfites; patients physically dependent on opioids and who have not been detoxified (may precipitate withdrawal).

Use Cautiously in: Head trauma; ↑ intracranial pressure; severe renal, hepatic, or pulmonary disease; hypothyroidism; adrenal insufficiency; alcoholism; undiagnosed abdominal pain; prostatic hyperplasia; patients who have recently received opioid agonists. OB: Has been used during labor but may cause respiratory depression in the newborn. Geri: Dose ↓ suggested.

Adverse Reactions/Side Effects (CAPITALS indicate life-threatening; <u>underlines</u> indicate most frequent.)

CNS: <u>dizziness</u>, <u>headache</u>, <u>sedation</u>, confusion, dysphoria, euphoria, floating feeling, hallucinations, unusual dreams. **EENT:** blurred vision, diplopia, miosis (high doses). **Resp:** respiratory depression. **CV:** hypertension, orthostatic hypotension, palpitations. **GI:** <u>dry mouth</u>, <u>nausea</u>, <u>vomiting</u>, constipation, ileus. **GU:** urinary urgency. **Derm:** <u>clammy feeling</u>, <u>sweating</u>. **Misc:** physical dependence, psychological dependence, tolerance.

Interactions

Drug–Drug: Use with extreme caution in patients receiving **MAO inhibitors** (may result in unpredictable, severe reactions; ↓ initial dose of nalbuphine to 25% of usual dose). Additive CNS depression with **alcohol**, **antihistamines**, and **sedative/hypnotics**. May precipitate withdrawal in patients who are physically dependent on **opioid agonists**. Avoid concurrent use with other **opioid analgesic agonists** (may diminish analgesic effect).

Drug–Natural: Concomitant use of **kava-kava**, **valerian**, **skullcap**, **chamomile**, or **hops** can ↑ CNS depression.

Route/Dosage

Analgesia

IM, SC, IV (adults): Usual dose is 10 mg q3–6h (maximum: 20 mg/dose or 160 mg/day).

IM, SC, IV (Children): 0.1–0.15 mg/kg q3–6h (maximum: 20 mg/dose or 160 mg/day).

Supplement to Balanced Anesthesia

IV (Adults): *Initial*—0.3 to 3 mg/kg over 10–15 min. *Maintenance*—0.25 to 0.5 mg/kg as needed.

Opioid-Induced Pruritus

IV (Adults): 2.5–5 mg; may repeat dose.

Availability (generic available)

Injection: 10 mg/mL, 20 mg/mL

Nursing Implications

Assessment

- Assess type, location, and intensity of pain before and 1 hr after IM or 30 min (peak) after IV administration. When titrating opioid doses, increases of 25%–50% should be administered until there is either a 50% reduction in the patient's pain rating on a numeric or visual analogue scale, or the patient reports satisfactory pain relief. A repeat dose can be safely administered at the time of the peak if previous dose is ineffective and side effects are minimal. Patients requiring doses higher than 20 mg should be converted to an opioid agonist. Nalbuphine is not recommended for prolonged use or as first-line therapy for acute or cancer pain.

- An equianalgesic chart should be used when changing routes or when changing from one opioid to another.

- Assess BP, pulse, and respirations before and periodically during administration. If respiratory rate is < 10/min, assess level of sedation. Physical stimulation may be sufficient to prevent significant hypoventilation. Dose may need to be decreased by 25%–50%. Nalbuphine produces respiratory depression, but this does not markedly increase with increased doses.

- Assess previous analgesic history. Antagonistic properties may induce withdrawal symptoms (vomiting, restlessness, abdominal cramps, and increased BP and temperature) in patients physically dependent on opioids.

- Although this drug has a low potential for dependence, prolonged use may lead to physical and psychological dependence and tolerance. This should not prevent patient from receiving adequate analgesia. Most patients who receive nalbuphine for pain do not develop psychological dependence. If tolerance develops, changing to an opioid agonist may be required to relieve pain.

- **Laboratory Test Considerations:** May cause ↑ serum amylase and lipase concentrations.

- **Toxicity and Overdose:** If an opioid antagonist is required to reverse respiratory depression or coma, naloxone (Narcan) is the antidote. Dilute the 0.4-mg ampule of naloxone in 10 mL of 0.9% NaCl, and administer 0.5 mL (0.02 mg) by direct IV push every 2 min. For children and patients weighing < 40 kg, dilute 0.1 mg naloxone in 10 mL of 0.9% NaCl for a concentration of 10 mcg/mL, and administer 0.5 mcg/kg every 2 min. Titrate dose to avoid withdrawal, seizures, and severe pain.

Potential Nursing Diagnoses
Acute pain (Indications)

Risk for injury (Side Effects)

Disturbed sensory perception (visual, auditory) (Side Effects)

Implementation
- **High Alert:** Accidental overdose of opioid analgesics has resulted in fatalities. Before administering, clarify all ambiguous orders; have second practitioner independently check original order, dose calculations, and infusion pump settings.

- Explain therapeutic value of medication before administration to enhance the analgesic effect.

- Regularly administered doses may be more effective than prn administration. Analgesic is more effective if administered before pain becomes severe.

- Coadministration with nonopioid analgesics may have additive effects and permit lower opioid doses.

- **IM:** Administer deep into well-developed muscle. Rotate sites of injections.

IV Administration
- **pH:** 3.0–4.5.

- **Direct IV:** May give IV undiluted.

- **Concentration:** 10–20 mg/mL.
  Rate: Administer slowly, each 10 mg over 3–5 min.

- **Syringe Compatibility:** atropine, cimetidine, diphenhydramine, droperidol, glycopyrrolate, hydroxyzine, lidocaine, midazolam, prochlorperazine, ranitidine, scopolamine

- **Syringe Incompatibility:** diazepam, ketorolac, pentobarbital
- **Y-Site Compatibility:** amifostine, aztreonam, bivalirudin, cisatracurium, cladribine, dexmedetomidine, etoposide phosphate, fenoldopam, filgrastim, fludarabine, gemcitabine, granisetron, lansoprazole, linezolid, melphalan, oxaliplatin, paclitaxel, propofol, remifentanil, teniposide, thiotepa, vinorelbine
- **Y-Site Incompatibility:** allopurinol, amphotericin B cholesteryl sulfate complex, cefepime, docetaxel, methotrexate, pemetrexed, piperacillin/tazobactam, sargramostim, sodium bicarbonate

Patient/Family Teaching
- Instruct patient on how and when to ask for pain medication.
- May cause drowsiness or dizziness. Advise patient to call for assistance when ambulating and to avoid driving or other activities requiring alertness until response to the medication is known.
- Caution patient to change positions slowly to minimize orthostatic hypotension.
- Advise patient that frequent mouth rinses, good oral hygiene, and sugarless gum or candy may decrease dry mouth.
- Encourage patient to turn, cough, and breathe deeply every 2 hr to prevent atelectasis.
- Advise patient to avoid concurrent use of alcohol or other CNS depressants with this medication.

Evaluation/Desired Outcomes
- Decrease in severity of pain without significant alteration in level of consciousness or respiratory status

High Alert
oxyCODONE (ox-i-**koe**-done)
Oxecta, OxyCONTIN, OxyIR, OxyNEO, Roxicodone, Supeudol

Classification
Therapeutic: opioid analgesics

Pharmacologic: opioid agonists/nonopioid analgesic combinations

Schedule II

Pregnancy Category B

Indications
Moderate-to-severe pain; extended-release product should be used for patients requiring around-the-clock management of chronic pain.

Action
Binds to opiate receptors in the CNS. Alters the perception of and response to painful stimuli, while producing generalized CNS depression. **Therapeutic Effects:** Decreased pain.

Pharmacokinetics
Absorption: Well absorbed from the GI tract.

Distribution: Widely distributed. Crosses the placenta; enters breast milk.

Protein Binding: 38%–45%

Metabolism and Excretion: Mostly metabolized by the liver by the CYP3A4 isoenzyme.

Half-life: 2–3 hr.

Time/Action Profile (analgesic effects)

ROUTE	ONSET	PEAK	DURATION
PO	10–15 min	60–90 min	3–6 hr
PO-CR*	10–15 min	3 hr	12 hr

*Controlled release.

Contraindications/Precautions

Contraindicated in: Hypersensitivity; some products contain alcohol or bisulfites and should be avoided in patients with known intolerance or hypersensitivity; significant respiratory depression; paralytic ileus; acute or severe bronchial asthma.

Use Cautiously in: Head trauma; ↑ intracranial pressure; Severe renal or hepatic disease; hypothyroidism; adrenal insufficiency; alcoholism; undiagnosed abdominal pain; prostatic hyperplasia; difficulty swallowing or GI disorders that may predispose patient to obstruction (↑ risk for GI obstruction). OB: Avoid chronic use; weigh maternal benefit against fetal risks. Lactation: Lactation. Geri: Elderly or debilitated patients (initial dose ↓ recommended).

Adverse Reactions/Side Effects (CAPITALS indicate life-threatening; <u>underlines</u> indicate most frequent.)

CNS: <u>confusion</u>, <u>sedation</u>, dizziness, dysphoria, euphoria, floating feeling, hallucinations, headache, unusual dreams. **EENT:** blurred vision, diplopia, miosis. **Resp:** RESPIRATORY DEPRESSION. **CV:** orthostatic hypotension. **GI:** <u>constipation</u>, dry mouth, choking, GI obstruction, nausea, vomiting. **GU:** urinary retention. **Derm:** flushing, sweating. **Misc:** physical dependence, psychological dependence, tolerance.

Interactions

Drug–Drug: Use with caution in patients receiving **MAO inhibitors** (may result in unpredictable reactions; ↓ initial dose of oxycodone to 25% of usual dose). Additive CNS depression with **alcohol**, **antihistamines**, and **sedative/hypnotics**. Administration of **partial-antagonist opioid analgesics** may precipitate withdrawal in physically dependent patients. **Nalbuphine**, **buprenorphine**, or **pentazocine** may ↓ analgesia. Potent **CYP3A4 inhibitors** including **erythromycin, ketoconazole, itraconazole, voriconazole, <u>or</u> ritonavir** may ↑ levels. Potent **CYP3A4 inducers** including **rifampin, carbamazepine**, and **phenytoin** may ↓ levels.

Route/Dosage

Larger doses may be required during chronic therapy.

PO (adults ≥50 kg): 5–10 mg q3–4h initially, as needed. Controlled-release tablets (OxyContin) may be given q12h.

PO (adults <50 kg): 0.2 mg/kg q3–4h initially, as needed.

PO (children): 0.05–0.15 mg/kg q4–6h as needed, as immediate-release product.

Rectal (adults): 10–40 mg 3–4 times daily initially, as needed.

Availability (generic available)

Tablets (Oxecta, Roxicodone): 5 mg, 7.5 mg, 15 mg, 30 mg. Cost: *Generic—* 5 mg $34.14/3010 mg $19.97/3015 mg $31.16/3030 mg $41.56/30. **Immediate-release capsules:** 5 mg. **Controlled-release tablets (OxyContin):** 10 mg,

15 mg, 20 mg, 30 mg, 40 mg, 60 mg, 80 mg. Cost: 10 mg $149.97/6015 mg $218.97/6020 mg $258.95/6030 mg $377.96/6040 mg $462.95/6060 mg $637.94/6080 mg $872.97/60. **Concentrated oral solution:** 20 mg/mL. **Suppositories:** 10 mg, 20 mg. *In combination with:* ibuprofen (Combunox), aspirin (Endodan, Percodan), acetaminophen (Endocet, Magnacet, Oxycet, Percocet, Roxicet, Tylox).

Nursing Implications

Assessment

- Assess type, location, and intensity of pain before and 1 hr (peak) after administration. When titrating opioid doses, increases of 25%–50% should be administered until there is either a 50% reduction in the patient's pain rating on a numerical or visual analogue scale, or the patient reports satisfactory pain relief. A repeat dose can be safely administered at the time of the peak if previous dose is ineffective and side effects are minimal.

- Patients taking controlled-release tablets may also be given supplemental short-acting opioid doses for breakthrough pain.

- An equianalgesic chart should be used when changing routes or when changing from one opioid to another.

- Assess BP, pulse, and respirations before and periodically during administration. If respiratory rate is <10/min, assess level of sedation. Physical stimulation may be sufficient to prevent significant hypoventilation. Dose may need to be decreased by 25%–50%. Initial drowsiness will diminish with continued use.

- Prolonged use may lead to physical and psychological dependence and tolerance. This should not prevent patient from receiving adequate analgesia. Most patients who receive oxycodone for pain do not develop psychological dependence. Progressively higher doses may be required to relieve pain with long-term therapy.

- Assess bowel function routinely. Prevention of constipation should be instituted with increased intake of fluids and bulk, and laxatives to minimize constipating effects. Stimulant laxatives should be administered routinely if opioid use exceeds 2–3 days, unless contraindicated.

- *Laboratory Test Considerations:* May ↑ plasma amylase and lipase levels.

- *Toxicity and Overdose:* If an opioid antagonist is required to reverse respiratory depression or coma, naloxone (Narcan) is the antidote. Dilute the 0.4-mg ampule of naloxone in 10 mL of 0.9% NaCl and administer 0.5 mL (0.02 mg) by direct IV push every 2 min. For children and patients weighing <40 kg, dilute 0.1 mg naloxone in 10 mL of 0.9% NaCl for a concentration of 10 mcg/mL and administer 0.5 mcg/kg every 2 min. Titrate dose to avoid withdrawal, seizures, and severe pain.

Potential Nursing Diagnoses

Acute pain (Indications)

Chronic pain (Indications)

Risk for injury (Side Effects)

Implementation

- *High Alert:* Accidental overdose of opioid analgesics has resulted in fatalities. Before administering, clarify all ambiguous orders; have second practitioner independently check original order and dose calculations.

- Do not confuse short-acting oxycodone with long-acting OxyContin. Do not confuse oxycodone with hydrocodone. Do not confuse OxyContin with MS Contin.
- Explain therapeutic value of medication before administration to enhance the analgesic effect.
- Regularly administered doses may be more effective than prn administration. Analgesic is more effective if given before pain becomes severe.
- Coadministration with nonopioid analgesics may have additive analgesic effects and may permit lower doses.
- Oxycodone should be discontinued gradually after long-term use to prevent withdrawal symptoms.
- **PO:** May be administered with food or milk to minimize GI irritation.
- Administer solution with properly calibrated measuring device.
- **Controlled Release:** Take 1 tablet at a time. Swallow controlled-release tablet whole; do not crush, break, or chew. Taking broken, chewed, crushed, or dissolved controlled-release tablets leads to rapid release and absorption of a potentially fatal dose of oxycodone. Advise patients not to presoak, lick, or wet controlled-release tablets before placing in the mouth. Take each tablet with enough water to ensure complete swallowing immediately after placing in mouth. Dose should be based on 24-hr opioid requirement determined with short-acting opioids, then converted to controlled-release form.
- Do not use *Oxceta* for administration via nasogastric, gastric, or other feeding tubes because it may cause obstruction of feeding tubes.

Patient/Family Teaching
- Instruct patient on how and when to ask for and take pain medication.
- Advise patient that oxycodone is a drug with known abuse potential. Protect it from theft, and never give to anyone other than the individual for whom it was prescribed.
- Medication may cause drowsiness or dizziness. Advise patient to call for assistance when ambulating or smoking. Caution patient to avoid driving and other activities requiring alertness until response to medication is known.
- Advise patients taking *OxyContin* tablets that empty matrix tablets may appear in stool.
- Advise patient to make position changes slowly to minimize orthostatic hypotension.
- Advise patient to avoid concurrent use of alcohol or other CNS depressants with this medication.
- Instruct patient to notify health-care professional of all Rx or OTC medications, vitamins, or herbal products being taken, and consult health-care professional before taking any new medications.
- Encourage patient to turn, cough, and breathe deeply every 2 hr to prevent atelectasis.
- Advise patient to notify health-care professional if pregnancy is planned or suspected, or if breastfeeding.

Evaluation/Desired Outcomes
- Decrease in severity of pain without a significant alteration in level of consciousness or respiratory status

HYDROmorphone (hye-droe-**mor**-fone)
Dilaudid, Dilaudid-HP, Exalgo, Hydromorph Contin, Jurnista

Classification
Therapeutic: allergy, cold, and cough remedies (antitussives), opioid analgesics

Pharmacologic: opioid agonists

Schedule II

Pregnancy Category C

Indications
Moderate-to-severe pain (alone and in combination with nonopioid analgesics); extended-release product for opioid-tolerant patients requiring around-the-clock management of persistent moderate-to-severe pain. Antitussive (lower doses).

Action
Binds to opiate receptors in the CNS. Alters the perception of and response to painful stimuli while producing generalized CNS depression. Suppresses the cough reflex via a direct central action. **Therapeutic Effects:** Decrease in moderate-to-severe pain. Suppression of cough.

Pharmacokinetics
Absorption: Well absorbed after oral, rectal, SC, and IM administration. Extended-release product results in an initial release of drug, followed by a second sustained phase of absorption.

Distribution: Widely distributed. Crosses the placenta; enters breast milk.

Metabolism and Excretion: Mostly metabolized by the liver.

Half-life: *Oral (immediate-release), or injection*—2–4 hr. *Oral (extended-release)*—8–15 hr.

Time/Action Profile (analgesic effect)

ROUTE	ONSET	PEAK	DURATION
PO-IR	30 min	30–90 min	4–5 hr
PO-ER	Unknown	Unknown	Unknown
SC	15 min	30–90 min	4–5 hr
IM	15 min	30–60 min	4–5 hr
IV	10–15 min	15–30 min	2–3 hr
Rectal	15–30 min	30–90 min	4–5 hr

Contraindications/Precautions
Contraindicated in: Hypersensitivity; some products contain bisulfites and should be avoided in patients with known hypersensitivity; severe respiratory depression (in absence of resuscitative equipment) (extended-release only). Paralytic ileus (extended-release only). Prior GI surgery or narrowing of GI tract (extended-release only). Opioid nontolerant patients (extended-release only). OB/Lactation: Avoid chronic use during pregnancy or lactation.

Use Cautiously in: Head trauma; ↑ intracranial pressure; severe renal, hepatic, or pulmonary disease; hypothyroidism; seizure disorder; adrenal insufficiency; alcoholism; undiagnosed abdominal pain; prostatic hypertrophy; biliary tract disease (including pancreatitis). Geri: Geriatric and debilitated patients may be more susceptible to side effects; dose ↓ recommended.

Adverse Reactions/Side Effects (CAPITALS indicate life-threatening; underlines indicate most frequent.)

CNS: <u>confusion</u>, <u>sedation</u>, dizziness, dysphoria, euphoria, floating feeling, hallucinations, headache, unusual dreams. **EENT:** blurred vision, diplopia, miosis. **Resp:** respiratory depression. **CV:** <u>hypotension</u>, bradycardia. **GI:** <u>constipation</u>, dry mouth, nausea, vomiting. **GU:** urinary retention. **Derm:** flushing, sweating. **Misc:** physical dependence, psychological dependence, tolerance.

Interactions

Drug–Drug: Exercise extreme caution with **MAO inhibitors** (may produce severe, unpredictable reactions—reduce initial dose of hydromorphone to 25% of usual dose, discontinue MAO inhibitors 2 wk before hydromorphone). ↑ risk for CNS depression with **alcohol**, **antidepressants**, **antihistamines**, and **sedative/hypnotics** including **benzodiazepines** and **phenothiazines**. Administration of partial antagonists (**buprenorphine**, **butorphanol**, **nalbuphine**, or **pentazocine**) may precipitate opioid withdrawal in physically dependent patients. **Nalbuphine** or **pentazocine** may ↓ analgesia.

Drug–Natural: Concomitant use of **kava-kava**, **valerian**, **chamomile**, or **hops** can ↑ CNS depression.

Route/Dosage

Doses depend on level of pain and tolerance. Larger doses may be required during chronic therapy

Analgesic

PO (adults ≥50 kg): *Immediate release*—4 to 8 mg q3–4h initially (some patients may respond to doses as small as 2 mg initially); *or* once 24-hr opioid requirement is determined, convert to *extended release* by administering total daily oral dose once daily.

PO (adults and children < 50 kg): 0.06 mg/kg q3–4h initially, younger children may require smaller initial doses of 0.03 mg/kg. Maximum dose, 5 mg.

IV, IM, SC (adults ≥50 kg): 1.5 mg q3–4h as needed initially; may be ↑.

IV, IM, SC (adults and children < 50 kg): 0.015 mg/kg mg q3–4h as needed initially; may be ↑.

IV (adults): *Continuous infusion (unlabeled)*—0.2–30 mg/hr depending on previous opioid use. An initial bolus of twice the hourly rate in milligrams may be given with subsequent breakthrough boluses of 50%–100% of the hourly rate in milligrams.

Rectal (Adults): 3 mg q6–8h initially as needed.

Antitussive

PO (adults and children > 12 yr): 1 mg q3–4h.

PO (children 6–12 yr): 0.5 mg q3–4h.

Availability (generic available)

Immediate-release tablets: 2 mg, 3 mg, 4 mg, 8 mg, **Extended-release tablets:** 4 mg, 8 mg, 12 mg, 16 mg, 32 mg, 64 mg. **Oral solution:** 5 mg/5 mL. **Injection:** 1 mg/mL, 2 mg/mL, 4 mg/mL, 10 mg/mL. **Suppositories:** 3 mg.

Nursing Implications

Assessment

- Assess BP, pulse, and respirations before and periodically during administration. If respiratory rate is < 10/min, assess level of sedation. Dose may need to be decreased by 25%–50%. Initial drowsiness will diminish with continued use. Geri/Pedi: Assess geriatric and pediatric patients frequently; more sensitive to the effects of opioid analgesics and may experience side effects and respiratory complications more frequently.

- Assess bowel function routinely. Institute prevention of constipation with increased intake of fluids and bulk, and laxatives to minimize constipating effects. Administer stimulant laxatives routinely if opioid use exceeds 2–3 days, unless contraindicated.

- **Pain:** Assess type, location, and intensity of pain before and 1 hr after IM or PO and 5 min (peak) after IV administration. When titrating opioid doses, increases of 25%–50% should be administered until there is either a 50% reduction in the patient's pain rating on a numerical or visual analogue scale, or the patient reports satisfactory pain relief. When titrating doses of short-acting hydromorphone, a repeat dose can be safely administered at the time of the peak if previous dose is ineffective and side effects are minimal.

- Patients on a continuous infusion should have additional bolus doses provided every 15–30 min, as needed, for breakthrough pain. The bolus dose is usually set to the amount of drug infused each hour by continuous infusion.

- Patients taking sustained-release hydromorphone may require additional short-acting opioid doses for breakthrough pain. Doses should be equivalent to 10%–20% of 24-hr total and given every 2 hr as needed.

- An equianalgesic chart should be used when changing routes or when changing from one opioid to another.

- Prolonged use may lead to physical and psychological dependence and tolerance. This should not prevent patient from receiving adequate analgesia. Most patients who receive hydromorphone for pain do not develop psychological dependence. Progressively higher doses may be required to relieve pain with long-term therapy.

- **Cough:** Assess cough and lung sounds during antitussive use.

- **_Laboratory Test Considerations:_** May ↑ plasma amylase and lipase concentrations.

- **_Toxicity and Overdose:_** If an opioid antagonist is required to reverse respiratory depression or coma, naloxone (Narcan) is the antidote. Dilute the 0.4-mg ampule of naloxone in 10 mL of 0.9% NaCl, and administer 0.5 mL (0.02 mg) by direct IV push every 2 min. For children and patients weighing < 40 kg, dilute 0.1 mg naloxone in 10 mL of 0.9% NaCl for a concentration of 10 mcg/mL, and administer 0.5 mcg every 2 min. Titrate dose to avoid withdrawal, seizures, and severe pain.

Potential Nursing Diagnoses

Acute pain (Indications)

Chronic pain (Indications)

Risk for injury (Side Effects)

Implementation

- **_High Alert:_** Accidental overdosage of opioid analgesics has resulted in fatalities. Before administering, clarify all ambiguous orders; have second practitioner independently check original order, dose calculations, and infusion pump settings. Do not confuse with morphine; fatalities have occurred. Do not confuse high-potency (HP) dose forms with regular dose forms. Pedi: Medication errors with opioid analgesics are common in pediatric patients; do not misinterpret or miscalculate doses. Use appropriate measuring devices.

- Explain therapeutic value of medication before administration to enhance the analgesic effect.

- Regularly administered doses may be more effective than prn administration. Analgesic is more effective if given before pain becomes severe.
- Coadministration with nonopioid analgesics may have additive analgesic effects and permit lower opioid doses.
- Medication should be discontinued gradually after long-term use to prevent withdrawal symptoms.
- When converting from immediate-release to extended-release hydromorphone, administer total daily oral hydromorphone dose once daily; dose of extended-release product can be titrated q3–4days. To convert from another opioid to extended-release hydromorphone, convert to total daily dose of hydromorphone and then administer 50% of this dose as extended-release hydromorphone once daily; can then titrate dose q3–4days. When converting from transdermal fentanyl, initiate extended-release hydromorphone 18 hr after removing transdermal fentanyl patch; for each 25-mcg/hr fentanyl transdermal dose, the equianalgesic dose of extended-release hydromorphone is 12 mg once daily (should initiate at 50% of this calculated total daily dose given once daily).
- **PO:** May be administered with food or milk to minimize GI irritation.
- Swallow extended-release tablets whole; do not break, crush, dissolve, or chew (could result in rapid release and absorption of a potentially toxic dose).

IV Administration
- **pH:** 4.0–5.5.
- **Direct IV: *Diluent:*** Dilute with at least 5 mL of sterile water or 0.9% NaCl for injection. Inspect solution for particulate matter. Slight yellow color does not alter potency. Store at room temperature.
  Rate: Administer slowly, at a rate not to exceed 2 mg over 3–5 min. **High Alert:** Rapid administration may lead to increased respiratory depression, hypotension, and circulatory collapse.
- **Y-Site Compatibility:** acyclovir, alemtuzumab, allopurinol, amifostine, amikacin, aminocaproic acid, aminophylline, amphotericin B colloidal, amphotericin B lipid complex, amphotericin B liposome, ampicillin/sulbactam, amsacrine, anidulafungin, argatroban, atracurium, atropine, aztreonam, bivalirudin, bleomycin, bumetanide, busulfan, calcium chloride, calcium gluconate, carboplatin, carmustine, caspofungin, cefepime, cefoperazone, cefotaxime, cefoxitin, ceftaroline, ceftazidime, ceftriaxone, cefuroxime, chloramphenicol, chlorpromazine, ciprofloxacin, cisatracurium, cisplatin, cladribine, clindamycin, cyclophosphamide, cyclosporine, cytarabine, dactinomycin, daptomycin, dexamethasone, dexmedetomidine, digoxin, diltiazem, diphenhydramine, dobutamine, docetaxel, dopamine, doripenem, doxacurium, doxorubicin, doxorubicin liposome, doxycycline, droperidol, enalaprilat, ephedrine, epinephrine, epirubicin, eptifibatide, ertapenem, erythromycin lactobionate, esmolol, etoposide, etoposide phosphate, famotidine, fenoldopam, fentanyl, filgrastim, fluconazole, fludarabine, fluorouracil, foscarnet, furosemide, ganciclovir, gemcitabine, gentamicin, glycopyrrolate, granisetron, haloperidol, heparin, hydralazine, hydrocortisone, idarubicin, ifosfamide, imipenem/cilastatin, insulin, irinotecan, isoproterenol, kanamycin, ketorolac, labetalol, levofloxacin, lidocaine, linezolid, lorazepam, magnesium sulfate, mannitol, mechlorethamine, melphalan, meropenem, methohexital, methotrexate, methyldopate, methylprednisolone, metoclopramide, metoprolol, metronidazole, micafungin, midazolam, milrinone, mitoxantrone, morphine, mycophenolate, nafcillin, nesiritide, nicardipine, nitroglycerin, nitroprusside, norepinephrine, octreotide, ondansetron, oxacillin, oxaliplatin, oxytocin, paclitaxel, palonosetron, pamidronate, pancuronium, pantoprazole, pemetrexed, penicillin G potassium, pentamidine, pentobarbital, phenylephrine,

piperacillin/tazobactam, potassium acetate, potassium chloride, potassium phosphates, procainamide, prochlorperazine, promethazine, propofol, propranolol, quinupristin/dalfopristin, ranitidine, remifentanil, rituximab, rocuronium, scopolamine, sodium acetate, sodium phosphates, strepto-zocin, succinylcholine, tacrolimus, teniposide, theophylline, thiotepa, ticarcillin/clavulanate, tigecycline, tirofiban, tobramycin, trastuzumab, trimethoprim/sulfamethoxazole, vancomycin, vasopressin, vecuronium, verapamil, vincristine, vinorelbine, zidovudine, zoledronic acid

- **Y-Site Incompatibility:** amphotericin B cholesteryl, dantrolene, pheny-toin, sargramostim, thiopental
- **Solution Compatibility:** D5W, D5/0.45% NaCl, D5/0.9% NaCl, D5/LR, D5/Ringer's solution, 0.45% NaCl, 0.9% NaCl, Ringer's , LR

Patient/Family Teaching

- Instruct patient on how and when to ask for pain medication.
- May cause drowsiness or dizziness. Advise patient to call for assistance when ambulating or smoking. Caution patient to avoid driving or other activities requiring alertness until response to medication is known.
- Advise patient to change positions slowly to minimize orthostatic hypotension.
- Instruct patient to avoid concurrent use of alcohol or other CNS depressants.
- Encourage patient to turn, cough, and breathe deeply every 2 hr to prevent atelectasis.
- **Home-Care Issues:** Explain to patient and family how and when to admin-ister hydromorphone, discuss safe storage of the medication, and how to care for infusion equipment properly. Pedi: Teach parents or caregivers how to accurately measure liquid medication and to use only the measur-ing device dispensed with the medication.
- Emphasize the importance of aggressive prevention of constipation with the use of hydromorphone.

Evaluation/Desired Outcomes

- Decrease in severity of pain without a significant alteration in level of consciousness or respiratory status
- Suppression of cough

ibuprofen (oral) (eye-byoo-**proe**-fen)

Advil, Advil Migraine Liqui-Gels, Children's Advil, Children's Motrin, Excedrin IB, Genpril, Haltran, Junior Strength Advil, Menadol, Medipren, Midol Maximum Strength Cramp Formula, Motrin, Motrin Drops, Motrin IB, Motrin Junior Strength, Motrin Migraine Pain, Nu-Ibuprofen, Nuprin, PediaCare Children's Fever

ibuprofen (injection)

Caldolor

Classification

Therapeutic: antipyretics, antirheumatics, nonopioid analgesics, nonsteroidal anti-inflammatory agents

Pharmacologic: nonopioid analgesics

Pregnancy Category C (up to 30 wk gestation), D (starting at 30 wk gestation)

Indications

PO, IV: Treatment of mild-to-moderate pain, fever. **PO:** Treatment of in-flammatory disorders including rheumatoid arthritis (including juvenile) and osteoarthritis; dysmenorrhea. **IV:** Moderate-to-severe pain with opioid analgesics.

Action
Inhibits prostaglandin synthesis. **Therapeutic Effects:** Decreased pain and inflammation. Reduction of fever.

Pharmacokinetics

Absorption: Oral formulation is well absorbed (80%) from the GI tract; IV administration results in complete bioavailability.

Distribution: Does not enter breast milk in significant amounts.

Protein Binding: 99%.

Metabolism and Excretion: Mostly metabolized by the liver; small amounts (1%) excreted unchanged by the kidneys.

Half-life: Children: 1–2 hr; Adults: 2–4 hr.

Time/Action Profile

ROUTE	ONSET	PEAK	DURATION
PO (antipyretic)	0.5–2.5 hr	2–4 hr	6–8 hr
PO (analgesic)	30 min	1–2 hr	4–6 hr
PO (anti-inflammatory)	≤7 days	1–2 wk	Unknown
IV (analgesic)	Unknown	Unknown	6 hr
IV (antipyretic)	Within 2 hr	10–12 hr*	4–6 hr

*With repeated dosing.

Contraindications/Precautions

Contraindicated in: Hypersensitivity (cross-sensitivity may exist with other NSAIDs, including aspirin); active GI bleeding or ulcer disease; chewable tablets contain aspartame and should not be used in patients with phenylketonuria; perioperative pain from coronary artery bypass graft (CABG) surgery. OB: Avoid after 30 wk gestation (may cause premature closure of fetal ductus arteriosus).

Use Cautiously in: Cardiovascular disease (may ↑ risk for cardiovascular events); renal or hepatic disease, dehydration, or patients on nephrotoxic drugs (may ↑ risk for renal toxicity); aspirin triad patients (asthma, nasal polyps, and aspirin intolerance); can cause fatal anaphylactoid reactions. Geri: ↑ risk for adverse reactions secondary to age-related ↓ in renal and hepatic function, concurrent illnesses, and medications; chronic alcohol use/abuse; coagulation disorders. OB: Use cautiously up to 30 wk gestation; avoid after that. Lactation: Use cautiously. Pedi: Safety not established for infants < 6 mo (oral) and children < 17 yr (IV).

Exercise Extreme Caution in: History of GI bleeding or GI ulcer disease.

Adverse Reactions/Side Effects (CAPITALS indicate life-threatening; underlines indicate most frequent.)

CNS: headache, dizziness, drowsiness, psychic disturbances. **EENT:** amblyopia, blurred vision, tinnitus. **CV:** arrhythmias, edema, hypertension. **GI:** GI BLEEDING, HEPATITIS, constipation, dyspepsia, nausea, vomiting, abdominal discomfort. **GU:** cystitis, hematuria, renal failure. **Derm:** EXFOLIATIVE DERMATITIS, STEVENS–JOHNSON SYNDROME, TOXIC EPIDERMAL NECROLYSIS, rashes. **Hemat:** anemia, blood dyscrasias, prolonged bleeding time. **Misc:** ALLERGIC REACTIONS INCLUDING ANAPHYLAXIS.

Interactions

Drug–Drug: May limit the cardioprotective effects of low-dose **aspirin**. Concurrent use with **aspirin** may ↓ effectiveness of ibuprofen. Additive adverse GI side effects with **aspirin**, **oral potassium**, other **NSAIDs**, **corticosteroids**, or **alcohol**. Chronic use with **acetaminophen** may ↑ risk for adverse renal reactions. May ↓ effectiveness of **diuretics**, **ACE inhibitors**, or other **antihypertensives**. May ↑ hypoglycemic effects of **insulin** or **oral hypoglycemic agents**. May ↑ serum **lithium** levels and risk for toxicity. ↑ risk for toxicity from **methotrexate**. **Probenecid** ↑ risk for toxicity from ibuprofen. ↑ risk for bleeding with **cefotetan**, **cefoperazone**, **corticosteroids**, **valproic acid**, **thrombolytics**, **warfarin**, and **drugs affecting platelet function** including **clopidogrel**, **ticlopidine**, **abciximab**, **eptifibatide**, or **tirofiban**. ↑ risk for adverse hematologic reactions with **antineoplastics** or **radiation therapy**. ↑ risk for nephrotoxicity with **cyclosporine**.

Drug–Natural: ↑ bleeding risk with, **arnica**, **chamomile**, **feverfew**, **garlic**, **ginger**, **ginkgo**, **Panax ginseng**, and others.

Route/Dosage

Analgesia

PO (adults): *Anti-inflammatory*—400–800 mg 3–4 times daily (not to exceed 3200 mg/day). *Analgesic/antidysmenorrheal/antipyretic*—200–400 mg q4–6h (not to exceed 1200 mg/day).

PO (children 6 mo–12 yr): *Anti-inflammatory*—30–50 mg/kg/day in 3–4 divided doses (maximum dose: 2.4 g/day). *Antipyretic*—5 mg/kg for temperature <102.5°F (39.17°C) or 10 mg/kg for higher temperatures (not to exceed 40 mg/kg/day); may be repeated q4–6h. *Cystic fibrosis (unlabeled)*—20–30 mg/kg/day divided twice daily.

PO (infants and children): *Analgesic*—4–10 mg/kg/dose q6–8h.

IV (adults): *Analgesic*—400–800 mg q6h as needed (not to exceed 3200 mg/day); *Antipyretic*—400 mg initially, then 400 mg q4–6h or 100–200 mg q4h as needed (not to exceed 3200 mg/day).

Pediatric OTC Dosing

PO (children 11 yr/72–95 lb): 300 mg q6–8h

PO (children 9–10 yr/60–71 lb): 250 mg q6–8h

PO (children 6–8 yr/48–59 lb): 200 mg q6–8h

PO (children 4–5 yr/36–47 lb): 150 mg q6–8h

PO (children 2–3 yr/24–35 lb): 100 mg q6–8h

PO (children 12–23 mo/18–23 lb): 75 mg q6–8h

PO (infants 6–11 mo/12–17 lb): 50 mg q6–8h

Availability *(generic available)*

Tablets: 100 mg^OTC, 200 mg^OTC, 300 mg, 400 mg, 600 mg, 800 mg. **Capsules (liqui-gels):** 200 mg^OTC. **Chewable tablets (fruit, grape, orange, and citrus flavor):** 50 mg^OTC, 100 mg^OTC. **Liquid (berry flavor):** 100 mg/5 mL^OTC. **Oral suspension (fruit, berry, grape flavor):** 100 mg/5 mL^OTC, 100 mg/2.5 mL^OTC. **Pediatric drops (berry flavor):** 50 mg/1.25 mL^OTC. **Solution for injection:** 100 mg/mL. *In combination with:* decongestants^OTC, hydrocodone (Vicoprofen), oxycodone (Combunox), famotidine (Duexis).

Nursing Implications

Assessment

- Patients who have asthma, aspirin-induced allergy, and nasal polyps are at increased risk for development of hypersensitivity reactions. Assess for rhinitis, asthma, and urticaria.

- Assess for signs and symptoms of GI bleeding (tarry stools, lightheadedness, hypotension), renal dysfunction (elevated BUN and creatinine levels, decreased urine output), and hepatic impairment (elevated liver enzymes, jaundice). Geri: Higher risk for poor outcomes or death from GI bleeding. Age-related renal impairment increases risk for hepatic and renal toxicity.

- Assess patient for skin rash frequently during therapy. Discontinue ibuprofen at first sign of rash; may be life-threatening. Stevens–Johnson syndrome or toxic epidermal necrolysis may develop. Treat symptomatically; may recur once treatment is stopped.

- **Pain:** Assess pain (note type, location, and intensity) before and 1–2 hr after administration.

- **Arthritis:** Assess pain and range of motion before and 1–2 hr after administration.

- **Fever:** Monitor temperature; note signs associated with fever (diaphoresis, tachycardia, malaise).

- *Laboratory Test Considerations:* BUN, serum creatinine, CBC, and liver function tests should be evaluated periodically in patients receiving prolonged therapy.

- Serum potassium, BUN, serum creatinine, alkaline phosphatase, LDH, AST, and ALT may show ↑ levels. Blood glucose, hemoglobin, and hematocrit concentrations, leukocyte and platelet counts, and CCr may be ↓.

- May cause prolonged bleeding time; may persist for < 1 day after discontinuation.

Potential Nursing Diagnoses
Acute pain (Indications)

Impaired physical mobility (Indications)

Ineffective thermoregulation (Indications)

Implementation
- Do not confuse Motrin (ibuprofen) with Neurontin (gabapentin).

- Administration of higher than recommended doses does not provide increased pain relief but may increase incidence of side effects.

- Patient should be well hydrated before administration to prevent renal adverse reactions.

- Use lowest effective dose for shortest period of time, especially in the elderly.

- Coadministration with opioid analgesics may have additive analgesic effects and may permit lower opioid doses.

- **PO:** For rapid initial effect, administer 30 min before or 2 hr after meals. May be administered with food, milk, or antacids to decrease GI irritation. Tablets may be crushed and mixed with fluids or food; 800-mg tablet can be dissolved in water.

- **Dysmenorrhea:** Administer as soon as possible after the onset of menses. Prophylactic treatment has not been shown to be effective.

IV Administration
- **Intermittent Infusion: Diluent:** 0.9% NaCl, D5W, or LR. **Concentration:** Dilute the 800 mg dose in at least 200 mL and the 400-mg dose in at least 100 mL for a concentration of 4 mg/mL. Do not administer solutions that are discolored or contain particulate matter. Stable for up to 24 hr at room temperature.
  Rate: Infuse over at least 30 min.

- Advise patients to take ibuprofen with a full glass of water and to remain in an upright position for 15–30 min after administration.

- Instruct patient to take medication as directed. Take missed doses as soon as remembered but not if almost time for next dose. Do not double doses. Pedi: Teach parents and caregivers to calculate and measure doses accurately, and to use measuring device supplied with product.

- May cause drowsiness or dizziness. Advise patient to avoid driving or other activities requiring alertness until response to medication is known.

- Caution patient to avoid the concurrent use of alcohol, aspirin, acetaminophen, and other OTC or herbal products without consulting health-care professional.

- Advise patient to inform health-care professional of medication regimen before treatment or surgery.

- Instruct patients not to take OTC ibuprofen preparations for >10 days for pain or >3 days for fever, and to consult health-care professional if symptoms persist or worsen. Many OTC products contain ibuprofen; avoid duplication.

- Caution patient that use of ibuprofen with ≥3 glasses of alcohol per day may increase the risk for GI bleeding.

- Advise patient to consult health-care professional if rash, itching, visual disturbances, tinnitus, weight gain, edema, epigastric pain, dyspepsia, black stools, hematemesis, persistent headache, or influenza-like syndrome (chills, fever, muscle aches, pain) occurs.

- Pedi: Advise parents or caregivers not to administer ibuprofen to children who may be dehydrated (can occur with vomiting, diarrhea, or poor fluid intake); dehydration increases risk for renal dysfunction.

- Advise female patients to notify health-care professional if pregnancy is planned or suspected.

Evaluation/Desired Outcomes

- Decrease in severity of pain.

- Improved joint mobility. Partial arthritic relief is usually seen within 7 days, but maximum effectiveness may require 1–2 wk of continuous therapy. Patients who do not respond to one NSAID may respond to another.

- Reduction in fever.

ERYTHROMYCIN

(eh-rith-roe-**mye**-sin)

erythromycin base

E-Mycin, Erybid, Eryc, Ery-Tab, Erythro-EC, PCE

erythromycin ethylsuccinate

E.E.S, EryPed, Erythro-ES, Pediazole

erythromycin lactobionate

Erythrocin

erythromycin stearate

Erythrocin, Erythro-S

erythromycin (topical)

Akne-Mycin, Erygel, Erysol

Classification
Therapeutic: anti-infectives

Pharmacologic: macrolides

Pregnancy Category B

Indications
IV, PO: Infections caused by susceptible organisms, including upper and lower respiratory tract infections, otitis media (with sulfonamides), skin and skin structure infections, pertussis, diphtheria, erythrasma, intestinal amebiasis, pelvic inflammatory disease, nongonococcal urethritis, syphilis, Legionnaires' disease, rheumatic fever. Useful when penicillin is the most appropriate drug but cannot be used because of hypersensitivity, including streptococcal infections, treatment of syphilis or gonorrhea. **Topical:** Treatment of acne.

Action
Suppresses protein synthesis at the level of the 50S bacterial ribosome. **Therapeutic Effects:** Bacteriostatic action against susceptible bacteria. **Spectrum:** Active against many gram-positive cocci, including Streptococci, Staphylococci. Gram-positive bacilli, including *Clostridium*, *Corynebacterium*. Several gram-negative pathogens, notably *Neisseria*, *Legionella pneumophila*. *Mycoplasma* and *Chlamydia* are also usually susceptible.

Pharmacokinetics
Absorption: Variable absorption from the duodenum after oral administration (dependent on salt form). Absorption of enteric-coated products is delayed. Minimal absorption may follow topical or ophthalmic use.

Distribution: Widely distributed. Minimal CNS penetration. Crosses placenta; enters breast milk.

Protein Binding: 70%–80%.

Metabolism and Excretion: Partially metabolized by the liver, excreted mainly unchanged in the bile; small amounts excreted unchanged in the urine.

Half-life: Neonates: 2.1 hr; Adults: 1.4–2 hr.

Time/Action Profile (blood levels)

ROUTE	ONSET	PEAK	DURATION
PO	1 hr	1–4 hr	6–12 hr
IV	Rapid	End of infusion	6–12 hr

Contraindications/Precautions
Contraindicated in: Hypersensitivity; concurrent use of pimozide, ergotamine, dihydroergotamine, procainamide, quinidine, dofetilide, amiodarone, or sotalol. Known alcohol intolerance (most topicals); tartrazine sensitivity (some products contain tartrazine—FDC yellow dye #5). Products containing benzyl alcohol should be avoided in neonates.

Use Cautiously in: Liver/renal disease. OB: May be used in pregnancy to treat chlamydial infections or syphilis; myasthenia gravis (may worsen symptoms). Geri: ↑ risk for ototoxicity if parenteral dose >4 g/day, ↑ risk for QTc interval prolongation.

Adverse Reactions/Side Effects (CAPITALS indicate life-threatening; underlines indicate most frequent.)

CNS: seizures (rare). **EENT:** ototoxicity. **CV:** TORSADE DE POINTES, VENTRICULAR ARRHYTHMIAS, QT interval prolongation. **GI:** PSEUDOMEMBRANOUS COLITIS, nausea, vomiting, abdominal pain, cramping, diarrhea, hepatitis, infantile hypertrophic pyloric stenosis, pancreatitis (rare). **GU:** interstitial nephritis. **Derm:** rash. **Local:** phlebitis at IV site. **Misc:** allergic reactions, superinfection.

Interactions

Drug–Drug: Concurrent use with **pimozide** may ↑ levels and the risk for serious arrhythmias (concurrent use contraindicated); similar effects may occur with **diltiazem, verapamil, ketoconazole, itraconazole, nefazodone,** and **protease inhibitors;** avoid concurrent use. May ↑ levels of **ergotamine** and **dihydroergotamine,** and risk for acute ergot toxicity; concurrent use contraindicated. May ↑ **verapamil** levels and the risk for hypotension, bradycardia, and lactic acidosis. ↑ blood levels and effects of **sildenafil, tadalafil,** and **vardenafil;** use lower doses. Concurrent **rifabutin** or **rifampin** may ↓ effect of erythromycin and ↑ risk for adverse GI reactions. ↑ levels and risk for toxicity from **alfentanil, alprazolam, bromocriptine, carbamazepine, cyclosporine, cilostazol diazepam disopyramide, ergot alkaloids, felodipine, methylprednisolone, midazolam, quinidine, rifabutin, tacrolimus, triazolam,** or **vinblastine.** May ↑ levels of **lovastatin** and **simvastatin,** and ↑ the risk for myopathy/rhabdomyolysis. May ↑ serum **digoxin** levels. **Theophylline** may ↓ blood levels. May ↑ **colchicine** levels and the risk for toxicity; use lower starting and maximum dose of colchicine. May ↑ **theophylline** levels and the risk for toxicity; ↓ theophylline dose. May ↑ **warfarin** levels and the risk for bleeding.

Route/Dosage

250 mg erythromycin base or stearate = 400 mg erythromycin ethylsuccinate.

Most Infections

PO (adults): *Base, stearate*—250 mg q6h, *or* 333 mg q8h, *or* 500 mg q12h. *Ethylsuccinate*—400 mg q6h *or* 800 mg q12h.

PO (children >1 mo): *Base and ethylsuccinate*—30–50 mg/kg/day divided q6–8h (maximum 2 g/day as base or 3.2 g/day as ethylsuccinate). *Stearate*—30–50 mg/kg/day divided q6h (maximum 2 g/day).

PO (neonates): *Ethylsuccinate*—20–50 mg/kg/day divided q6–12h.

IV (adults): 250–500 mg (up to 1 g) q6h.

IV (children > 1 mo): 15–50 mg/kg/day divided q6h, maximum 4 g/day.

Acne

Topical (adults and children > 12 yr): 2% ointment, gel, solution, or pledgets twice daily.

Availability (generic available)

Erythromycin Base

Enteric-coated tablets: 250 mg, 333 mg. **Tablets with polymer-coated particles:** 333 mg, 500 mg. **Film-coated tablets:** 500 mg. **Delayed-release capsules:** 250 mg.

Erythromycin Ethylsuccinate

Chewable tablets (fruit flavor): 200 mg. **Tablets:** 400 mg, 600 mg. **Oral suspension (fruit flavor, cherry):** 200 mg/5 mL. **Oral suspension (orange, banana flavors):** 400 mg/5 mL. **Drops (fruit flavor):** 100 mg/2.5 mL.

Erythromycin Lactobionate

Powder for injection: 500 mg, 1 g

Erythromycin Stearate
Film-coated tablets: 250 mg, 500 mg

Topical Preparations
Ointment: 2%, **Gel:** 2%, **Solution:** 2%, **Pledgets:** 2%. *In combination with:* sulfisoxazole (generic only) and benzoyl peroxide (Benzamycin).

Nursing Implications

Assessment

- Assess for infection (vital signs; appearance of wound, sputum, urine, and stool; white blood cell) at beginning of and during therapy.

- Obtain specimens for culture and sensitivity before initiating therapy. First dose may be given before receiving results.

- Monitor bowel function. Diarrhea, abdominal cramping, fever, and bloody stools should be reported to health-care professional promptly as a sign of pseudomembranous colitis. May begin up to several weeks after cessation of therapy.

- *Laboratory Test Considerations:* Monitor liver function tests periodically on patients receiving high-dose, long-term therapy.

- May cause ↑ serum bilirubin, AST, ALT, and alkaline phosphatase concentrations.

- May cause false ↑ of urinary catecholamines.

Potential Nursing Diagnoses
Risk for infection (Indications, Side Effects)

Noncompliance (Patient/Family Teaching)

Implementation

- **PO:** Administer around the clock. *Erythromycin film-coated tablets (base and stearate)* are absorbed better on an empty stomach, at least 1 hr before or 2 hr after meals; may be taken with food if GI irritation occurs. *Enteric-coated erythromycin (base)* may be taken without regard to meals. *Erythromycin ethylsuccinate* is best absorbed when taken with meals. Take each dose with a full glass of water.

- Use calibrated measuring device for liquid preparations. Shake well before using.

- Chewable tablets should be crushed or chewed and not swallowed whole.

- Do not crush or chew delayed-release capsules or tablets; swallow whole. *Erythromycin base delayed-release capsules* may be opened and sprinkled on applesauce, jelly, or ice cream immediately before ingestion. Entire contents of the capsule should be taken.

IV Administration

- **IV:** Add 10 mL sterile water for injection without preservatives to 250- or 500-mg vials and 20 mL to 1-g vial. Solution is stable for 7 days after reconstitution if refrigerated.

- **Intermittent Infusion: *Diluent:*** Dilute in 0.9% NaCl or D5W. ***Concentration:*** 1–5 mg/mL.
  Rate: Administer slowly over 20–60 min to avoid phlebitis. Assess for pain along vein; slow rate if pain occurs; apply ice and notify health-care professional if unable to relieve pain.

- **Continuous Infusion:** May also be administered as an infusion over 4 hr. ***Diluent:*** 0.9% NaCl, D5W, or LR. ***Concentration:*** 1 g/L.

Erythromycin Lactobionate

- **Y-Site Compatibility:** acyclovir, alemtuzumab, alfentanil, amikacin, aminocaproic acid, aminophylline, amiodarone, anidulafungin, atracurium, atropine, azathioprine, benztropine, bivalirudin, bleomycin, bumetanide, buprenorphine, butorphanol, calcium chloride, calcium gluconate, carboplatin, carmustine, caspofungin, cefotaxime, ceftriaxone, cefuroxime, chlorpromazine, cisplatin, cyanocobalamin, cyclophosphamide, cyclosporine, cytarabine, dactinomycin, daptomycin, dexmedetomidine, digoxin, diltiazem, diphenhydramine, dobutamine, docetaxel, dopamine, doxacurium, doxapram, doxorubicin, enalaprilat, ephedrine, epinephrine, epirubicin, epoetin alfa, eptifibatide, ertapenem, esmolol, etoposide, etoposide phosphate, famotidine, fenoldopam, fentanyl, fluconazole, fludarabine, fluorouracil, folic acid, foscarnet, gemcitabine, gentamicin, glycopyrrolate, granisetron, hetastarch, hydrocortisone, hydromorphone, idarubicin, ifosfamide, imipenem/cilastatin, insulin, irinotecan, isoproterenol, labetalol, levofloxacin, lidocaine, lorazepam, mannitol, mechlorethamine, meperidine, methotrexate, methoxamine, methyldopa, methylprednisolone, metoclopramide, metronidazole, midazolam, milrinone, mitoxantrone, morphine, multivitamins, mycophenolate, nafcillin, nalbuphine, naloxone, nesiritide, nicardipine, nitroglycerin, norepinephrine, octreotide, ondansetron, oxacillin, oxaliplatin, oxytocin, paclitaxel, palonosetron, pamidronate, papaverine, pentamidine, pentazocine, perphenazine, phentolamine, phenylephrine, phytonadione, piperacillin/tazobactam, potassium acetate, procainamide, prochlorperazine, promethazine, propranolol, protamine, pyridoxine, ranitidine, sodium acetate, sodium bicarbonate, streptokinase, succinylcholine, sufentanil, tacrolimus, teniposide, theophylline, thiamine, thiotepa, tigecycline, tirofiban, tobramycin, tolazoline, trimetaphan, vancomycin, vasopressin, vecuronium, verapamil, vincristine, vinorelbine, vitamin B complex with C, voriconazole, zidovudine, zoledronic acid

- **Y-Site Incompatibility:** amphotericin B colloidal, amphotericin B lipid complex, amphotericin B liposome, ascorbic acid, aztreonam, cefazolin, cefepime, cefotetan, cefoxitin, chloramphenicol, dantrolene, dexamethasone, diazepam, diazoxide, doxycycline, furosemide, ganciclovir, indomethacin, ketorolac, metaraminol, nitroprusside, pemetrexed, penicillin G, pentobarbital, phenobarbital, phenytoin, ticarcillin/clavulanate, trimethoprim/sulfamethoxazole

- **Topical:** Cleanse area before application. Wear gloves during application.

Patient/Family Teaching

- Instruct patient to take medication around the clock and to finish the drug completely as directed, even if feeling better. Take missed doses as soon as remembered, with remaining doses evenly spaced throughout day. Advise patient that sharing of this medication may be dangerous.

- May cause nausea, vomiting, diarrhea, or stomach cramps; notify healthcare professional if these effects persist or if severe abdominal pain, yellow discoloration of the skin or eyes, darkened urine, pale stools, or unusual tiredness develops. May cause infantile hypertrophic pyloric stenosis in infants; notify health-care professional if vomiting and irritability occur.

- Caution patient to notify health-care professional if fever and diarrhea occur, especially if stool contains blood, pus, or mucus. Advise patient not to treat diarrhea without consulting health-care professional. May occur up to several weeks after discontinuation of medication.

- Advise patient to report signs of superinfection (black, furry overgrowth on the tongue; vaginal itching or discharge; loose or foul-smelling stools).

- Instruct patient to notify health-care professional if symptoms do not improve.

Evaluation/Desired Outcomes

- Resolution of the signs and symptoms of infection; length of time for complete resolution depends on the organism and site of infection

- Improvement of acne lesions

Index

Page numbers followed by "f" denote figures, "t" denote tables, and "b" denote boxes